Modern Urology

Modern Urology

Edited by Ezra Martin

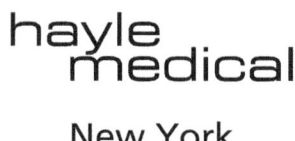

hayle
medical

New York

Hayle Medical,
750 Third Avenue, 9th Floor,
New York, NY 10017, USA

Visit us on the World Wide Web at:
www.haylemedical.com

ISBN: 978-1-63241-919-4

Cataloging-in-Publication Data

Modern urology / edited by Ezra Martin.
    p. cm.
Includes bibliographical references and index.
ISBN 978-1-63241-919-4
1. Urology. 2. Genitourinary organs--Diseases. I. Martin, Ezra.
RC871 .M63 2020
616.6--dc23

Table of Contents

Preface

Urology is a branch of medicine which focuses on the diagnosis, treatment and prevention of the diseases of the male and female urinary-tract system, and the defects of the male reproductive system. The organs studied in urology are the kidneys, ureters, adrenal glands, urethra, urinary bladder, and the male reproductive organs. The field of urology is closely associated with the fields of gynecology, nephrology, oncology, colorectal surgery, endocrinology, gastroenterology, pediatric surgery and andrology. Urology is a broad discipline with a number of significant sub-disciplines, chief among which are endourology, neurourology, urologic oncology and reconstructive urology. Some of the surgical procedures in urology include bladder augmentation, Burch colposuspension, cystectomy, ileal conduit urinary diversion, intersex medical interventions, nephrotomy, nephrectomy, urostomy, etc. This book is compiled in such a manner, that it will provide in-depth knowledge about the theory and practice of modern urology. The aim of this book is to present researches that have transformed this discipline and aided its advancement. For someone with an interest and eye for detail, this book covers the most significant topics in this field.

After months of intensive research and writing, this book is the end result of all who devoted their time and efforts in the initiation and progress of this book. It will surely be a source of reference in enhancing the required knowledge of the new developments in the area. During the course of developing this book, certain measures such as accuracy, authenticity and research focused analytical studies were given preference in order to produce a comprehensive book in the area of study.

This book would not have been possible without the efforts of the authors and the publisher. I extend my sincere thanks to them. Secondly, I express my gratitude to my family and well-wishers. And most importantly, I thank my students for constantly expressing their willingness and curiosity in enhancing their knowledge in the field, which encourages me to take up further research projects for the advancement of the area.

Editor

Preface

The postoperative morbidity index: a quantitative weighing of postoperative complications applied to urological procedures

Jonathan Beilan[1†], Ruth Strakosha[1†], Diego Aguilar Palacios[1†] and Charles J Rosser[2*]

Abstract

Background: The reporting of post-operative complications in the urological field is lacking of a uniform quantitative measure to assess severity, which is essential in the analysis of surgical outcomes. The purpose of this study was to evaluate the feasibility of estimating quantitative severity weighing of post-operative complications after common urologic procedures.

Methods: Using a large healthcare system's quality database, complications were identified in eleven common urologic procedures (*e.g.,* insertion or replacement of inflatable penile prosthesis, nephroureterectomy, partial nephrectomy, percutaneous nephrostomy tube placement, radical cystectomy, radical prostatectomy, renal/ureteral/bladder extracorporeal shockwave lithotripsy (ESWL), transurethral destruction of bladder lesion, transurethral prostatectomy, transurethral removal of ureteral obstruction, and ureteral catheterization) from January 1, 2011 to December 31, 2011. Complications were classified by the Expanded Accordion Severity Grading System, which was then quantified by validated severity weighting scores. The Postoperative Morbidity Index (PMI) for each procedure was calculated where an index of 0 would indicate no complication in any patient and an index of 1 would indicate that all patients died.

Results: This study included 654 procedures of which 148 (22%) had one or more complications. As would be expected, a more complex procedure like radical cystectomy possessed a higher PMI (0.267), while a simpler procedure like percutaneous nephrostomy tube placement possessed a lower PMI (0.011). The PMI of the additional nine procedures fell within the range of these PMIs. These PMIs could be used to compare surgeons, hospitals or procedures.

Conclusions: Quantitative severity weighing of post-operative complications for urologic procedures is feasible and may provide exceptionally informative data related to outcomes.

Keywords: Complication, Index, Postoperative, Quantitative, Urology

Background

The concept of outcomes measurement was first described by Dr. E. Codman in the early 1900's and has now become a national incentive set forth by the Centers for Medicare and Medicaid Services and other organizations [1]. Although there are many well-designed programs currently in place to monitor the quality and outcomes of care in certain specialties or institutions, they tend to be complex and therefore unlikely to be effectively implemented at a national or global level [2]. One of the major outcomes to report in any surgical field is post-operative complications. The Clavien complication grading system is a severity grading system developed by Clavien *et al.*, and published in 1992. This complication grading system ranks complications based on the magnitude of the intervention(s) required for their treatment and whether the complications cause permanent injury or death [3]. In 2004, the Clavien complication grading system was modified to add more detail to the more serious complications, however, with it has come inconsistencies in the application of this grading system, *e.g.*, non-uniform grade contraction [4].

As a result of these inconsistencies, the grading system was extensively modified (renamed Accordion Severity Grading System) in 2009. Specifically, the Accordion

* Correspondence: deacdoc@aol.com
†Equal contributors
²Clinical and Translational Program, University of Hawaii Cancer Center, 701 Ilalo St, Honolulu, HI 96814, USA
Full list of author information is available at the end of the article

Severity Grading System added flexibility to the grading system by introducing an expandable classification, and clarity was improved by introducing rigorously defined qualitative terms [5]. However, to date, all complication severity grading systems, *e.g.,* Memorial Sloan Kettering Severity Grading System and Accordion Severity Grading System [6]. are key short-term outcomes measures of operative procedures and lack robust quantitative measure of the severity of surgical complications, which would allow comparison between two health states.

Recently, severity weighting of the Accordion Severity Grading System led to a) correction of criteria for two of the higher grades of severity and b) severity scores with weight for each of the six severity levels, enabling for the first time a way to quantify complications. Specifically, the application of severity weights to Accordion Severity Grading System (postoperative morbidity index, PMI) was applied to data gathered from American College of Surgeons (ACS) National Surgical Quality Improvement Program (NSQIP) program for the year 2007 and demonstrated that weighting of complications provided new insights into the burden contributed by specific types of complications [7,8].

Straberg *et al.* evaluated and reported the feasibility of PMI, which applied to general surgery estimates quantitative morbidity scores after surgical procedures including laparoscopic colectomy, appendectomy, and pancreaticoduodenectomy, by taking into consideration validated weighted values in post-operative complications [9]. Based on these encouraging results from our general surgery colleagues, we report on the feasibility of applying Accordion Severity Grading System and PMI in a large urologic cohort (n = 654) that underwent 11 common urologic procedures. To date the expansion of PMI as an estimation of postoperative complication of urologic procedures has not been explored.

Methods

This study was approved by Orlando Health Inc. (Orlando, FL) Institutional Review Board with a waiver of consent. Orlando Health Inc. is a large healthcare system (> 1,000 beds) comprised of eight facilities in central Florida, affiliated with the University of Central Florida College of Medicine and Florida State University School of Medicine. Complications identified within the American College of Surgeons National Surgical Quality Improvement Program (ACS-NSQIP) within the Department of Urology in Orlando Health Inc. were queried retrospectively to gather information regarding patient outcomes to urologic surgeries performed from January 1, 2011 to December 31, 2011. Based on the number of procedures performed in 2011, the location of the procedures (in-patient and outpatient) and the difficulty of the procedures, CPT codes associated with 11 diverse procedures covering a wide range of urologic procedures [*e.g.,* insertion or replacement of inflatable penile prosthesis, nephroureterectomy, partial nephrectomy, percutaneous nephrostomy tube placement, radical cystectomy, radical prostatectomy, renal/ureteral/bladder extracorporeal shockwave lithotripsy (ESWL), transurethral destruction of bladder lesion, transurethral prostatectomy, transurethral removal of ureteral obstruction, and ureteral catheterization] were queried and included for analysis. All patients identified in each of the 11 procedures were evaluated (*i.e.,* no patient was excluded from analysis). To establish the true PMI of a procedure in an institution one would expect that >25 patients per group would be needed although the study has not yet been done to determine the exact number.

Individual medical records of the patients who underwent the above procedures were reviewed to determine the incidence of post-operative complications as defined by American College of Surgery National Surgical Quality Improvement Program (ACS NSQIP) within 30 days (any NSQIP 30-day morbidity). The ACS NSQIP complications that were noted included bleeding, superficial wound infection, deep wound infection, organ space infection, wound dehiscence, acute renal failure, progressive renal insufficiency, urinary tract infection, prolonged ileus, pneumonia, failure to wean from ventilator, unplanned intubation, pneumothorax, pulmonary embolus, cardiac arrest, exacerbation of heart failure, deep venous thrombosis, cerebrovascular accident, transient ischemic attack, sepsis, septic shock, and death (all-cause 30-day mortality). The severity of each complication was graded independently by two clinicians (JAB and RS) according to the recently validated Accordion Severity Grading System (Table 1). A third investigator (CJR) reviewed discrepancies and rendered a final score. In cases with multiple ACS NSQIP complications, the case was assigned a grade corresponding to the highest graded complication.

Next, a weighted postoperative morbidity index (PMI) was calculated as previously described [8] (*i.e.,* to calculate the PMI for each operative procedure, the weights of all the complications for all patients who underwent the corresponding procedure were summed and divided by the total number of patients undergoing that procedure). A PMI of 0 would indicate that no patient having the procedure had any postoperative complications, while on the other hand, and a PMI of 1.000 would indicate that every patient having the procedure suffered postoperative death. In order to analyze complication severity, the sum of severity weights for all patients having any complication after a procedure were divided by the total number of patients with complications in the group (*i.e.,* the denominator was the number of patients having a complication after the procedure, rather than the total number of patients having the procedure). Descriptive statistics were performed in Excel 2007 (Microsoft Corp).

Table 1 Accordion classification system with severity weights

Grade	Description	Severity weight
1	Treatment of complication requires only minor invasive procedures that can be done at the bedside, such as insertion of intravenous lines, urinary catheters, and nasogastric tubes, and drainage of wound infections. Physiotherapy and antiemetics, antipyretics, analgesics, diuretics, electrolytes, and physiotherapy are permitted.	0.110
2	Complication requires pharmacologic treatment with drugs other than such allowed for minor complications, e.g. antibiotics. Blood transfusions and total parenteral nutrition are also included.	0.260
3	No general anesthesia is required to treat the complication: requires management by an endoscopic, interventional procedure, or reoperation without general anesthesia.	0.370
4	General anesthesia is required to treat complication. Alternately, single-organ failure has developed.	0.600
5	General anesthesia is required to treat complication and single organ failure has developed. Alternately, multisystem organ failure (2 or more organ systems) has developed.	0.790
6	Postoperative death occurred.	1.000

Results

Of the 11 procedures queried for inclusion into this study, a total of 654 corresponding surgical procedures performed by 25 attending physicians were identified. Table 2 (Additional file 1: Figure S1A) shows the number of cases and severity grade of each complication by procedure. Of the 654 surgical procedures, 506 procedures did not have an associated complication noted, thus 148 procedures were noted to be associated with a post-operative complication. Grade one complications were the most common (47%). There were no perioperative deaths (grade 6) reported. It is important to note the great variability in the distribution of the number of cases in each procedure, ranging from 13 radical cystectomies to 159 transurethral removal of ureteral obstruction.

Table 3 (Additional file 2: Figure S1B) shows the complications classified by a weighted severity grade. By reporting these data, it was possible to understand the burden of complications in a given procedure and to compare the burden between two procedures that have similar PMIs.

While Grade 1 complications made up 47% of the total complication (Table 2), it only accounted for 18% of the complication burden. The largest burden of complications was associated with Grade 4 complications, which comprised 26% of the total complications, but accounted for 53% of the complication burden. Grade 2 complications comprised 22% of the total complications and accounted for 20% of the complication burden. Grade 3, 5 and 6 complications were the least reported (total < 6%), accounting for a total complication burden of < 10%.

Table 4 depicts the calculated PMI of the 11 reported procedures. As would be expected, a more complex procedure like radical cystectomy possessed a higher PMI (0.267), while a simpler procedure like percutaneous nephrostomy tube placement possessed a lower PMI (0.011). Thus the morbidity index associated with radical cystectomy was 24 times greater than the morbidity index associated with percutaneous nephrostomy tube placement. The PMI of the additional nine procedures fell within the range of the above PMIs. Table 4 also

Table 2 Complications classified by unweighted severity grades

Procedure	0*	Severity grade						n
		1	2	3	4	5	6	
Inflatable penile prosthesis	13	2	1		2			18
Nephrourete rectomy	42	2	9	1	4	1		59
Partial nephrectomy	8		3		2			13
Percutaneous nephrostomy tube	31	1	1					33
Radical cystectomy	3	3	3	1	2	1		13
Radical prostatectomy	101	10	5	1	1			118
ESWL	33	2			1			36
Transurethral destruction of bladder lesion	32	2			4	1		39
Transurethral prostatectomy	56	15	5	1	10			87
Transurethral removal of ureteral obstruction	120	24	3		12			159
Ureteral catheterization	67	8	3	1				79
Subtotal by grade	506	69	33	5	38	3	0	654
Subtotal by grade (%)		47%	22%	3%	26%	2%	0%	

*"0" means no complications.

Table 3 Complications classified by weighted severity grades

Procedure	Severity grade						
	1	2	3	4	5	6	Total
Inflatable penile prosthesis	0.22	0.26		1.2			1.68
Nephroureterectomy	0.22	2.34	0.37	2.4	0.79		6.12
Partial nephrectomy		0.78		1.2			1.98
Percutaneous nephrostomy tube	0.11	0.26					0.37
Radical cystectomy	0.33	0.78	0.37	1.2	0.79		3.47
Radical prostatectomy	1.1	1.3	0.37	0.6			
ESWL	0.22			0.6			
Transurethral destruction of bladder lesion	0.22			2.4	0.79		3.41
Transurethral prostatetomy	1.65	1.3	0.37	6			9.32
Transurethral removal of ureteral obstruction	2.64	0.78		7.2			10.62
Ureteral catheterization	0.88	0.78	0.37				
Subtotal by grade	7.59	8.58	1.85	22.8	2.37	0	43.19
Subtotal by grade (%)	18%	20%	4%	53%	5%	0%	

shows the complication rate and the severity of complication per case. For example, the complication rate of partial nephrectomy was about 38.46%, but if a complication occurs, its severity index was 0.396, which was about two times more severe than any complication that occurred during a ureteral catheterization.

Discussion

The volume of surgery over the past several decades has increased dramatically in all parts of the world, with an estimated 234 million operations performed annually, making safe delivery of surgical care a major

Table 4 Postoperative morbidity index (PMI), complication rate and severity of complication by procedure

Procedure	Complication rate (%)	PMI*	Severity of complication**
Percutaneous nephrostomy tube	6.06	0.011	0.185
ESWL	8.33	0.023	0.273
Ureteral catheterization	15.19	0.026	0.169
Radical prostatectomy	14.41	0.029	0.198
Transurethral removal of ureteral obstruction	24.53	0.067	0.272
Transurethral destruction of bladder lesion	17.95	0.087	0.487
Inflatable penile prosthesis	27.78	0.093	0.336
Nephroureterectomy	28.81	0.104	0.360
Transurethral prostatetomy	35.63	0.107	0.301
Partial nephrectomy	38.46	0.152	0.396
Radical cystectomy	76.92	0.267	0.347

*Severity points per case where 0 = no complication and 1 death.
**Severity points per case with complication.

public health concern [10]. From the early 1900's, it has been a tenet of the surgical profession that the careful tracking and analysis of outcomes is essential to provide safe, high-quality care [1]. A simple, low-cost metric assessing post-operative complications, capable of providing rapid feedback to the surgical teams in any setting could therefore aid clinical care and quality improvement efforts.

The concept of severity weighting used to calculate the PMI is derived from utility weighting, which is the mathematical method of assigning value weights to multidimensional outcomes states to reflect overall impact [9]. The value of severity weights used in the current study comes from a well-validated study where 50 surgical experts were asked to evaluate and score 12 clinical vignettes [11]. Thus the PMI is an index, which might be most useful in detecting trends and serve as a point of reference in the surgical field. Considering this, the PMI numbers generated in the present study should be only taken as a starting point. For example, as shown in Additional file 1: Figure S1A, the PMI could be used to follow trends in complications for any particular urological procedure at the institutional level over months or years. As demonstrated in Table 3, when using the PMI, we are no longer simply analyzing the incidence rate of complications for a particular procedure, but we are also estimating the severity score of these respective complications. Furthermore, we can analyze the expected and actual severity grades of each complication that occurs. For instance, the post-operative complication rate of a transurethral prostatectomy was 35.63%, which could be further sub-classified into severity grades and compared to the complication grades with other procedures. This can be a valuable tool in standardizing practice or research, but also can be useful in properly counseling patients of their surgical risks. For example, one can advise that the severity of complications after a transurethral prostatectomy are approximately five times higher than the severity of a complication following a ureteral catheterization (PMI 0.10 *vs.* PMI 0.02, respectively).

It is evident that radical cystectomy at our institution had the most frequent complication rate and that most of the morbidity related to radical cystectomy was due to Grade 4 and Grade 5 complications, as shown in Additional file 1: Figure S1A. This high complication rate was noted by other investigators [12-14]. Specifically, DeNuzio and colleagues reported 415 complications in 302 patients undergoing cystectomy and classified these complications as Clavien type I (109 patients), II (220 patients), IIIa (45 patients), IIIb (22 patients), IV (11 patients) and V (8 patients) [14]. Furthermore, ureteral catheterization and ESWL had similar PMIs, but closer analysis shows that the burden of complications of ESWL came from Grade 4 complications, making it more severe than the burden from ureteral catheterization. Another important application of the PMI is to detect trends in deterioration or improvement in surgical outcomes, particularly after the institution of corrective measures or protocols. When analyzing this data and comparing with the curves in Additional file 1: Figure S1A, which displays the percentages of complications using the unweighted severity grades by procedure, similar PMI scores show completely different severity grade distributions. For example, when comparing nephroureterectomy and transurethral prostatectomy, both procedures have similar PMI scores (0.104 *vs.* 0.107), however transurethral prostatectomy has a greater number of grade 1 complications. In contrast, comparison of the curves in Additional file 2: Figure S1B, which shows the burden of weighted severity grades by procedure group, we can observe that most of the severity score for the transurethral prostatectomy is derived from grade 4 complications rather than from grade 1 as observed in the unweighted plot. In our series, we realized that almost all grade 4 complications in the transurethral prostatectomy were secondary to the need of a further resection of the prostate (data not shown). It would then be possible to further examine the indications for reoperation in our case series. Furthermore, this information can be used to compare surgeons, hospitals and procedures as well as initiate studies in order to determine the causes of such complications in that particular procedure. This technique of assessment then quality improvement could ultimately enhance the level of care provided to the urologic patient.

One limitation of this method is that it still lacks absolute objectivity in rating complications. For instance, there is no way to factor in whether the high reoperation rate after transurethral prostatectomy was due to the natural disease process of prostatic hypertrophy or to inadequate gland resection. Furthermore, we applied the severity weights of these ACS NSQIP 30-day morbidity derived from our general surgery colleagues. We believe these weights should be transferrable to the urologic patient, seeing that they are based on general medical/surgical tenets, but a follow-up study will validate these findings with urologic surgeons. Next, the patient population may have a higher comorbidity or some other factor that predisposes them to have a higher post-operative risk profile. These are important factors that must be factored into such a comprehensive system, however they are beyond the scope of this project. Thus, the technique utilized by our study of calculating PMI scores has limitations that must be considered before it can be applied in any institution or in any clinical situation. In concordance with Strasberg *et al.*, we believe that a) the simplicity of the PMI makes it an easy tool to implement but at the same time, a tool lacking the ability to perform individual risk adjustment, b) the fact that only the most serious complication in each patient is considered in order to calculate the PMI may tend to lose certain information when a patient presents with multiple complications, c) the PMI might be less useful for detecting differences across urological care providers at any point in time and d) the application of the PMI should be adequate for the majority of procedures, except for that ones with unusual complication, for example in the area of transplantation where the death of a living donor must receive a special severity weight.

Conclusions

Based on the above results, quantitative severity weighing of post-operative complications of urologic procedures is feasible and may provide exceptionally informative data related to outcomes. As our national healthcare system continues to search for uniform yet applicable ways to measure and report quality care of the surgical patient, attention should be given to PMI.

Additional files

Additional file 1: Figure S1A. The burden of unweighted severity grades by procedure group (the y-axis is percentage of complication or the complication rate per 100 procedures).

Additional file 2: Figure S1B. The burden of weighted severity grades by procedure group (the y-axis is the complication rate per 100 procedures multiplied per the weighting factor).

Abbreviations
PMI: Postoperative morbidity index; ACS: American college of surgeons; NSQIP: National surgical quality improvement program.

Competing interests
The authors declare that they have no competing interests.

Authors' contributions

All authors have read and approved the final manuscript. JB, MD - Study concept and design, data collection, data analysis, drafting of manuscript. RS, MD – Study concept and design, data collection, data analysis, drafting of manuscript. DAP, MD, PhD – Statistical analysis and drafting of manuscript. CJR, MD, MBA - Study concept and design, drafting of manuscript. All authors read and approved the final manuscript.

Author details

[1]University of Central Florida College of Medicine, Orlando, FL, USA. [2]Clinical and Translational Program, University of Hawaii Cancer Center, 701 Ilalo St, Honolulu, HI 96814, USA.

References

1. Donabedian A: **The end results of health care: Ernest Codman's contribution to quality assessment and beyond.** *Milbank Q* 1989, **67**:233.
2. Fink AS, Campbell DA, Mentzer RM, *et al*: **The National Surgical Quality Improvement Program in non-veterans administration hospitals: initial demonstration of feasibility.** *Ann Surg* 2002, **236**:344.
3. Clavien PA, Sanabria JR, Strasberg SM: **Proposed classification of complications of surgery with examples of utility in cholecystectomy.** *Surgery* 1992, **111**:518.
4. Dindo D, Demartines N, Clavien PA: **Classification of surgical complications: a new proposal with evaluation in a cohort of 6336 patients and results of a survey.** *Ann Surg* 2004, **240**:205.
5. Strasberg SM, Linehan DC, Hawkins WG: **The accordion severity grading system of surgical complications.** *Ann Surg* 2009, **250**:177.
6. Yoon PD, Chalasani V, Woo HH: **Use of Clavien-Dindo Classification in reporting and grading of complications after urologic surgical procedures; Analysis of 2010–2012.** *J Urol* 2013. 10.1016/j.juro.2013.04.025.
7. Jung MR, Park YK, Seon JW, *et al*: **Definition and classification of complications of gastrectomy for gastric cancer based on the accordion severity grading system.** *World J Surg* 2012, **36**:2400.
8. Asbun HJ, Stauffer JA: **Laparoscopic vs. open pancreaticoduodenectomy: overall outcomes and severity of complications using the Accordion Severity Grading System.** *J Am Coll Surg* 2012, **215**:810–819. 10.1016/j.jamcollsurg.2012.0.
9. Strasberg SM, Hall BL: **Postoperative morbidity index: a quantitative measure of severity of postoperative complications.** *J Am Coll Surg* 2011, **213**:616.
10. Weiser TG, Rgenbogen SE, Thompson KD, *et al*: **An estimation of the global volume of surgery: a modeling strategy based on available data.** *Lancet* 2008, **372**:139.
11. Porembka MR, Hall BL, Hirbe M, *et al*: **Quantitative weighting of postoperative complications based on the accordion severity grading system: demonstration of potential impact using the american college of surgeons national surgical quality improvement program.** *J Am Coll Surg* 2010, **210**:286.
12. Trinh VQ, Trinh QD, Tian Z, *et al*: **In-hospital mortality and failure-to-rescue rates after radical cystectomy.** *BJU Int* 2013, **112**:20.
13. Roghmann F, Trinh QD, Braun K, *et al*: **Standardized assessment of complications in a contemporary series of European patients undergoing radical cystectomy.** *Int J Urol* 2013. 10.1111/iju.12232.
14. De Nunzio C, Cindolo L, Leonardo C, *et al*: **Analysis of radical cystectomy and urinary diversion complications with the Clavien classification system in an Italian real life cohort.** *Eur J Surg Oncol* 2013, **39**(7):792–798.

2

Outcomes of experimental rat varicocele with and without microsurgery

Tie Zhou[1,2†], Huan Cao[1,2†], Guanghua Chen[1†], Bo Yang[1*] and Yinghao Sun[1*]

Abstract

Background: Experimental rat varicocele was usually developed by the conventional technique but with varied success; and microsurgical rat varicocele model was an effective alternative. In this study we further analyzed differential outcome of experimental rat model with and without microsurgery.

Methods: One hundred and twenty male Sprague-Dawley rats were randomly assigned to two groups. In Group A, experimental rat varicocele model was developed with conventional technique. The left renal vein was partially ligated with concurrent ligation of communicating branches between the left spermatic vein and common iliac vein. In Group B, all the above procedures were finished with microsurgical manipulation under operating microscope. Before and after model development, the mean diameter of the left internal spermatic vein was compared; and at 8 weeks after initial surgery the mean sperm concentration and motility in both groups was analyzed.

Results: The baseline mean diameter of the left internal spermatic vein in Group A and Group B was 0.14 ± 0.04 and 0.15 ± 0.03 mm, respectively ($P = 0.3157$). In Group A 9 rats had severe complications resulting in model failure; while in Group B all rats had successful model except for one died of anesthetic accident ($P = 0.008$). At 8 weeks after initial surgery the mean left internal spermatic vein, sperm concentration and motility in both groups was 1.65 mm, 321.5×10^6/gm and 51.9%; and 1.65 mm, 318.9×10^6/gm and 53.5% respectively. There was nonsignificant difference of internal spermatic vein diameter, sperm concentration and motility between two groups.

Conclusions: Microsurgery makes developing experiment rat varicocele model easy. Compared with conventional technique, microsurgical rat varicocele model has higher success rate and less complication.

Keywords: Varicocele, Microsurgery, Rat

Background

Varicocele is believed to be associated with subfertility and has been found in 15% of normal male population [1]. Also, varicocele is an underlying cause in 41% of male patients with primary infertility and 75-81% of male patients with secondary infertility [2]. Although testicular hypoxia, hormonal dysfunction, elevated testicular temperature and spermatic veins hypertension have been considered to be involved in varicocele-related testicular dysfunction [1,3], the exact pathophysiologic mechanism is not yet completely understood.

Experimental rat varicocele is the most common animal model to investigate the molecular mechanism of varicocele induced male infertility. But developing rat model with the conventional technique has varied success [4-6]. Recently microsurgical rat varicocele model has been considered to be effective in dilation of spermatic vein and reduction of sperm concentration as well as motility [7]. In this study we further analyzed differential outcome of experimental rat model with and without microsurgery.

Methods

Study design

One hundred and twenty male Sprague-Dawley rats weighing 250-300 g were selected and randomly assigned to Group A (conventional technique) and Group B (microsurgery technique) with the method of random digits table. A sample size of 60 rats per group was sufficient according to the calculation formula when 80% power and a = 0.05 were

* Correspondence: wenzhoutie@163.com; sunyh@medmail.com
†Equal contributors
[1]Department of Urology, Changhai Hospital, The Second Military Medical University, 168 Changhai Road, 200433 Shanghai, PR China
Full list of author information is available at the end of the article

considered. The study was approved by the Animal Care and Ethics Committee of SHANGHAI CHANGHAI hospital. Animals were housed under standard conditions in controlled environment with free access to food and water under a 12-hour day/night cycle.

Surgery

1. Experimental rat varicocele model with conventional technique (Group A)

The model was induced according to the procedure described by Saypol and associates [8], with minor modifications. After 12 hours fasting, the rat was anesthetized by pentobarbital sodium (50 mg/kg) through intraperitoneal injection. The rat was fixed in supine position and the abdominal cavity was entered through a midline laparotomy incision. The abdominal contents were pushed to the right to identify the left kidney, the left renal vein and the left spermatic vein. The external diameter of the left internal spermatic vein was measured using micrometers at level of crossing iliolumbar vein. A metal probe 0.85 mm in diameter was placed on the left renal vein and a 4-0 silk suture tied around the vein and metal probe, medial to the adrenal and internal spermatic veins. The probe was removed, and the vein expanded against the limit of the suture loop. Subsequently, communicating branches between the left spermatic vein and common iliac vein were dissected and fully ligated using a 4-0 silk suture. Finally, the midline incision was closed in two layers with 3-0 silk suture. Eight weeks after initial surgery, the rat was anesthetized and a midline abdominal incision was again made. The external diameter of the left internal spermatic vein was measured again at the similar level to that of initial surgery. All measurements were confirmed by 2 investigators.

2. Experimental rat varicocele model with microsurgery (Group B)

Similarly, the rat was anesthetized by pentobarbital sodium (50 mg/kg) and the midline incision was made. The following manipulation was performed under operating microscope with 16× (Yi Guang Instrument company, Shanghai, China). Under magnification, the tunnel around the renal vein was easily dissected, and partial ligation of left renal vein was easily performed (Figure 1). Also, the left internal spermatic vein with branch to the common iliac vein and the adjacent ureter were clearly identified (Figure 2a). The branch to the common iliac vein was ligated with 10-zero nylon (Figure 2b). The remainder of the procedure was identical to that of Group A.

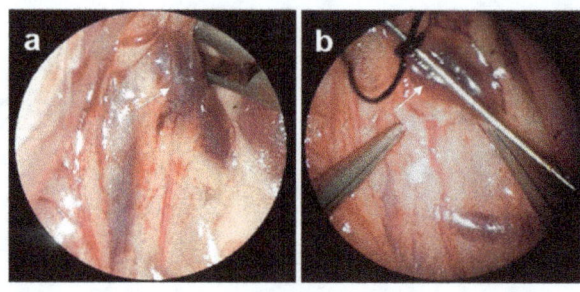

Figure 1 Under enlarged field by operation microscopy, the tunnel around the renal vein was easily dissected (a), and partial ligation of left renal vein was easily performed (b). Arrow: renal vein.

Sperm evaluation

The cauda epididymis from each testis was weighed and minced in 5 ml of the media (Hank's solution containing 0.5% bovine serum albumin) at 37°C. Solution was then placed on a slide glass that was warmed to 37°C for observation of sperm motility. Sperm motility was determined by counting >200 spermatozoa in randomly selected fields under a light microscope. The sperm count was calculated as the number of spermatozoa per gram of cauda epididymis. Sperm concentration and motility were evaluated by two licensed clinical andrology laboratory technologist blinded to the specimen group simultaneously and the average value was adopted.

Statistical analysis

We calculated descriptive statistics for each variable. Before analysis we examined each variable for its distributional characteristics. All data are shown as the mean ± SD. Statistical significance was defined as $P < 0.05$ for a two-tailed test. Calculation was done using SAS® 9.1.

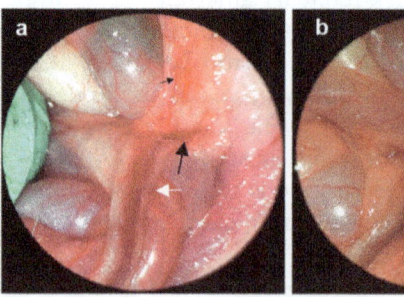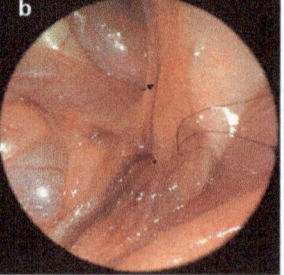

Figure 2 Under operation microscope, the left internal spermatic vein with branch to the common iliac vein and the adjacent ureter were clearly identified (a); and the branch to the common iliac vein was ligated with 10-zero nylon (b). Small black arrow: internal spermatic vein; big black arrow: branch to the common iliac vein; big white arrow: ureter.

Results

The mean baseline total body weight of rats in Group A and Group B was 274.8 ± 13.1 and 271.4 ± 12.4 gm, respectively (P = 0.1432). Baseline mean diameter of the internal spermatic vein in Group A and Group B was 0.14 ± 0.04 and 0.15 ± 0.03 mm, respectively (P =0.3157).

In Group A 9 rats had severe complications resulting in model failure; while in Group B no severe complication happened, and all rats had successful model except for one died of anesthetic accident (85% VS 98.3%, p = 0.008). Of 9 rats in Group A with model failure, 3 rats had injury of common iliac vein and 2 rats had injury of left renal vein immediately at developing the model. At eight weeks after surgery, another 4 rats' left internal spermatic vein could not be identified because of adhesion from pyonephrosis (3 rats) or abdomen abscess (1 rat).

At 8 weeks after initial surgery the mean internal spermatic vein diameter, sperm concentration and motility in both groups were shown in Table 1. There was nonsignificant difference of internal spermatic vein diameter, sperm concentration and motility between two groups.

Discussion

Varicocele has been considered to be closely associated with male infertility, but involved mechanism is not yet completely understood. Difficult tissue acquisition from human, forbidden invasive experiment in human and indefinite patient characteristics made the mechanism study in human is impossible. Thus animal models have been playing an important role in studying pathophysiology of varicocele.

Initially Kay and associates induced varicocele in rhesus monkey by partially ligating the left renal vein [9]. The first animal model reported decreased sperm counts and bilateral elevated testicular temperature. Harisson and co-workers conducted a similar animal model and reported bilateral impairment of lymphatic drainage and decreased testicular blood flow [10]. Subsequently Saypol et al extended the monkey model to dogs, followed by Cockett et al. and Dandia et al. [8,11,12] But in above animal models the reversion of abnormalities in semen characteristics and reduction of dilation degree in spermatic vein has occurred. Also, in 1981 Saypol et al introduced rat experimental model by partially ligating the left renal vein [8]. Since then experimental rat varicocele has become the most common animal model because of similar venous anatomy between human and rat when left varicocele occurs.

Even so, vascular variation adds indefinite factors to successful development of rat varicocele model. Similar to human anatomy, experimental rat varicocele accompanies dilation of the pampiniform plexus, the spermatic vein, and the collaterals leading to the iliac. In most rats more thinner internal spermatic vein from the pampiniform plexus drains into the left renal vein while more thicker branch vein into left common iliac. This pelvic venous drainage can negate the increased venous pressure proximal to partial occlusion of the left renal vein. Thus in this study we ligated the branch veins to the left common iliac besides partially ligating left renal vein. Such a modification has been demonstrated to be important for success of varicocele induction in rats by Turner et al and Najari et al. [7,13]

Although experimental rat varicocele model is widely used, rare report has referred to the complications of developing rat varicocele model. In this study we found success rate of rat varicocele model with conventional technique is only 85%. Except for variation of veinous anatomy, complication may be also the main factor. Vascular injury and pyonephrosis are the most common complications. Vascular injury often happens just when ligating the left renal vein or branches to left common iliac vein. Inadvertent puncture or tear of the vein from blind dissection behind the vein is the possible reason. Pyonephrosis is mainly ascribed to accident ligation of ureter adjacent to spermatic vein, followed by obstructive hydronephrosis and infection.

Comparison of the mean left internal spermatic vein diameter and sperm parameters between two groups shows no significant difference, but there was less complication and higher success in Group B. Addition of microsurgery to conventional technique results in less invasiveness in developing model. Operating microscope with 16× magnification will provide clear and enlarged visual field; and, combined with microsurgical instruments, make the dissection of blood vessel, even tiny branch, easy and safe. Moreover, microsurgical modeling of rat varicocele can easily identify the ureter adjacent to left internal spermatic vein and make ligation of tiny branch to common iliac vein with 10-zero nylon possible, which avoids injuring the ureter.

There are some limitations in this study. Microsurgical rat model needs special training and instruments, which are not commonly used in laboratories. Although the effect of our models on sperm parameters has been referred to in this study, the models as the platform of studying infertility are still further evaluated in the future study.

Table 1 The mean diameter of internal spermatic vein and sperm concentration and motility in both groups at 8 weeks after surgery

Group (n)	Diameter of internal spermatic vein (mm)	Sperm	
		Concentration (10^6/gm)	Motility (%)
A (51)	1.65 ± 0.29	321.5 ± 19.9	51.9 ± 4.8
B (59)	1.65 ± 0.25	318.9 ± 13.6	53.5 ± 5.5
P value	0.9465	0.4076	0.1114

Conclusion

With operating microscope, developing experimental rat varicocele model becomes easy and safe. Compared with conventional technique, microsurgical rat varicocele model has high success rate and less complication.

Competing interests
The authors declare that they have no competing interests.

Authors' contributions
TZ, FG, AB, HC, AB, GC, ES, BY, ES, AB, YS, FG. All authors read and approved the final manuscript.

Author details
[1]Department of Urology, Changhai Hospital, The Second Military Medical University, 168 Changhai Road, 200433 Shanghai, PR China. [2]Department of Urology, Haining People's Hospital, 2 QianJiang West Road, 314400 Haining City, ZheJiang Province, PR China.

References
1. Naughton CK, Nangia AK, Agarwal A. Pathophysiology of varicoceles in male infertility. Hum Reprod Update. 2001;7:473–81.
2. Eisenberg ML, Lipshultz LI. Varicocele-induced infertility: newer insights into its pathophysiology. Indian J Urol. 2011;27:58–64.
3. Brown JS, Dubin L, Hotchkiss RS. The varicocele as related to fertility. Fertil Steril. 1967;18:46–56.
4. Li H1, Dubocq F, Jiang Y, Tiguert R, Gheiler EL, Dhabuwala CB. Effect of surgically induced varicocele on testicular blood flow and Sertoli cell function. Urology. 1999;53:1258–62.
5. Hsu HS, Chang LS, Chen MT, Wei YH. Decreased blood flow and defective energy metabolism in the varicocele-bearing testicles of rats. Eur Urol. 1994;25:71–5.
6. Pascual JA, Lemmi C, Rajfer J. Variability of venous anatomy of rat testis: application to experimental testicular surgery. Microsurgery. 1992;13:335–7.
7. Najari BB, Li PS, Ramasamy R, Katz M, Sheth S, Robinson B, et al. Microsurgical rat varicocele model. J Urol. 2014;191:548–53.
8. Saypol DC, Howards SS, Turner TT, Miller Jr ED. Influence of surgically induced varicocele on testicular blood flow, temperature, and histology in adult rats and dogs. J Clin Invest. 1981;68:39–45.
9. Kay R, Alexander NJ, Baugham WL. Induced varicoceles in rhesus monkeys. Fertil Steril. 1979;31:195–9.
10. Harrison RM, Lewis RW, Roberts JA. Testicular blood flow and fluid dynamics in monkeys with surgically induced varicoceles. J Androl. 1983;4:256–60.
11. Cockett AT, Al-Juburi A, Altebarmakian V, Vergamini RF, Caldamone AA. The varicocele: new experimental and clinical data. Urol. 1980;15:492–5.
12. Dandia SD, Bagree MM, Vyas CP, Singh H, Pendse AK, Joshi KR. Experimental production of varicocele and its effects on testis. JAP J Sur. 1979;4:372–8.
13. Turner TT, Caplis LA, Brown KJ. Vascular anatomy of experimentally induced left varicocele in the rat. Lab Anim Sci. 1996;46:206–10.

3

Use of buccal mucosa grafts for urethral reconstruction in children

Emilie K Johnson[*], Spencer I Kozinn, Kathryn L Johnson, Sohee Kim, David A Diamond and Alan B Retik

Abstract

Background: The use of buccal mucosa grafts (BMG) for urethral reconstruction has increased in popularity over the last several decades. Our aim was to describe our institutional experience with and outcomes after BMG urethroplasty.

Methods: We conducted a retrospective cohort study of boys undergoing BMG urethral reconstruction. Preoperative and perioperative characteristics and postoperative outcomes were evaluated.

Results: Twenty-nine patients (median age 8.2 years) underwent BMG urethroplasty from 1995–2012. Of the 10 patients undergoing 1-stage repairs, 6 had tubularized grafts, the last of which was performed in 2000 due to an unacceptably high revision rate (100%). A 2-stage approach was elected for 19 patients (median follow-up 21.3 months). Complications including stricture, fistula, or chordee were seen in 60% of patients completing both stages and 32% required ≥1 revision. However, 71% of 2-stage patients were free of significant problems at last follow-up.

Conclusions: We found BMG to be a reasonable option for use in complex pediatric urethral reconstruction. Tubularized grafts had poor results, and we no longer use them. We favor a 2-stage approach for all patients except those with "simple" non-hypospadiac strictures. Although revision procedures were not uncommon, the majority of patients were ultimately free of long-term problems.

Keywords: Stricture, Hypospadias, Urethroplasty, Buccal mucosa, Oral mucosa

Background

Urethral pathology in children is generally comprised of complex hypospadias cases and other causes of urethral stricture disease, which include traumatic, iatrogenic, and idiopathic etiologies. In many situations, these abnormalities can be reconstructed primarily. For hypospadias, most cases can be corrected via chordee release and local tissue rearrangement such as in the tubularized incised plate repair [1]. Short strictures less than 1–2 cm in length due to other causes are often amenable to direct visualization internal urethrotomy or primary anastomotic urethroplasty [2].

Hypospadias is most often repaired in the first 6–12 months of life with short-term success rates approaching 90% [3,4]. However, long-term complication rates may

be much higher, particularly for patients with severe hypospadias where complication rates approaching 30% have been reported [5]. Complications include urethrocutaneous fistula, diverticulum, residual chordee, breakdown of the repair, and urethral stricture, all requiring further surgical intervention. Subsequent attempts at repair are less likely to succeed than primary intervention due to tissue loss and scarred, hypovascular, immobile skin. Additionally, patients with strictures longer than 1–2 cm and/or multiple strictures may require augmentation or replacement of the diseased urethral tissue to achieve a successful surgical result.

Over the last 2 decades, the use of replacement grafts has become an increasingly popular choice for cases with complex urethral pathology. In particular, buccal mucosa grafting (BMG) is an attractive option because the buccal surface is non-hair bearing, it normally exists in a moist environment, and the tissue is abundant and readily

* Correspondence: emilie.johnson@childrens.harvard.edu
Department of Urology, Boston Children's Hospital, 300 Longwood Ave, Boston, MA 02115, USA

accessible. There is a robust body of literature regarding the use of oral mucosa in the adult urethral stricture population [6-8]. Both single and multi-staged approaches have been described with favorable outcomes thus far. However, less data exists for the use of BMG in the repair of complex urethral stricture disease pediatric patients. The aim of our study was to investigate and describe the Boston Children's Hospital experience with BMG for urethral reconstruction.

Methods

Patient identification

We conducted a retrospective cohort study of all patients treated for urethral pathology at Boston Children's Hospital whose repair required the use of BMG. Patients were initially identified via the presence of a Current Procedural Terminology (CPT) billing code for a complicated hypospadias repair (54340, 54344 or 54348), repair of hypospadias cripple (54352), first stage urethral revision (53400) and/or excision of oral mucosa for graft (40818). Patient operative notes were then screened to identify the use of a BMG during at least 1 urethral reconstruction procedure at our hospital.

Data abstraction

Retrospective chart abstraction was performed for each patient in our cohort. Variables collected included demographics, urologic and non-urologic comorbidities, initial diagnoses, and pre-buccal repair characteristics (if applicable). We also collected perioperative data including type of repair, number of stages necessary, indication for the repair that included buccal mucosa, graft characteristics, immediate complications, and length of time between stages. We recorded duration of follow-up for each patient, need for (and types of) revision after buccal repair, assessed the proportion and types of long-term complications (e.g. stricture, fistula, chordee, etc.) and determined whether these problems persisted at the time of last visit to our clinic. Failure was identified by clinical history and examination, and (in some cases) flow rate. For 1-stage repairs, follow-up time was calculated as time since the BMG repair. For patients undergoing 2-stage repairs, follow-up time was calculated as the time since their 2nd stage.

Analysis

Descriptive statistics were used to characterize our population of patients undergoing BMG urethroplasty. Surgical characteristics and postoperative outcomes were evaluated for patients undergoing 1-stage and 2-stage repairs. Data analysis was conducted using IMB SPSS Statistics© Version 19, 2012, Somers, NY. The study was reviewed and approved by the Boston Children's Hospital institutional review board. The protocol number is IRB-P00006955.

Results

Patient cohort

We identified 29 patients who underwent urethral reconstruction using buccal mucosa from 1995–2012 at Boston Children's Hospital by a total of 11 surgeons. The demographic characteristics of these patients are illustrated in Table 1. For those who underwent an initial repair prior to their buccal urethroplasty, their median age at the time of first repair was 9.9 months. Seven patients had urologic comorbidities, including 1 with an unspecified 46 XY disorder of sexual differentiation and 4 patients with isolated cryptorchidism.

Table 2 illustrates the characteristics of our patients prior to their buccal urethroplasty. The initial diagnosis was hypospadias in 24/29 patients (83%) and the initial meatal opening was proximal (proximal shaft, penoscrotal or perineal) in 18/24 cases (75%). Two patients with urethral strictures had a buccal urethroplasty as their first repair. Of the patients with prior repairs, 23/27 (81%) had at least one revision of their initial repair prior to BMG and 6/27 (22%) had 4 or more revisions.

One-stage repairs

A 1-stage repair was elected for 10 patients in total. The clinical characteristics of these patients are illustrated in Table 3. For 6 patients, a tube graft was performed. All of these patients developed complications, with stricture being the most common, and all required at least 1 open revision. Due to these suboptimal outcomes, the last tube graft was performed at our institution in 2000. Since then,

Table 1 Patient demographics (N = 29)

Characteristic	N (%) or median [IQR]
Age at initial repair in months	9.9 [6.8-18.6]
Race	
White	18 (62.1)
Black	4 (13.8)
Asian	1 (3.4)
Other or mixed	3 (10.3)
Unknown	3 (10.3)
Urologic comorbidities (N = 7)	
UDT	5 (71.4)
DSD	1 (14.3)
Vesicoureteral reflux	2 (28.6)
Medical comorbidities (N = 14)	
Pulmonary	4 (28.6)
GI	4 (28.6)
Cardiac	4 (28.6)
Endocrine	3 (21.4)
Other	2 (14.3)

Table 2 Pre-buccal graft repair characteristics

Characteristic	N (%)
Initial diagnosis (N = 29)	
Hypospadias	24 (82.8)
Urethral stricture	3 (10.3)
Urethral duplication	1 (3.4)
Chordee	1 (3.4)
Initial hypospadias location (N = 24)	
Distal	4 (16.7)
Midshaft	2 (8.3)
Proximal	18 (75.0)
Initial type of repair (N = 27)	
1 stage flap	4 (14.8)
1 stage tube	2 (7.4)
1 stage, unspecified type	1 (3.7)
First stage	1 (3.7)
Multistage	8 (29.6)
Unknown	5 (18.5)
Other	6 (22.2)
Number of procedures prior to buccal grafting (N = 29)	
0	2 (6.9)
1	5 (17.2)
2	5 (17.2)
3	5 (17.2)
4+	12 (41.4)
Endoscopic management attempted prior to buccal grafting (N = 29)	
Yes	12 (41.4)
No	17 (58.6)
Buccal graft surgical approach	
1-stage tube	6 (31.6)
1-stage onlay	4 (21.1)
2-stage	19 (65.5)

4 patients have undergone 1-stage onlay BMG (3 ventral and 1 dorsal) with better results. Although ¾ have had a recurrent stricture, the only subsequent procedures required have been endoscopic stricture management in 2 patients.

Two-stage repairs

A 2-stage approach was selected for 19 patients, whose clinical characteristics are illustrated in Table 4. Three patients are still awaiting their second stage procedures and 2 were recently completed with follow-up pending, so results are reported for the 14 patients who have undergone both stages and have subsequent follow-up. The median interval between stages was 9 months, and

Table 3 Clinical characteristics of patients undergoing 1-stage BMG urethroplasty (N = 10)

Characteristic	N (%) or median [IQR]
Age at surgery in years	9.6 [3.7-16.3]
Duration of follow-up in months	50.1 [10.6-120.2]
Age at follow-up in years	17.0 [11.3-19.7]
Indication(s) for buccal repair[a]	
Stenosis/Stricture	6 (60)
Breakdown	2 (20)
Diverticulum	1 (10)
Chordee	5 (50)
Fistula	1 (10)
Graft length in cm	3.5 [3.0-4.2]
Surgical approach	
Onlay	4 (40)
Tubularized graft – buccal only	5 (50)
Tubularized graft composite with bladder	1 (10)

[a]Numbers add to >100% due to patients with multiple indications for repair.

median follow-up was 21.3 months for patients undergoing both stages.

Early complications (within 30 days of surgery) were seen in 3 patients after their 1st stage and in 5 patients after their 2nd stage. After the 1st stage, we observed 1 patient with urinary retention, 1 with pyelonephritis, and 1 with a bolster (compressive dressing designed to protect graft) that became dislodged and required replacement under anesthesia. For the 2nd stage, 2 patients had postoperative abscesses, and 1 had an early fistula.

When we defined a long-term complication as a problem such as stricture, fistula, diverticulum and/or chordee, 9/14 (60%) of patients undergoing a 2-stage repair had at least one of these over the course of their follow-up, with

Table 4 Clinical characteristics of patients undergoing 2-stage BMG urethroplasty (N = 19)

Characteristic	N (%) or median [IQR]
Age at 1st stage surgery	8.1 [2.8-16.0]
Duration of follow-up in months[a]	8.2 [5.4-18.3]
Age at follow-up in years[a]	21.3 [6.9-37.7]
Indication(s) for buccal repair[b]	
Stenosis/Stricture	15 (79.0)
Breakdown	6 (31.6)
Diverticulum	5 (26.3)
Chordee	2 (10.5)
Fistula	6 (31.6)
Graft length in cm	3.8 [2.0-4.3]

[a]N = 14 patients who underwent both stages and had follow-up.
[b]Numbers add to >100% due to patients with multiple indications for repair.

stricture being the most common. One patient undergoing a 2-stage repair required revision of the 1st stage to correct glandular graft contracture at 9 months postoperatively, and 5/14 patients (36%) required at least 1 revision of their 2nd stage repair, at a median of 13 months (range 10–37 months) after surgery. Median graft length was 3.0 cm in patients without vs. 3.5 cm in patients with a long-term complication. At the time of last visit to our clinic, 10/14 (71%) of patients were free of any complications such as stricture, fistula, or chordee.

Surgical technique

Surgical technique was somewhat surgeon-specific; however, there were several common themes. The graft was secured to the recipient site with fine, absorbable suture, either running or interrupted based on surgeon preference. When possible, a vascularized interposition graft was used to cover the repair; 27% were dartos flaps and 73% required a tunica vaginalis flap for coverage. For 2-stage repairs the graft was secured in place with a bolster dressing, which was left in place for a median of 7 days. Urinary drainage was with a foley or urethral stent in 75%, a suprapubic catheter in 11%, and both a urethral and suprapubic catheter in the remainder (14%).

Donor site

The BMG was harvested from the cheek in 27/29 (93%), 2 of whom had extension of the graft onto the lip. All grafts were harvested by the urologic surgeon. The remaining 2 patients had their graft harvested from the lip alone. All cheek donor sites were closed, and all lip donor sites were left open, a decision that was made by the surgeon to allow for potential re-harvest from the cheek if necessary in the future. No patient developed symptomatic donor site sequelae.

Discussion

In this report, we detail our institutional experience with the use of BMG for urethral reconstruction, which spans nearly 3 decades. The majority of our patients had an initial diagnosis of hypospadias and required multiple reconstructions prior to presentation at our institution. Nearly 2/3 of patients underwent a 2-stage repair, and we favored this approach over time. Tube grafts were abandoned relatively early in our experience due to an unacceptably high re-stricture rate, which we hypothesize is due to circumferential graft contracture. Long-term complications were seen in 47% of patients undergoing 2-stage repairs and 32% required at least 1 revision of their BMG. However, 68% were free of significant problems at the time of last follow-up.

Buccal mucosa first gained popularity as an option for complex urethral reconstructions in the early 1990s [9,10]. BMG is an attractive option due to the fact that it is a mucosal, non-hair bearing surface with fast uptake and vascularization after free grafting for urethral substitution [10,11]. BM tissue is abundant and accessible and the donor site morbidity is acceptably low [12,13], although contractures have been reported with lip donor sites [14], as well as with large cheek grafts [15].

Multiple previous authors have reported their institutional experiences with buccal mucosa grafting for complex hypospadias. These reports have noted complication rates ranging from 14-57% [16-20], with most complications occurring early (within 6–12 months) after buccal repair [19,20]. Although our early experience with buccal grafts had a complication rate higher than the range previously noted in the literature, our more recent experience is congruent with that of other centers.

In addition to the learning curve inherent with a new technique, our suboptimal early results are reflective of the lack of success of tube grafting compared with other approaches. A consensus is forming in the literature that buccal tube grafts represent a less successful strategy than onlay BMG. Consistent with our experience, Hensle and colleagues' report of a 50% complication rate with tube grafts [19], comparable to our rate of 100%. Surprisingly, Metro and colleagues noted opposite results in their series of 29 patients, where 42% of patients with onlay grafts developing postoperative strictures compared with only 6.3% of tube grafts [17].

Given our disappointing experience with tube grafts, we have adopted a philosophy of using onlay grafts for "simple" strictures, and have come to favor a 2-stage repair for the majority of patients requiring a revision urethroplasty. Newer approaches to onlay grafting, such as the widely anchored patch recently suggested by Djordjevic and colleagues may improve the results of a 1-stage approach for these complicated patients [21]. Thus far, we have found buccal mucosal grafting to be unnecessary for primary hypospadias repairs, although other authors have reported success with this technique for cases of hypospadias with severe chordee [22].

Alternatives to BMG do exist for patients with complex urethral stricture disease where local tissue is not available or suitable for reconstruction. For example, one alternative is to use a posterior auricular full-thickness skin graft as a material for urethral substitution. Our group has recently explored this concept for patients who require reconstruction of the distal penile urethra where buccal mucosa from the cheek might be thicker than desired. Additionally, the use of posterior auricular grafting has been reported in adults where the oral mucosa was unsuitable due to fibrotic changes [23].

Our study has several limitations that warrant mention. Although our experience spans a significant timeframe, it represents a single-institution, retrospective description that may have limited generalizability outside of the complex group of patients treated at our tertiary care academic pediatric hospital. Additionally, this series represents the experience of 11 different surgeons (average cases 2.6/surgeon), underscoring the fact that complex urethral pathology is relatively rare and difficult to manage even in a tertiary care setting. It is also difficult to make specific conclusions regarding the role of a specific surgeon on outcomes due to the small number of patients per surgeon. Also, our patient cohort was identified using billing data, so we could have unintentionally omitted patients undergoing buccal grafting at our institution. To mitigate this limitation, we were purposely broad in the initial billing codes included, and then manually screened patients to exclude them from the final study population. Due to the retrospective nature of our study, we were also limited in the outcome data that could be collected from the patient record; the same outcome measures were not necessarily reported in all encounters for each patient, and we were unable to systematically assess patient-reported outcomes such as quality of life (QOL) and sexual function, which have only been comprehensively reported by one previous group [14,24]. Although these studies suggest that QOL and sexual function was favorable among patients at a single center, the incorporation of patient-reported outcome data from additional centers into future reports is paramount. In particular, assessment of post-pubertal outcomes will be of great interest. Finally, our series represents a heterogeneous group of patients, surgeons, and approaches. While this allowed a basic evaluation of several surgical approaches, this heterogeneity of our patients made a detailed determination of specific patient-and surgeon-level factors predicting complications after surgery challenging.

Despite these limitations, our study provides additional insight into the experience using BMG for reconstruction in patients with complex urethral pathology treated at a specialized academic center. Specifically, our series adds to the knowledge regarding complication rates and particular difficulties with tubularized 1-stage repairs. Our data should help to facilitate appropriate expectation setting for patients and families regarding complications and the potential for revision after buccal urethroplasty, and highlights the importance of long-term follow-up.

Conclusions

At our institution, we have found BMG to be a reasonable option for use in complex urethral reconstruction in children where local tissue is not available or suitable. Tubularized grafts had poor results in our series, and we no longer use them. Currently we favor a 2-stage approach for all patients except for those with "simple" urethral strictures due to causes other than hypospadias. Although many patients required revision procedures after BMG, the majority were free of long-term problems at the time of last follow-up.

Consent

This study was reviewed and approved by our hospital's institutional review board. The results are reported in aggregate, and no individual case details were reported. Therefore a waiver of informed consent was granted for this study.

Abbreviations
BMG: Buccal mucosa graft; QOL: Quality of life.

Competing interests
The authors declare that they have no competing financial or non-financial interests.

Authors' contributions
EKJ contributed to the study design, performed data collection, planned and executed the analysis, drafted and revised the manuscript and approved the final version. SIK contributed to the study design, performed data collection, and assisted with drafting and revising the manuscript and approved the final version. KLJ performed data collection, preliminary data analyses, assisted with drafting and revising the manuscript and approved the final version. SK contributed to the study design, performed data collection, and assisted with drafting and revising the manuscript and approved the final version. DAD supervised the study design and interpretation of results, assisted with drafting and revising the manuscript and approved the final version. ABR supervised the study design, data collection and interpretation of results, assisted with drafting and revising the manuscript and approved the final version.

References
1. Snodgrass W: **Tubularized, incised plate urethroplasty for distal hypospadias.** *J Urol* 1994, **151**(2):464–465.
2. Wright JL, Wessells H, Nathens AB, Hollingworth W: **What is the most cost-effective treatment for 1 to 2-cm bulbar urethral strictures: societal approach using decision analysis.** *Urology* 2006, **67**(5):889–893.
3. Borer JG, Bauer SB, Peters CA, Diamond DA, Atala A, Cilento BG Jr, Retik AB: **Tubularized incised plate urethroplasty: expanded use in primary and repeat surgery for hypospadias.** *J Urol* 2001, **165**(2):581–585.
4. Snodgrass WT, Bush N, Cost N: **Tubularized incised plate hypospadias repair for distal hypospadias.** *J Pediatr Urol* 2010, **6**(4):408–413.
5. Wilcox D, Snodgrass W: **Long-term outcome following hypospadias repair.** *World J Urol* 2006, **24**(3):240–243.
6. Morey AF, McAninch JW: **When and how to use buccal mucosal grafts in adult bulbar urethroplasty.** *Urology* 1996, **48**(2):194–198.
7. Mangera A, Patterson JM, Chapple CR: **A systematic review of graft augmentation urethroplasty techniques for the treatment of anterior urethral strictures.** *Eur Urol* 2011, **59**(5):797–814.
8. Markiewicz MR, Lukose MA, Margarone JE 3rd, Barbagli G, Miller KS, Chuang SK: **The oral mucosa graft: a systematic review.** *J Urol* 2007, **178**(2):387–394.
9. Brock JW 3rd: **Autologous buccal mucosal graft for urethral reconstruction.** *Urology* 1994, **44**(5):753–755.
10. Duckett JW, Coplen D, Ewalt D, Baskin LS: **Buccal mucosal urethral replacement.** *J Urol* 1995, **153**(5):1660–1663.
11. Mokhless IA, Kader MA, Fahmy N, Youssef M: **The multistage use of buccal mucosa grafts for complex hypospadias: histological changes.** *J Urol* 2007, **177**(4):1496–1499. discussion 1499–1500.
12. Cohen SD, Armenakas NA, Light DM, Fracchia JA, Glasberg SB: **Single-surgeon experience of 87 buccal mucosal graft harvests.** *Plast Reconstr Surg* 2012, **130**(1):101–104.
13. Tolstunov L, Pogrel MA, McAninch JW: **Intraoral morbidity following free buccal mucosal graft harvesting for urethroplasty.** *Oral Surg Oral Med Oral Pathol Oral Radiol Endod* 1997, **84**(5):480–482.
14. Nelson CP, Bloom DA, Kinast R, Wei JT, Park JM: **Long-term patient reported outcome and satisfaction after oral mucosa graft urethroplasty for hypospadias.** *J Urol* 2005, **174**(3):1075–1078.

15. Meeks JJ, Erickson BA, Gonzalez CM: **Staged reconstruction of long segment urethral strictures in men with previous pediatric hypospadias repair.** *J Urol* 2009, **181**(2):685–689.

16. Ahmed S, Gough DC: **Buccal mucosal graft for secondary hypospadias repair and urethral replacement.** *Br J Urol* 1997, **80**(2):328–330.

17. Metro MJ, Wu HY, Snyder HM 3rd, Zderic SA, Canning DA: **Buccal mucosal grafts: lessons learned from an 8-year experience.** *J Urol* 2001, **166**(4):1459–1461.

18. Leslie B, Lorenzo AJ, Figueroa V, Moore K, Farhat WA, Bagli DJ, Pippi Salle JL: **Critical outcome analysis of staged buccal mucosa graft urethroplasty for prior failed hypospadias repair in children.** *J Urol* 2011, **185**(3):1077–1082.

19. Hensle TW, Kearney MC, Bingham JB: **Buccal mucosa grafts for hypospadias surgery: long-term results.** *J Urol* 2002, **168**(4 Pt 2):1734–1736. discussion 1736–1737.

20. Fichtner J, Filipas D, Fisch M, Hohenfellner R, Thuroff JW: **Long-term followup of buccal mucosa onlay graft for hypospadias repair: analysis of complications.** *J Urol* 2004, **172**(5 Pt 1):1970–1972. discussion 1972.

21. Djordjevic ML, Kojovic V, Bizic M, Majstorovic M, Vukadinovic V, Korac G: **"Hanging" of the buccal mucosal graft for urethral stricture repair after failed hypospadias.** *J Urol* 2011, **185**(6 Suppl):2479–2482.

22. Macedo A Jr, Liguori R, Ottoni SL, Garrone G, Damazio E, Mattos RM, Ortiz V: **Long-term results with a one-stage complex primary hypospadias repair strategy (the three-in-one technique).** *J Pediatr Urol* 2011, **7**(3):299–304.

23. Manoj B, Sanjeev N, Pandurang PN, Jaideep M, Ravi M: **Postauricular skin as an alternative to oral mucosa for anterior onlay graft urethroplasty: a preliminary experience in patients with oral mucosa changes.** *Urology* 2009, **74**(2):345–348.

24. Nelson CP, Bloom DA, Kinast R, Wei JT, Park JM: **Patient-reported sexual function after oral mucosa graft urethroplasty for hypospadias.** *Urology* 2005, **66**(5):1086–1089. discussion 1089–1090.

4

The impact of fellowship training on pathological outcomes following radical prostatectomy

Jasmir G Nayak[1], Darrel E Drachenberg[1], Elke Mau[1], Derek Suderman[2], Oliver Bucher[2], Pascal Lambert[2] and Harvey Quon[2]*

Abstract

Background: Radical prostatectomy (RP) is a common treatment for prostate cancer (PCa). Morbidity, mortality and pathological outcomes may be superior in academic institutions. One explanation may be the involvement of oncology fellowship trained urologists within academic institutions. The literature examining pathological outcomes often lacks individual surgeon data. The objective of this study was to compare pathological outcomes following RP between fellowship trained and non-fellowship trained urologists.

Methods: Population-based, retrospective chart review of men diagnosed with PCa between 2003 and 2008, the majority treated with open approach RP (>99%). Pathological outcomes were compared between oncology fellowship trained academic (FTA), non-fellowship trained academic (NFTA) and non-academic (NA) urologists. Relationships with pathological outcomes were examined utilizing multivariable logistic regression.

Results: 83.1% of eligible patients were included in our analysis resulting in 1075 patients. In multivariable analysis, surgeon group was an independent predictor of positive surgical margin (PSM) (p < 0.0001). NFTA and NA urologists were more likely to have PSM compared to FTA urologists (OR 2.50; 95% CI: 1.44 - 4.35 and OR 2.10; 95% CI: 1.53 - 2.88, respectively). However, the proportion of PSM between NFTA and NA urologists was not significant (p = 0.492). In addition, pathological stage (p = 0.0004), Gleason sum (p < 0.0001), and surgeon volume (p = 0.017) were associated with PSM. Limitations include retrospective design and lack of clinical and functional outcomes.

Conclusions: Uro-oncology fellowship trained surgeons had significantly lower rates of PSM than non-fellowship trained surgeons in this population based cohort. This study demonstrates the importance of surgeon-related variables on pathological outcomes and highlights the value of additional urologic oncology fellowship training.

Keywords: Education, Fellowship, Pathology, Prostatectomy, Prostatic neoplasms

Background

Prostate adenocarcinoma (PCa) is a prevalent disease with an estimated 256,600 cases expected to be diagnosed in Canada and the US in 2014 alone [1,2]. A significant proportion of patients diagnosed with PCa will undergo a radical prostatectomy (RP). Although a complex issue, it is generally believed that hospitals and surgeons with increased caseloads have reduced rates of post-operative complications, including lower urinary complications and improved oncological outcomes [3-12]. Furthermore,

numerous clinical and pathological factors have been shown to be associated with disease recurrence following RP including clinical stage, biopsy Gleason sum, final Gleason sum, pre-treatment prostate-specific antigen (PSA) and surgical margin status [13,14]. Positive surgical margins (PSM) are associated with increased risks of biochemical recurrence after RP and currently represent a potentially modifiable variable to improve oncological control [7,13,15-18]. Furthermore, PSM is one of the very few quality indicators of surgery. It has previously been shown that substantial variation exists in PSM rates between individual surgeons. Even among experienced surgeons, others have shown that PSM rates range from

* Correspondence: harvey.quon@cancercare.mb.ca
[2]CancerCare Manitoba, Winnipeg, Manitoba, Canada
Full list of author information is available at the end of the article

10-48% in men with organ confined disease, suggesting that the individual surgeon may be an independent risk factor for PSM [5,7].

Earlier studies have demonstrated that after adjusting for annual hospital caseload, better outcomes were achieved following RP in academically affiliated institutions [19]. Specifically, RP performed in academic institutions were associated with fewer blood transfusions, fewer post-operative complications and shorter lengths of stay in hospital [20]. The authors postulated that this might be due to increased caseloads, continual peer-review through the decision-making process and/or multi-disciplinary team approaches to patients. Unfortunately, this study was limited by lack of individual surgeon data and information on clinic-pathological outcomes. Another potential reason for superior outcomes may be the involvement of uro-oncology trained clinicians within these institutions. Generally speaking, supporters of sub-specialization claim that fellowship training translates into improved outcomes. Urologic oncology fellowship programs provide intensive training with a concentrated surgical experience focusing on oncological theory and skills. In fact, it has been shown in a small prospective, cohort study, that fellowship training can abbreviate the learning curve associated with RP [21]. However, to the authors' knowledge there have been no studies investigating the impact of oncology fellowship training on pathological outcomes following RP in a population-based cohort.

It is well documented that PSM have negative prognostic implications including increased rates of biochemical recurrence and disease progression [7,13,15-18]. Thus, PSM may be used as a surrogate measure of oncological outcomes. As such, we sought to determine the impact of urological oncology fellowship training on PSM rates following RP.

Methods

The study was approved by the University of Manitoba Research Ethics Board. As this was a retrospective study, informed consent was not obtained from patients.

Study population

We performed a retrospective population-based study, utilizing a provincial cancer registry to identify all men who were diagnosed with PCa between 2003 and 2008 in whom the vast majority were treated with open approach RP (>99%). A small number of RP's were performed laparoscopically (estimated, approximately <10) and were included within this study cohort. Robotic assisted RP were not available at the time of our study. All malignancies are mandatorily reported to the provincial cancer registry. The pathological records of these patients are stored in a central location and were reviewed manually.

Data collection

For all patients, age, year of diagnosis of prostate cancer, year of surgery, surgeon characteristics, and pathological outcomes following RP were obtained. Surgeons were classified as either: fellowship trained academic (FTA), non-fellowship trained academic (NFTA) or non-academic (NA) urologists based on the highest level of training achieved. For the purpose of our study, fellowship training refers exclusively to surgeons who completed accredited Urologic Oncology programs according to the Society of Urological Oncology. Academic urologists who completed other fellowships (e.g. endourology) were considered as 'non-fellowship' for the purpose of this study. A hospital was considered an academic centre if associated with an accredited residency training program. There was no cross-over between surgeons and their respective institutions. No non-academic surgeons had accredited oncology fellowship training. Pathological reports were reviewed and the following variables were identified: Gleason sum, margin positivity, and lymph node status. Positive margins were defined as cancer at the inked resection margin.

Statistical analysis

The primary purpose of our study was to evaluate the relationship between the PSM rates following RP and surgeon training. Surgeons were grouped into three categories as previously described (FTA, NFTA, and NA). Age was analyzed as a continuous variable. Annual volume was not linearly related to the outcome. As such, annual surgeon volume was analyzed as a categorical variable, defined as the average number of cases per year over the study period (low: <10 cases/year, medium: 10–20 cases/year, high: >20 cases/year). As these were patients diagnosed with PCa between 2003 and 2008, the patients may have undergone their treatment in a different year than they were diagnosed. Thus, the annual volume was assessed over 2004–2008 as a representation of the surgeons RP practice. Pathological outcomes that were analyzed as categorical variables included: Gleason sum (≤6, 7 (3 + 4, 4 + 3), ≥8) and stage (pT2, pT3a, pT3b, pT4). Nodal status was categorized as presence or absence of pathologically involved lymph nodes.

Logistic regression was conducted to examine factors related to positive margins following radical prostatectomy. The surgeon group variable (FTA, NFTA, NA), as well as the covariates of surgeon volume, pathological stage, Gleason sum, and node status were examined as potential predictors of PSM. Associations between predictor variables of interest and PSM were initially evaluated with univariable models. Variables were considered significant and eligible for inclusion in a multivariable model if p-values ≤0.2. This p-value was chosen to help prevent the inadvertent exclusion of variables whose effect may be masked by another variable (i.e. the effect of a predictor only becomes apparent after controlling for a confounder). Correlation between variables was assessed by Spearman's Rank correlation test, variance inflation factor and tolerance statistics. Correlation coefficients ≥0.80, variance inflation factor values ≥10, and/or tolerance values ≤0.2 were considered indicative of multi-colinearity. All significant, non-correlated predictor variables were considered for inclusion in a multivariable model using a manual forward, then backward selection. Variables were considered significant if p-value ≤0.05. All model building analyses were performed with Stata statistical software (version 11.0; Stata Corp, College Station, TX).

Results

Between 2003 and 2008, 1294 patients were identified as meeting our study criteria. 1080 patients were ultimately deemed eligible and included in descriptive analyses, while incomplete pathological reports led to a small number of additional exclusions. The subsequent multivariable modeling was base on 1075 patients, representing 83.1% of all eligible RP's. Baseline characteristics of patients undergoing RP are in Table 1. Fifteen surgeons were divided according to their fellowship training and academic affiliation resulting in three groups: FTA (n = 2), NFTA (n = 3) and NA (n = 10). The average number of annual RP's per group was: FTA 20.5 (range: 13.4-27.6), NFTA 4.3 (range: 0.2-11.4) and NA 12.1 (range: 0.2-51.6). 7 of 15 surgeons averaged less than 5 RP's per year (2 of 3 within NFTA group and 5 of 10 within the NA group). In our cohort, the majority of RP's were performed in non-academic centers (70.1%). The median age of the study population was 62 years. The majority of patients had organ-confined disease (71.5%) with a Gleason Sum of 7 (60.5%). 3.1% of patients had positive lymph nodes on final

pathology. Overall PSM rates for organ confined disease were 28.1%, 49.2% and 47.9% for FTA, NFTA and NA groups accordingly.

On univariable analysis, age, pathological stage, Gleason score, and surgeon group were all statistically significant predictors of PSM (Table 2). Multivariable results are presented in Table 3. Surgeon volume was an independent predictor of margin positivity, with low and medium volumes being associated with lower rates of PSM (p = 0.0166). Pathological stage and Gleason sum were also independent predictors of PSM (p = 0.0004 and p < 0.0001, respectively). After controlling for surgeon volume, pathological stage and Gleason sum, the surgeon group remained independently associated with PSM (p < 0.0001). Overall, NFTA surgeons were associated with a higher rate of PSM than FTA surgeons (OR 2.5, 95% CI: 1.44 – 4.35, p = 0.001). Similarly, NA urologists were also associated with a higher rate of PSM following RP compared to the FTA group (OR 2.1, 95% CI: 1.53 – 2.88, p < 0.001). The difference between NFTA and NA urologists was not significant (OR =1.09; 95% CI 0.64 - 1.88, p = 0.492).

Discussion

In our population-based cohort, we have shown that surgeon group was an independent predictor of obtaining PSM following RP, after adjusting for annual volume, pathological stage, and Gleason sum. RP is a complex procedure that has a steep learning curve associated with it (>250 cases) [22]. Individual surgeon experience and annual volume are important variables that have been previously shown to be associated with PSM [3-12]. Interestingly, in a small, prospective, cohort study, two newly graduated surgeons who completed formal urological oncology

Table 1 Patient characteristics (n = 1080)

| | All groups (%) | Surgeon affiliation (%) | | | p-value |
		FTA, n=238 (22.0)	NFTA, n=85 (7.9)	NA, n=757 (70.1)	
Age*	62 (9.3)	60 (8.4)	62 (8.6)	64 (9.0)	<0.01
Pathological Stage					0.38
pT2	772 (71.5)	160 (67.2)	65 (76.5)	547 (72.3)	
pT3a	168 (15.6)	39 (16.4)	14 (16.5)	115 (15.2)	
pT3b	121 (11.2)	34 (14.3)	6 (7.1)	81 (10.7)	
pT4	19 (1.8)	5 (2.1)	0 (0.0)	14 (1.9)	
Gleason Sum					0.04
≤ 6	295 (27.4)	64 (26.9)	16 (19.3)	215 (28.5)	
7	653 (60.7)	147 (61.8)	63 (75.9)	443 (58.8)	
≥ 8	127 (11.8)	27 (11.3)	4 (4.8)	96 (12.7)	
Node Status					0.06
Positive	30 (3.1)	12 (5.4)	1 (1.3)	17 (2.5)	
Negative	945 (96.9)	210 (94.6)	76 (98.7)	659 (97.5)	

*Median (inter-quartile range).

Table 2 Univariable analysis examining predictors of positive surgical margins

Variable	Odds ratio	95% CI	P-value
Age	1.02	1.00 – 1.04	0.066
Surgeon affiliation			<0.0001
FTA	Reference		
NFTA	1.83	1.11 – 3.02	
NA	1.93	1.43 – 2.60	
Pathological stage			<0.0001
pT2	Reference		
pT3a	2.36	1.67 – 3.34	
pT3b	2.08	1.41 – 3.09	
pT4	1.76	0.70 – 4.42	
Gleason score (sum)			<0.0001
≤6	Reference		
7	2.04	1.54 – 2.72	
≥8	3.46	2.24 – 5.36	
Node status			0.053
Negative	Reference		
Positive	2.09	0.97 – 4.51	
Volume of surgeries			0.113
Low (<10 cases/year)	Reference		
Med (10–20 cases/year)	0.83	0.54 – 1.28	
High (>20 cases/year)	1.10	0.73 – 1.65	

FTA: fellowship trained, academic; NFTA: non-fellowship trained, academic; NA: non-academic.

Table 3 Multivariable analysis of factors predictive of positive surgical margins

Variable	Odds ratio	95% CI	P-value
Surgeon affiliation			<0.0001
FTA	Reference	-	
NFTA	2.50	1.44 – 4.35	
NA	2.10	1.53 – 2.88	
Surgical volume			0.0170
High (>20 cases/year)	Reference	-	
Medium (10–20 cases/year)	0.65	0.487 – 0.878	
Low (<10 cases/year)	0.77	0.503 – 1.199	
Pathological stage			0.0004
pT2	Reference	-	
pT3a	2.08	1.45 – 2.99	
pT3b	1.63	1.06 – 2.53	
pT4	1.51	0.58 – 3.91	
Gleason score			<0.0001
≤6	Reference	-	
7	1.90	1.41 – 2.56	
≥8	2.66	1.64 – 4.31	

FTA: fellowship trained, academic; NFTA: non-fellowship trained, academic; NA: non-academic.

fellowship training at M.D. Anderson Cancer Center, showed that their results were comparable to results of RP's performed by very experienced surgeons in larger series [21]. In this study, their first 66 consecutive patients undergoing RP were assessed from a tertiary, academic referral center. Their overall PSM rate was commendable at 14% while achieving a 94% 5-year biochemical, disease free survival rate. The author's highlight that a strong urological residency combined with their surgically intense (approximately 87 RP's) clinical fellowship likely enhanced their proficiency in performing RP. As a growing number of urologic oncology fellowship trained surgeons enter academia, the impact of oncology-specific fellowship training on pathological outcomes is important to address as it represents an objective means of evaluating this additional training. Certainly, the concept that specialization may improve outcomes is not novel, yet our study is the first to show in a population-based design, that urological oncology fellowship training is associated with improved rates of PSM. The reason for this is unclear however others have suggested this difference may be due to improved surgical technique or perhaps that those who undergo fellowship training are more critical of their own surgical approach [23].

In addition, there is a paucity of population-based literature examining pathological outcomes following RP and we have also shown that PSM rates are likely higher in "real-life" which may suggest that studies based out of tertiary cancer centers may not necessarily hold true at the population-based level. In another population-based study, the rate of PSM after RP in organ-confined disease was 33% [18], comparatively lower than our NFA and NA groups in our study, but higher than our FTA group. However, even amongst experienced surgeons, the rates of PSM shows considerable variability, ranging from 10-48% [7]. Many studies examining PSM rates are from tertiary cancer centers and may not truly represent the "real world" which endorses the importance of conducting population-based studies. Regardless, the rates of PSM in our study are high. The reasons for this are unclear but are likely multi-factorial. One explanation may be the significant heterogeneity within each surgeon groups. Almost half of surgeons included in this population averaged less than 5 RP's per year (2 of 3 NFTA surgeons, and 5 of 10 NA surgeons) that may have affected outcomes, particularly given the small group sizes. Their inclusion adds variability to the results, but highlights the "real-world" urologic practice. In fact, a study based out of the UK revealed that 54% of 212 urologic surgeons performed less than 10 RP's per year, in keeping with our results [24]. Similarly, there were four surgeons (2

NFTA and 2 NA) who stopped performing RP's midway through the study period around the same time that the FTA surgeons volume began to increase which may suggest a generational change in practice that may be confounded by the fellowship training. Although experience is an invaluable asset in performing RP, we were unable to account for this in our analysis.

There are several limitations to our study. Firstly, a significant proportion of patients (16.9%) were excluded from our analysis due to unavailable pathological reports. The inclusion of these missing patients potentially could affect our models and outcomes. However, for a population-based study, the inclusion of over 80% of patients may also be viewed as strength, as other similar studies have drawn conclusions from a notably smaller proportion of patients [18]. Another perceived limitation of our study may be the lack of follow-up to assess disease-specific and overall survival. Data availability precluded this. However, the study was not designed to assess clinical outcomes but rather to examine differences in PSM rates. Others have already shown that PSM may be a surrogate for oncological outcomes [7,13,15-18]. In contrast to previously published literature, we also found that low and medium volume surgeon groups were associated with reduced PSM. This may be due to the relatively small number of surgeons practicing in this region (n = 15), making the results for each group easily influenced by a limited number of individuals. In fact, although the FTA group consisted of surgeons with moderate-high average annual RP volumes (median 21.5, range 13.4-27.6), overall 70% of RP's were performed in non-academic centers where the average number of RP's per year ranged from 0.2-51.6. In addition, our study did not have central pathology review. The histo-pathological interpretation of RP specimens is inherently subjective, yet although inter-observer variability exists, it has been shown that concordance between expert urological pathologists regarding PSM are excellent [25]. Others have also shown that the location, length, and Gleason sum of the PSM has prognostic significance [26], and that not all PSM carry the same risk of developing biochemical recurrence [27,28]. Unfortunately, data constraints prevented us from assessing this. Further, we did not have data on other potentially confounding variables such as nerve-sparing status, prostate volume, tumor volume or patient factors including body-mass index or comorbidities. The majority of RP's described within this study were by traditional open approach and may not apply to contemporary, minimally invasive techniques. Additionally, functional outcomes are another measure of successful surgery but were unable to be captured in the present study. Finally, our data apply to groups of urologists categorized by fellowship training and academic practice, and should not be extrapolated to individual surgeon performance.

Despite these limitations, our study shows that in this population-based cohort treated in the contemporary PSA era, academic surgeons with fellowship training were associated with a reduced risk of PSM. This finding highlights an important surgeon related factor that should be considered but requires further investigation in larger studies.

Conclusion

After adjusting for pathological stage, Gleason sum and surgeon volume, RP performed by oncology fellowship trained urologists were associated with significantly lower rates of PSM. This training may provide additional knowledge and skills to shorten the learning curve associated with RP. Furthermore, our results suggest that surgeon level of training be considered in future studies examining outcomes post-RP.

Abbreviations
RP: Radical prostatectomy; PCa: Prostate adenocarcinoma; PSA: Prostate specific antigen; PSM: Positive surgical margin; FTA: Fellowship-trained, academic; NFTA: Non-fellowship-trained, academic; NA: Non-academic.

Competing interests
The authors declare that they have no competing interests.

Authors' contributions
HQ, DD, JN, and DS participated in the design and co-ordination of the study. JN, EM, and DS were involved in data acquisition. OB and PL carried out statistical analysis. JN and HQ drafted the manuscript. All authors read and approved the final manuscript.

Acknowledgements
The authors would like to thank Cheryl Clague for her timely assistance in arranging for the data acquisition.

Author details
[1]Section of Urology, Department of Surgery, University of Manitoba, Winnipeg, Manitoba, Canada. [2]CancerCare Manitoba, Winnipeg, Manitoba, Canada.

References
1. **Canadian Cancer Statistics.** 2014. [http://www.cancer.ca/~/media/cancer.ca/CW/cancer%20information/cancer%20101/Canadian%20cancer%20statistics/Canadian-Cancer-Statistics-2014-EN.pdf]
2. **Cancer Facts & Figures.** 2014. [http://www.cancer.org/acs/groups/content/@research/documents/webcontent/acspc-042151.pdf]
3. Begg CB, Cramer LD, Hoskins WJ, Brennan MF: **Impact of hospital volume on operative mortality for major cancer surgery.** *JAMA* 1998, **280:**1747–1751.
4. Ellison LM, Heaney JA, Birkmeyer JD: **The effect of hospital volume on mortality and resource use after radical prostatectomy.** *J Urol* 2000, **163:**867–869.
5. Begg CB, Riedel ER, Bach PB, Kattan MW, Schrag D, Warren JL, Scardino PT: **Variations in morbidity after radical prostatectomy.** *N Engl J Med* 2002, **346:**1138–1144.
6. Birkmeyer JD, Siewers AE, Finlayson EV, Stukel TA, Lucas FL, Batista I, Welch HG, Wennberg DE: **Hospital volume and surgical mortality in the United States.** *N Engl J Med* 2002, **346:**1128–1137.
7. Eastham JA, Kattan MW, Riedel E, Begg CB, Wheeler TM, Gerigk C, Gonen M, Reuter V, Scardino PT: **Variations among individual surgeons in the rate of positive surgical margins in radical prostatectomy specimens.** *J Urol* 2003, **170:**2292–2295.

8. Joudi FN, Konety BR: The impact of provider volume on outcomes from urological cancer therapy. *J Urol* 2005, 174:432–438.

9. Chun FK, Briganti A, Antebi E, Graefen M, Currlin E, Steuber T, Schlomm T, Walz J, Haese A, Friedrich MG, Ahyai SA, Eichelberg C, Salomon G, Gallina A, Erbersdobler A, Perrotte P, Heinzer H, Huland H, Karakiewicz PI: Surgical volume is related to the rate of positive surgical margins at radical prostatectomy in European patients. *BJU Int* 2006, 98:1204–1209.

10. Alibhai SM, Leach M, Tomlinson G: Impact of hospital and surgeon volume on mortality and complications after prostatectomy. *J Urol* 2008, 180:155–162.

11. Briganti A, Capitanio U, Chun FK, Gallina A, Suardi N, Salonia A, Da Pozzo LF, Colombo R, Di Girolamo V, Bertini R, Guazzoni G, Karakiewicz PI, Montorsi F, Rigatti P: Impact of surgical volume on the rate of lymph node metastases in patients undergoing radical prostatectomy and extended pelvic lymph node dissection for clinically localized prostate cancer. *Eur Urol* 2008, 54:794–802.

12. Budäus L, Abdollah F, Sun M, Morgan M, Johal R, Thuret R, Zorn KC, Isbarn H, Shariat SF, Montorsi F, Perrotte P, Graefen M, Karakiewicz PI: Annual surgical caseload and open radical prostatectomy outcomes: improving temporal trends. *J Urol* 2010, 184:2285–2290.

13. Hong SK, Han BK, Lee ST, Kim SS, Min KE, Jeong SJ, Jeong H, Byun SS, Lee HJ, Choe G, Lee SE: Prediction of Gleason score upgrading in low-risk prostate cancers diagnosed via multi (> or =12)-core prostate biopsy. *World J Urol* 2009, 27:271–276.

14. Hull GW, Rabbani F, Abbas F, Wheeler TM, Kattan MW, Scardino PT: Cancer control with radical prostatectomy alone in 1,000 consecutive patients. *J Urol* 2002, 167:528–534.

15. Swindle P, Eastham JA, Ohori M, Kattan MW, Wheeler T, Maru N, Slawin K, Scardino PT: Do margins matter? The prognostic significance of positive surgical margins in radical prostatectomy specimens. *J Urol* 2005, 174:903–907.

16. Karakiewicz PI, Eastham JA, Graefen M, Cagiannos I, Stricker PD, Klein E, Cangiano T, Schröder FH, Scardino PT, Kattan MW: Prognostic impact of positive surgical margins in surgically treated prostate cancer: multi-institutional assessment of 5831 patients. *Urology* 2005, 66:1245–1250.

17. Swindle P, Eastham JA, Ohori M, Kattan MW, Wheeler T, Maru N, Slawin K, Scardino PT: Do margins matter? The prognostic significance of positive surgical margins in radical prostatectomy specimens. *J Urol* 2008, 179(Suppl 5):S47–S51.

18. Lawrentschuk N, Evans A, Srigley J, Chin JL, Bora B, Hunter A, McLeod R, Fleshner NE: Surgical margin status among men with organ-confined (pT2) prostate cancer: a population-based study. *Can Urol Assoc J* 2011, 5:161–166.

19. Yuan Z, Cooper GS, Einstadter D, Cebul RD, Rimm AA: The association between hospital type and mortality and length of stay: a study of 16.9 million hospitalized Medicare beneficiaries. *Med Care* 2000, 38:231–245.

20. Trinh QD, Schmitges J, Sun M, Shariat SF, Sukumar S, Bianchi M, Tian Z, Jeldres C, Sammon J, Perrotte P, Graefen M, Peabody JO, Menon M, Karakiewicz PI: Radical prostatectomy at academic versus nonacademic institutions: a population based analysis. *J Urol* 2011, 186:1849–1854.

21. Rosser CJ, Kamat AM, Pendleton J, Robinson TL, Pisters LL, Swanson DA, Babaian RJ: Impact of fellowship training on pathologic outcomes and complication rates of radical prostatectomy. *Cancer* 2006, 107:54–59.

22. Klein EA, Bianco FJ, Serio AM, Eastham JA, Kattan MW, Pontes JE, Vickers AJ, Scardino PT: Surgeon experience is strongly associated with biochemical recurrence after radical prostatectomy for all preoperative risk categories. *J Urol* 2008, 179:2212–2216.

23. Bianco FJ, Cronin AM, Klein EA, Pontes JE, Scardino PT, Vickers AJ: Fellowship training as a modifier of the surgical learning curve. *Acad Med* 2010, 85:863–868.

24. Vesey SG, McCabe JE, Hounsome L, Fowler S: UK radical prostatectomy outcomes and surgeon case volume: based on an analysis of the British Association of Urological Surgeons Complex Operations Database. *BJU Int* 2012, 109:346–354.

25. Evans AJ, Henry PC, Van der Kwast TH, Tkachuk DC, Watson K, Lockwood GA, Fleshner NE, Cheung C, Belanger EC, Amin MB, Boccon-Gibod L, Bostwick DG, Egevad L, Epstein JI, Grignon DJ, Jones EC, Montironi R, Moussa M, Sweet JM, Trpkov K, Wheeler TM, Srigley JR: Interobserver variability between expert urologic pathologists for extraprostatic extension and surgical margin status in radical prostatectomy specimens. *Am J Surg Pathol* 2008, 32:1503–1512.

26. Eastham JA, Kuroiwa K, Ohori M, Serio AM, Gorbonos A, Maru N, Vickers AJ, Slawin KM, Wheeler TM, Reuter VE, Scardino PT: Prognostic significance of location of positive margins in radical prostatectomy specimens. *Urology* 2007, 70:965–969.

27. Kordan Y, Chang SS, Salem S, Cookson MS, Clark PE, Davis R, Herrell SD, Baumgartner R, Phillips S, Smith JA Jr, Barocas DA: Pathological stage T2 subgroups to predict biochemical recurrence after prostatectomy. *J Urol* 2009, 182:2291–2295.

28. Emerson RE, Koch MO, Jones TD, Daggy JK, Juliar BE, Cheng L: The influence of extent of surgical margin positivity on prostate specific antigen recurrence. *J Clin Pathol* 2005, 58:1028–1032.

5

Targeted salvage lymphadenectomy in patients treated with radical prostatectomy with biochemical recurrence: complete biochemical response without adjuvant therapy in patients with low volume lymph node recurrence over a long-term follow-up

Alexander Winter[1][*], Rolf-Peter Henke[2] and Friedhelm Wawroschek[1]

Abstract

Background: Choline positron emission tomography/computed tomography (PET/CT) represents an option in restaging of prostate cancer patients with disease relapse after local treatment. The present study assess whether salvage resection of lymph node metastases detected on choline PET/CT imaging in prostate cancer patients with biochemical recurrence after radical prostatectomy can result in a long-term complete biochemical remission, without adjuvant therapy.

Methods: We analysed 13 patients with prostate specific antigen (PSA) recurrence (PSA median 1.64 ng/ml, range 0.5-9.55) after radical prostatectomy and suspicious lymph nodes (median 1; range 1–3) detected on [11C]choline and [18F] fluoroethylcholine PET/CT scans. An open salvage lymphadenectomy of positive lymph nodes in a PET/CT scan and nearby lymph nodes was carried out. We examined PSA outcome without adjuvant therapy; defined complete biochemical remission as PSA <0.01 ng/ml. Histological and PET/CT findings were compared.

Results: Ten of 11 patients with histologically confirmed lymph node metastases showed a PSA response. Three of ten patients with single lymph node metastases had a complete biochemical remission (median follow-up 72 months, range 31.0-83). In five cases with single lymph node metastasis PSA decreased <0.02 ng/ml. Histologically confirmed 13 of 16 metastasis suspicious lymph nodes. No lymph node metastases were detected in two patients. All of the additionally removed 30 lymph nodes were correctly negative.

Conclusions: This is the first confirmation of a complete biochemical remission after PET/CT guided secondary resection of a single lymph node metastasis in prostate cancer patients with biochemical recurrence after radical prostatectomy, over the long-term (>6.5 years), without adjuvant therapy. In order to improve these promising results, longer-term studies with more patients are required.

Keywords: Prostate cancer, Choline positron emission tomography/computed tomography, Biochemical recurrence, Salvage lymphadenectomy, Lymph node metastases

* Correspondence: winter.alexander@klinikum-oldenburg.de
[1]University Hospital for Urology, Klinikum Oldenburg, School of Medicine and Health Sciences, Carl von Ossietzky University Oldenburg, Rahel-Straus-Straße 10, 26133 Oldenburg, Germany
Full list of author information is available at the end of the article

Background

Biochemical recurrence following surgical treatment of prostate cancer is a common event. The introduction of new functional imaging developments have improved the detection of the site of small volume lymph node (LN) recurrence in prostate cancer patients. This raises now the question if there is a role for secondary targeted surgery of small volume LN recurrences. In recent years, different research groups have published data on positron emission tomography/computed tomography (PET/CT) guided salvage LN dissection in patients with biochemical recurrence and nodal recurrence after a radical prostatectomy [1-3]. Based on this data situation, salvage lymphadenectomy is seen as a possible option for patients with disease relapse limited to the LNs after radical prostatectomy [4]. Integrated [11C]choline or [18F]fluoroethylcholine PET/CT scans, despite their limitations [5], have exhibited good sensitivity and specificity for detecting small (>5 mm) LN metastases after radical prostatectomy. In patients with biochemical failure after local treatment with curative intent, actual meta-analysis results showed pooled sensitivity, specificity, and a diagnostic odds ratio of 85%, 88%, and 41.4 respectively, on a per-patient basis [6]. In contrast, CT and conventional magnetic resonance imaging (MRI) are not definitive for early detection of LNs recurrence. Lymphotropic nanoparticle enhanced MRI can detect smaller LN metastases (>2 mm) but has not been approved for routine diagnostics [7].

Long-term follow-up studies have shown relapse-free survival after radical prostatectomy in patients with minimal lymphatic dissemination, even without adjuvant therapy [8,9]. These data suggest that resection of LN metastases in selected patients in a secondary situation is also beneficial. However, most prior studies dealing with salvage LN dissection provide no evidence on long-term complete PSA response without adjuvant therapy. These patients were either treated after the secondary resection of LN metastases with hormones or radiation therapy [1,10] or were monitored without adjuvant therapy, mostly over a short period [11]. Moreover, these studies and Rigatti et al. [2] defined the biochemical response to treatment only as prostate specific antigen (PSA) <0.2 ng/ml.

Our group has already published promising initial results of patients with relapse-free survival after secondary LN surgery without adjuvant therapy [3]. The aim of the present study with more patients and a longer follow-up is to evaluate whether solely secondary resection of LN metastases in patients with biochemical recurrence or PSA persistence after radical prostatectomy can result in a complete long-term biochemical remission (PSA <0.01 ng/ml). The PSA outcome after targeted resection of LN metastases detected on choline PET/CT scans was analysed over the long-term in patients with biochemical recurrence or persistence after radical prostatectomy, without adjuvant therapy after salvage lymphadenectomy.

Methods
Patient population

This study included 13 patients with PSA recurrence or persistence after radical prostatectomy, performed within the previous three months to 10 years. A retropubic radical prostatectomy with pelvic lymphadenectomy was performed on 12 patients and a radical retropubic prostatectomy only on one patient. In our clinic, one patient underwent a sentinel guided LN dissection on both sides of the pelvic and an extended LN dissection on the right side, because of an advanced tumour; another one underwent only a sentinel guided LN dissection. The remaining patients had undergone conventional LN dissections carried out at other institutions and in one case at our clinic. All patients had LN pathological uptake on [11C]choline or [18F]fluoroethylcholine PET/CT scans and no signs of any local recurrence or distant metastasis. Furthermore, none of the patients showed any signs of ossary metastases in the skeletal scintigraphy.

Integrated choline PET/CT imaging

All [11C]choline or [18F]fluoroethylcholine PET/CT studies were performed in four external centres by experts using integrated PET/CT systems. Experienced radiologists and nuclear medicine specialists evaluated the images to anatomically localise the sites of pathological choline uptake. The diagnosis of tumour positive LNs on PET/CT images was based on visual evidence of the presence of focal increased uptake on a choline PET scan, where the location corresponded to LNs on CT images (Figure 1).

Surgical procedure, PSA evaluation, histological evaluation

Two highly experienced surgeons performed open secondary LN dissections at one centre on patients in the study, between September 2004 and February 2013. They dissected pathological LNs detected on choline PET/CT scans and nearby LNs. Clavien-Dindo grading system was used to classify complications. The PSA development was monitored postoperatively without adjuvant therapy.

Androgen ablation was not continued in those patients who did have androgen ablation before the salvage surgery. Patients with PSA persistence or further PSA increase after the secondary LN surgery have been treated with hormone withdrawal in the further course and have been followed up in the study anymore. The primary histological diagnosis was made on haematoxylin and eosin-stained sections. Immunohistochemical staining of cytokeratins was performed to verify micrometastases.

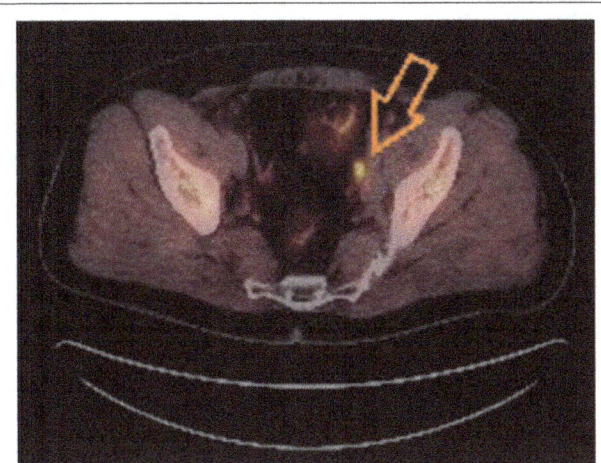

Figure 1 Integrated [18F]fluoroethylcholine PET/CT scan.
Integrated [18F]fluoroethylcholine PET/CT scan shows a single lymph node metastasis in the left iliac region (arrow). The lymph node metastasis was confirmed histopathologically after secondary lymph node surgery. (Source: Clinic for Nuclear Medicine, Pius Hospital Oldenburg, Germany).

In one case, additional antibodies against PSA, prostate-specific acid phosphatase, p504s, and the proliferation marker Ki67 were employed for typing the metastatic tissue. The histological findings were compared with the PET/CT findings.

Since only adjacent LNs were removed in addition to the PET/CT positive LNs and furthermore, no extended lymphadenectomy was performed, it was not possible to calculate the sensitivity of the PET/CT diagnostics for detecting metastases. Specificity was calculated according to its definition (true-negatives/true-negatives + false-positives).

Ethical approval

This study has been performed in accordance with the ethical standards and the German legislation. The current analysis represents a retrospective evaluation of a consecutive data bank, which was done by a separate unit. The data have already been made anonymous at the source. Therefore this retrospective analysis does not require formal ethical approval.

Results

A summary of patient characteristics is shown in Table 1. In 11 of 13 patients, metastasis-suspicious LNs detected by means of PET/CT images could be completely removed. These were also histologically positive. In one patient with two metastasis-suspicious LNs detected on PET/CT scans, only one histologically-negative LN could be resected, because of severe cicatrisation. A further 30 (mean 2.3, range 0 – 10) adjacent PET/CT negative LNs were dissected and found negative for cancer. In one case, the neighbouring LNs could not be removed, because just three months earlier this patient had undergone an sentinel guided and extended pelvic lymphadenectomy on the same affected side. In another patient, only cicatricial tissue could be removed in addition to one LN metastasis after radiotherapy. In the same patient, a small lesion of the ureter necessitated secondary ureteral stenting (Clavien-Dindo IIIb). In all other cases, the intra- and postoperative courses were without complications.

After the secondary LNs resection, ten of 11 patients with histologically-confirmed LN metastases showed a PSA response, without adjuvant therapy after secondary LN surgery. In five of ten patients with single LN metastases the PSA value decreased <0.2 ng/ml. Three patients with single metastases had a lasting complete PSA remission (<0.01 ng/ml). The maximum follow-up duration for these patients was 83 months (median 72 month, range 31.0 – 83). In one of the four cases with a single LN metastases and only a partial, incomplete remission local recurrence was detected in the course of the study by means of PET/CT and MRI. In the three other patients with incomplete remission, a tumorous infiltration of the adjacent tissue had already been detected histologically. In the patient without PSA response, three LN metastases were histologically confirmed. Table 1 shows the PSA outcome for all patients.

Discussion

The introduction of new functional imaging techniques improved detection of LN metastases in prostate cancer and opens new focal treatment options. For example studies with magnetic resonance lymphography guided intensity-modulated radiotherapy have shown to eliminate metastatic lymph nodes [12]. The role of secondary LN surgery in prostate cancer is still being debated. In recent years, an increasing number of publications have released data on secondary LN dissections in patients treated with radical prostatectomy and radiation therapy. However, the studies did not analyse the course of PSA or a complete remission after secondary resection of LNs metastases for longer than five years, without adjuvant therapy. Moreover, these studies defined a relapse-free condition as a PSA of only 0.2 ng/ml (Table 2). Ours is the first study that has been able to confirm complete PSA remission (<0.01 ng/ml) lasting over almost seven years, following secondary LN surgery of a patient with biochemical recurrence after radical prostatectomy, without adjuvant therapy. The median follow-up period was 72 months for three relapse-free patients, all of whom exhibited minimal lymphatic dissemination or a single LN metastasis.

The patients in the herein examined collective only show a comparatively low metastasis load, with an

Table 1 Summary of patient characteristics and PSA outcome after secondary resection of lymph node metastases without adjuvant therapy

Patient	Age (yr)	Primary treatment	Initial tumour stage	Gleason score	Hormonal therapy after primary treatment	Radio-therapy after primary treatment	PSA initial (ng/ml)	PSA1 (ng/ml)	[11C] choline PET/CT	[18F]fluoro-ethylcholine PET/CT	PET/CT positive LN	PSA2 (ng/ml)	Follow-up (month)
1	61	RRP + PLND	pT3a pN0 M0 R0	3 + 4	-	-	4.13	0.92	+	-	1	0.22	79
2	59	RRP + PLND	pT2c pN0 M0 R0	4 + 3	+	-	26.7	4.09	+	-	1	<0.01	83
3	64	RRP + PLND	pT3a pN1 M0 R0	4 + 3	-	-	16.0	2.45	+	-	1	<0.01	72
4	68	RRP	pT3a pNx M0 R0	-	-	+	9.9	1.64	-	+	1	<0.01	37
5	78	RRP + PLND	pT3b pN0 M0 R0	3 + 4	-	-	3.2	1.62	+	-	1	2.7	27
6	59	RRP + PLND	pT3a pN0 M0 R0	4 + 3	+	-	7.6	4.51	+	-	1	1.5	6
7	49	RRP + PLND	pT3b pN0 M0 R0	4 + 5	-	-	4.0	0.67	+	-	1	0.03	5
8	61	RRP + PLND	pT3a pN0 M0 R0	5 + 5	+	+	NA	9.55	+	-	3	54.46	12
9	53	RRP + PLND	pT3a pN0 M0 R1	4 + 4	-	+	36.0	3.54	-	+	1	0.4	7
10	75	RRP + PLND	pT3a pN0 M0 R1	4 + 3	-	+	5.94	3.77	+	-	1	10.3	2
11	75	RRP + PLND	pT3a pN0 M0 R0	3 + 3	-	+	7.14	0.94	-	+	1	0.01	10
12	55	RRP + PLND	pT3b pN1 M0 R0	4 + 3	-	-	5.08	0.5	+	-	2	no histologically confirmed LNM	
13	64	RRP + PLND	pT3a pN0 M0 R1	-	-	+	8.21	1.23	+	-	1	no histologically confirmed LNM	
Median	**61**							**1.64**			**1**		

RRP = radical retropubic prostatectomy; PLND = pelvic lymph node dissection; PSA initial = PSA at primary diagnosis; PSA1 = PSA at time of PET/CT diagnosis; PSA2 = PSA after resection of lymph node metastases; LNM = lymph node metastases. NA = not available.

Table 2 Biochemical response in prostate cancer patients after PET/CT guided salvage lymph node surgery

| Literature | Year | Patients or LN dissections | Patients or LN dissections with positive histology | Positive nodes (mean) | PSA at time of PET/CT diagnosis (mean, ng/ml) | Biochemical response (%) | Complete biochemical response without adjuvant therapy in patients with histologically confirmed LN metastases | | | | |
							PSA <0.2 ng/ml	follow-up (month, mean)	PSA <0.01 ng/ml	follow-up (month, mean)
Scattoni et al. [1]	2007	25	19 (76%)	8.8	1.98	NA	NA	NA	NA	NA
Rigatti et al. [2]	2011	72	60 (83%)	9.8	3.7	57	4 of 28 patients	38.9	NA	NA
Jilg et al. [10]	2012	52[†]	47 (90%)[†]	9.7	3.9	46	NA	NA	NA	NA
Martini et al. [13]	2012	8	6 (75%)	1.0	1.6	67	NA	NA	NA	NA
Winter et al.		13	11 (85%)	1.0	2.7	90	5 of 10 patients	41.4	3 of 10 patients	64 (max. 83)

[†]LN dissections.

LN = lymph node, NA = not available.

average of only one removed positive LN and an average PSA value of 2.7 ng/ml (Table 2). It is likely that the very good PSA response in our investigation also results from this. All patients with complete and thus far lasting remission were cases with only one LN metastasis. As shown previously by Rigatte et al. [2] and Jilg et al. [10], presurgical PSA levels and the number of removed positive LNs are independent predictors for clinical progression after secondary removal of the LNMs. Patients with low PSA levels (<4 ng/ml), well to moderately differentiated tumours (Gleason score ≤7); minimal or LN relapse limited to the pelvis only appear to be the best suited candidates for salvage LN dissection [4]. These factors also apply to the three patients with lasting complete PSA remission in our study.

Observations in the primary situation support a therapeutic benefit, especially for patients with minimal lymphatic dissemination, too. Several publications suggest that an extended pelvic lymphadenectomy increases the likelihood of finding positive nodes and improves biochemical relapse-free survival, particularly in patients with a maximum of two positive LNs [14-16].

One limitation of secondary LN surgery in prostate cancer patients is the constrained sensitivity of currently available imaging techniques, especially for detection of small LNs metastases. Contrary to conventional MRI and CT scans, PET ([11C]choline, [11F]choline) scans offer key benefits in detecting LN metastases, especially in case of restaging of patients with biochemical failure after local treatment with curative intent and prostate cancer foci of sizes up to 5 mm [6,17]. Nonetheless, the value of this method is limited because of the frequency of smaller metastases or micrometastases [18]. However, CT and MRI are far less reliable for detecting small metastases [19]. In future, diffusion-weighted MRI could provide additional information on tumour pathophysiology, in comparison with standardised uptake values (SUV) in choline PET/CT scans [20].

A debate is underway on whether choline PET/CT imaging offers the basis for early treatment decisions for patients with PSA failure after radical prostatectomy. Picchio et al. suggest that routine use of choline PET/CT scans cannot be recommended for PSA values <1 ng/ml [21]. However, patients with local recurrence after radical prostatectomy are best treated by salvage radiotherapy when the PSA serum level is <0.5 ng/ml. Our study detected positive findings with a very low PSA value (≥0.67 ng/ml). Also, Scattoni et al. [1] and others [22] have shown positive results in patients with very low PSA levels (<1 ng/ml). A study by Castellucci et al. detected recurrent disease in 28% of patients with PSA <1.5 ng/ml detected by PET/CT [23]. Distant unexpected metastases were detected by PET/CT scans in 21% of the patients, whereby unnecessary local radiotherapy could be avoided. Mamede

et al. [24] evaluate the role of ^{11}C-choline PET/CT imaging only in patients with biochemical recurrence after radical prostatectomy, showing PSA values below 0.5 ng/ml. The choline PET/CT scan was true positive in 15 of 71 (21.1%) cases. In seven of the 71 patients (9.9%), a choline uptake was observed in pelvic LNs. Nevertheless, it is evident that the positive detection rate of choline PET/CT scans depends on the PSA level and PSA kinetics. PSA and PSA doubling time are independent predictors of positive PET/CT findings. Accordingly, Giovacinni et al. observed a significant rise in positive findings, based on the PSA level (PSA 0.2 – 1 ng/ml: 19%; 1 – 3 ng/ml: 46%; >3 ng/ml: 82%) and the PSA doubling time (>6 months: 27%; 3 – 6 months: 61%; <3 months: 81%) [25]. Besides, another principal limitation of the method is the inhibitory effect of androgen deprivation therapy on choline uptake in patients with hormone sensitive prostate cancer [26]. A [68Ga] PSMA PET/CT scan appears to offer clear advantages over a choline PET/CT scan, particularly for small LN metastases. Compared to a choline PET/CT scan, a [68Ga] PSMA PET/CT scan shows LN metastases with significantly higher contrast, especially at low PSA levels [27].

Our study shows full correlation between [11C]choline PET/CT and [18F]fluoroethylcholine PET/CT images and histological findings in ten of eleven patients with a single LN metastasis (specificity 90.9%), and a specificity of 81.3% (13/16) across all patients. As far as the method is concerned, no conclusions can be drawn on the sensitivity of choline PET/CT imaging. On the contrary, Passoni et al. showed that [11C]choline PET/CT scans had a poor positive predictive value (24%) in identifying patients with single positive LNs at salvage LN dissections [28]. These patients also underwent a pelvic or pelvic and retroperitoneal LN dissection.

One limitation of the study is that no sufficient information on PSA kinetics (e.g. PSA doubling time) after radical prostatectomy was available for the included patients. However PSA doubling time coupled with the PSA parameter is an important predictor for positive PET/CT findings in a recurrence situation [25], which could not be taken into account accordingly in this analysis.

The small and heterogeneous sample size represent the main limitation of our study. Even among patients with a single LN metastasis (n= 10), only 30% of patients had a complete permanent remission (PSA <0.01 ng/ml) with undetectable PSA. However, in five (50%) of the patients with single LNs metastasis the PSA value decreased <0.2 ng/ml. Based on this data one cannot state with certainty whether patients with biochemical recurrence and minimal lymphatic dissemination after radical prostatectomy can be cured through surgery. Nonetheless, there is much to be said for this approach, considering one patient exhibited complete biochemical recurrence after secondary resection of a single LN metastases – for a period of over almost seven years by now. Hence, at least in such cases a therapeutic effect through secondary resection of LN metastases is likely. However, the results of studies with greater patient numbers and longer follow-up remain to be seen.

Conclusions

New functional imaging techniques have opened the door for new focal treatment options in prostate cancer recurrence. This is the first confirmation of a complete PSA remission (<0,01 ng/ml) after PET/CT guided secondary resection of single LNs metastases in patients with biochemical recurrence after radical prostatectomy, over the long-term (>6.5 years) and without adjuvant therapy after salvage lymphadenectomy. This approach at least offers a therapeutic benefit in selected cases with minimal lymphatic dissemination, possibly even a cure, through secondary dissection of LN metastases. Although choline PET/CT scans have their limitations, they are currently the most reliable and routinely available diagnostic tools for detecting LN metastases in prostate cancer with biochemical recurrence after radical prostatectomy. One can look forward to future improvements through the introduction of new tracers (e.g. 68Ga-labelled PSMA ligand), especially for detecting small LN metastases at low PSA values. In order to improve this promising results, multicenter studies are required.

Competing interests
The authors declare that they have no competing interests.

Authors' contributions
AW participated in the conception and design of the study, acquisition of data, analysis and interpretation of data and drafted the manuscript. RPH carried out histological examinations and have been involved in revising the manuscript critically for important intellectual content. FW participated in the conception and design of the study and interpretation of data and have been involved in revising the manuscript critically for important intellectual content. All authors read and approved the final manuscript.

Author details
[1]University Hospital for Urology, Klinikum Oldenburg, School of Medicine and Health Sciences, Carl von Ossietzky University Oldenburg, Rahel-Straus-Straße 10, 26133 Oldenburg, Germany. [2]Oldenburg Institute of Pathology, Oldenburg, Germany.

References
1. Scattoni V, Picchio M, Suardi N, Messa C, Freschi M, Roscigno M, et al. Detection of LN metastases with integrated [11C]choline PET/CT in patients with PSA failure after radical retropubic prostatectomy: Results confirmed by open pelvic retroperitoneal lymphadenectomy. Eur Urol. 2007;52:423–9.
2. Rigatti P, Suardi N, Briganti A, Da Pozzo LF, Tutolo M, Villa L, et al. Pelvic/retroperitoneal salvage LN dissection for patients treated with radical prostatectomy with biochemical recurrence and nodal recurrence detected by [11C]choline positron emission tomography/computed tomography. Eur Urol. 2011;60:935–43.
3. Winter A, Uphoff J, Henke RP, Wawroschek F. First results of [11C]choline PET/CT-guided secondary LN surgery in patients with PSA failure and single LN recurrence after radical retropubic prostatectomy. Urol Int. 2010;84:418–23.
4. Abdollah F, Briganti A, Montorsi F, Stenzl A, Stief C, Tombal B, et al. Contemporary role of salvage lymphadenectomy in patients with recurrence following radical prostatectomy. Eur Urol. 2014, doi:10.1016/j.eururo.2014.03.019, epub ahead of print.
5. Osmonov DK, Heimann D, Janßen I, Aksenov A, Kalz A, Juenemann KP. Sensitivity and specificity of PET/CT regarding the detection of lymph node metastases in prostate cancer recurrence. Springerplus. 2014;3:340. doi:10.1186/2193-1801-3-340.
6. Umbehr MH, Müntener M, Hany T, Sulser T, Bachmann LM. The role of 11C-choline and 18 F-fluorocholine positron emission tomography (PET) and PET/CT in prostate cancer: a systematic review and meta-analysis. Eur Urol. 2013;64:106–17.
7. Birkhäuser FD, Studer UE, Froehlich JM, Triantafyllou M, Bains LJ, Petralia G, et al. Combined ultrasmall superparamagnetic particles of iron oxide-enhanced and diffusion-weighted magnetic resonance imaging facilitates detection of metastases in normal-sized pelvic LNs of patients with bladder and prostate cancer. Eur Urol. 2013;64:953–60.
8. Withrow DR, DeGroot JM, Siemens DR, Groome PA. Therapeutic value of LN dissection at radical prostatectomy: a population-based case-cohort study. BJU Int. 2011;08:209–16.
9. Von Bodman C, Godoy G, Chade DC, Cronin A, Tafe LJ, Fine SW, et al. Predicting biochemical recurrence-free survival for patients with positive pelvic LNs at radical prostatectomy. J Urol. 2010;184:143–8.
10. Jilg CA, Rischke HC, Reske SN, Henne K, Grosu AL, Weber W, et al. Salvage LN dissection with adjuvant radiotherapy for nodal recurrence of prostate cancer. J Urol. 2012;188:2190–7.
11. Rinnab L, Mottaghy FM, Blumstein NM, Reske SN, Hautmann RE, Hohl K, et al. Evaluation of [11C]-choline positron emission/computed tomography in patients with increasing prostate-specific antigen levels after primary treatment for prostate cancer. BJU Int. 2007;100:786–93.
12. Meijer HJ, Debats OA, Kunze-Busch M, van Kollenburg P, Leer JW, Witjes JA, et al. Magnetic resonance lymphography-guided selective high-dose lymph node irradiation in prostate cancer. Int J Radiat Oncol Biol Phys. 2012;82:175–83.
13. Martini T, Mayr R, Trenti E, Palermo S, Comploj E, Pycha A, et al. The role of C-choline PET/CT guided secondary lymphadenectomy in patients with PSA failure after radical prostatectomy: Lessons Learned from Eight Cases. Adv Uro 2012; doi:10.1155/2012/601572.
14. Daneshmand S, Quek ML, Stein JP, Lieskovsky G, Cai J, Pinski J, et al. Prognosis of patients with lymph node positive prostate cancer following radical prostatectomy: long-term results. J Urol. 2004;172:2252–5.
15. Briganti A, Karnes JR, Da Pozzo LF, Cozzarini C, Gallina A, Suardi N, et al. Two positive nodes represent a significant cut-off value for cancer specific survival in patients with node positive prostate cancer. A new proposal based on a two-institution experience on 703 consecutive N+ patients treated with radical prostatectomy, extended pelvic LN dissection and adjuvant therapy. Eur Urol. 2009;55:261–70.
16. Touijer KA, Mazzola CR, Sjoberg DD, Scardino PT, Eastham JA. Long-term Outcomes of patients with lymph node metastasis treated with radical prostatectomy without adjuvant androgen-deprivation therapy. Eur Urol. 2014;65:20–5.
17. Hara T, Kosaka N, Kishi H. Pet imaging of prostate cancer using carbon-11-choline. J Nucl Med. 1998;39:990–5.
18. Husarik DB, Miralbell R, Dubs M, John H, Giger OT, Gelet A, et al. Evaluation of [(18)f]-choline PET/CT for staging and restaging of prostate cancer. Eur J Nucl Med Mol Imaging. 2008;35:253–63.
19. Hövels AM, Heesakkers RA, Adang EM, Jager GJ, Strum S, Hoogeveen YL, et al. The diagnostic accuracy of CT and MRI in the staging of pelvic lymph nodes in patients with prostate cancer: A meta-analysis. Clin Radiol. 2008;63:387–95.
20. Beer AJ, Eiber M, Souvatzoglou M, Holzapfel K, Ganter C, Weirich G, et al. Restricted water diffusibility as measured by diffusion-weighted MR imaging and choline uptake in (11)C-choline PET/CT are correlated in pelvic lymph nodes in patients with prostate cancer. Mol Imaging Biol. 2011;13:352–61.
21. Picchio M, Briganti A, Fanti S, Heidenreich A, Krause BJ, Messa C, et al. The role of choline positron emission tomography/computed tomography in the management of patients with prostate-specific antigen progression after radical treatment of prostate cancer. Eur Urol. 2011;59:51–60.

22. Vees H, Buchegger F, Albrecht S, Khan H, Husarik D, Zaidi H, et al. 18 F-choline and/or 11C-acetate positron emission tomography: detection of residual or progressive subclinical disease at very low prostate-specific antigen values (<1 ng/ml) after radical prostatectomy. BJU Int. 2007;99:1415–20.

23. Castellucci P, Fuccio C, Rubello D, Schiavina R, Santi I, Nanni C, et al. Is there a role for ^{11}C-choline PET/CT in the early detection of metastatic disease in surgically treated prostate cancer patients with a mild PSA increase <1.5 ng/ml? Eur J Nucl Med Mol Imaging. 2011;38:55–63.

24. Mamede M, Ceci F, Castellucci P, Schiavina R, Fuccio C, Nanni C, et al. The role of 11C-choline PET imaging in the early detection of recurrence in surgically treated prostate cancer patients with very low PSA level <0.5 ng/ml. Clin Nucl Med. 2013;38:342–5.

25. Giovacchini G, Picchio M, Scattoni V, Garcia Parra R, Briganti A, Gianolli L, et al. PSA doubling time for prediction of [(11)C]choline PET/CT findings in prostate cancer patients with biochemical failure after radical prostatectomy. Eur J Nucl Med Mol Imaging. 2010;37:1106–16.

26. Fuccio C, Schiavina R, Castellucci P, Rubello D, Martorana G, Celli M, et al. Androgen deprivation therapy influences the uptake of 11C-choline in patients with recurrent prostate cancer: the preliminary results of a sequential PET/CT study. Eur J Nucl Med Mol Imaging. 2011;38:1985–9.

27. Afshar-Oromieh A, Zechmann CM, Malcher A, Eder M, Eisenhut M, Linhart HG, et al. Comparison of PET imaging with a 68Ga-labelled PSMA ligand and 18 F-choline-based PET/CT for the diagnosis of recurrent prostate cancer. Eur J Nucl Med Mol Imaging. 2014;41:11–20.

28. Passoni NM, Suardi N, Abdollah F, Picchio M, Giovacchini G, Messa C, et al. Utility of [11C]choline PET/CT in guiding lesion-targeted salvage therapies in patients with prostate cancer recurrence localised to a single lymph node at imaging: Results from a pathologically validated series. Urol Oncol. 2014;32:38. e9-38.e16.

6

The effect of smoking on spontaneous passage of distal ureteral stones

Adem Fazlioglu[1], Yilmaz Salman[1], Zafer Tandogdu[1*], Fatih Osman Kurtulus[1], Serap Bas[2] and Mete Cek[3]

Abstract

Background: Animal studies have shown that nicotine affects the peristalsis of the ureter. The aim of the study is to analyze the effect of smoking on spontaneous passage of distal ureteral stones.

Methods: 88 patients in whom distal ureteral stone below 10 mm diameter diagnosed with helical computerized tomography enhanced images were reviewed. Patients were grouped as either smokers (n:33) or non smokers (n:50). Follow-up for spontaneous passage of stones was limited with 4 weeks. Patients did not receive any additional medical treatment other than non-steroid anti inflamatory drugs only during painful renal colic episodes. Two groups were compared with the chi-square test in terms of passing the stone or not. Stone passage was confirmed with either the patient collecting the stone during urination or by helical CT.

Results: Smoking habits was present in 30(34%) patients and the frequency in both groups were similar (smokers: 23(76%) vs non-smokers: 46(79%)). Spontaneous passage of the stone was observed in 69(78%) patients. The two groups were comparable in terms of patien age, male to female ratio and stone size. Stone passage decreased as stone diameter increased. Total stone passage rates were similar in both groups (smokers: 76% vs. non-smokers: 79%) (p > 0.05). Passage of stones > 4 mm was observed in 46% and 67% of smokers and non-smokers respectively. However passage of stones with a diameter ≤ 4 mm were similar in both groups (smokers: 100% vs non-smokers: 92%) (p > 0.05).

Conclusion: Smoking has neither a favorable nor un-favorable effect on spontaneous passage of distal ureteral stones. However, spontaneous passage rates in patients with a stone diameter > 4 mm was lower in smokers. These results should be further confirmed with studies including larger numbers of patients.

Keywords: Ureteral stone, Smoking habits, Nicotine, Distal stones, Spontaneous passage

Background

The prevalence of urolithiasis within the urinary tract is 2-3%. According to the current literature we know that stone localization and size are the most important factors associated with spontaneous stone passage. According to the European Association of Urology urolithiasis guidelines the rate of spontaneous passage for stones < =5 mm was 68% independent of location within the ureter [1].

Most of the time patients develop a colic style pain during the spontaneous passage of a urinary stone. In addition to the colic type pain, spontaneous passage of stones have also been associated with deterioration in renal function and increased susceptibility to urinary tract infections in some patients. During the management of

* Correspondence: drzafer@gmail.com
[1]Department of Urology, Taksim Teaching Hospital, Istanbul, Turkey
Full list of author information is available at the end of the article

ureteral stone the aforementioned possible outcomes should be taken into consideration. Waiting for the spontaneous passage of the stone with or without additional medical treatment is an option for a significant number of patients. In such cases the time frame suggested for the spontaneous passage is 4 weeks [1].

Many studies in the past have exploited various medical treatment options that could assist the spontaneous passage of distal ureteral stones. Alfa adrenergic receptor blockers, prostaglandin inhibitors, steroid treatment (e.g. Deflazacort 30 mg daily, methylprednisolone) and calcium channel blockers are some examples of the research undertaken [2,3]. Studies have shown that alfa-1 adrenergic receptor blockers inhibit the peristaltic activity and basal tonus of the ureter and increase the spontaneous passage rates significantly [4].

Nicotine, one of the major components of cigarettes, activates the sympathetic nervous system by acting on the nicotinic acetylcholine (ach) receptors. Boyarsky et al. hypothesized that nicotine may affect the ureteral peristalsis by the mentioned induction of the ach receptors. They tried to answer this question by exposing dogs to nicotine and have shown that inhaled, intravenous and topical nicotine all increase the peristalsis of dog's ureter [5].

As mentioned before nicotine has a possible effect on ureteral peristalsis. We hypothised that absorbed nicotine in cigarette smokers would influence peristalsis of the ureter and affect the spontaneous passage of ureteral stones. In this study the effect of smoking on spontaneous passage of distal ureteral stones smaller than 10 mm has been evaluated.

Patients and method

After ethical board approval from Gaziosmanpasa Hospital, we retrospectively analyzed the charts of patients who were diagnosed with ureteral stone between February 2008 – September 2008. We evaluated patients diagnosed with a single distal ureteral stone which was shown with CT (n:148). Patient charts were evaluated and patients with peptic ulcer, urinary tract infection in diabetics, spontaneous stone passage history, long term colic pain and antihypertensive drug usage were not included. Stones with a diameter of 10 mm or below identified with CT were included into the evaluation. No patient with alpha blocker treatment was included in the study. Patients with missing data were not included and finally 88 patients were included and were grouped as smokers or non-smokers.

CT was performed using a MDCT (somatom sensation cardiac 64, Siemens Medical Solutions). Non-contrast images were obtained in prone position. The spiral scan time was 10–15 seconds, rotation time 0,5 seconds, slice width 1,5 mm and pitch factor was 1,2. Images were obtained from the diaphragms to the symphysis pubis. Stone diameter was calculated using the benchmark software of the CT. The longest diameter was taken into consideration.

The policy of our department is to follow patients with ureteral stones with the previously mentioned criteria for 4 weeks. During the 4 week period patients are asked to come weekly for evaluations and during this time they are asked to void in a separate container. At the end of 4 weeks if spontaneous passage does not occur we suggest a definitive treatment option. All patients included in the study had a record of weekly evaluation during the 4 week period. Non-steroid antiinflamatory drugs (diclophenac sodium 75 mg) was used only during painful renal colic episodes. The weekly check-up charts were controlled for stone passage, pain and NSAID consumption. Stone passage was defined as radiological proof of no stone or patient record of proof of the stone.

The effect of the stone size and smoking status on spontaneous passage was analyzed using multivariate and univariate analysis.

Results

Total number of patients included in the study was 88. Female to male ratio was 2/7 (female: 20, male: 68) and median age was 40 (range: 17–77). Smoking habits was present in 30 (34%) patients (mean 13.7 pack-per-year). Spontaneous passage of the stone was observed in 69 (78%) patients. Mean age of patients with smoking habits was 42 ± 12 and female to male ratio was 0.33. In the group of patients without smoking habits the mean age was 43 ± 13 and female to male ratio was 0.34. The mean diameter of stones was similar in both groups of patients (smoking +: 4.7 ± 2.3 mm vs smoking -:4.7 ± 2.2 mm) ($p > 0.05$).

Spontaneous passage of stones, located at the distal portion of the ureter, within 4 weeks of follow-up was observed in 78% of patients. Spontaneous passage rates decreased as the stone burden increased. A detailed explanation of the stone passage rates according to stone burden and smoking habits is shown in Table 1.

Spontaneous passage rates were 76% and 79% in patients with smoking habits and no smoking habits respectively. There was no statistical difference between the two groups of patients ($p > 0.05$). Further analysis was made according to stone diameter. None of the patients with smoking habits who had a stone diameter between 8 and 10 mm were able to pass their stones within 4 weeks of follow-up. On the other hand patients with no smoking habits had an 80% passage rate of

Table 1 Spontaneous passage rates of distal ureteral stones according to stone burden, location and smoking habits

	Spontaneous passage number (total number)	Spontaneous passage percentage	p Value
All patients	69 (88)	78%	
1- 4 mm	42 (44)	95%	<0.05
4,1-8 mm	23 (36)	63%	
8,1-10 mm	4 (8)	50%	
Patients with smoking habits	23 (30)	76%	
1- 4 mm	17 (17)	100%	<0.05
4,1-8 mm	6 (10)	60%	
8,1-10 mm	0 (3)	0%	
Patients without smoking habits	46 (58)	79%	
1- 4 mm	25 (27)	92%	<0.05
4,1-8 mm	17 (26)	65%	
8,1-10 mm	4 (5)	80%	

stones between 8 and 10 mm. However due to the low number of patients (smokers n:3 vs non-smokers n:5) in this group the differences could not be proven statistically. Spontaneous stone passage rates of stones between 1-4 mm and 4-8 mm showed no difference when patients were compared according to smoking habits (p > 0.05). Smoking density did not differ in smokers who required an intervention (mean 14 pack-per-year) for their stone or who passed their stone without any intervention (mean 13.7 pack-per-year) (p > 0.05).

Discussion

According to the data of the World Health Organization (WHO), the mean frequency of tobacco smoking in Turkey was 31,2% (49,4% males & 17,6% females) in 2003 [6]. With such high smoking rates it is obvious that smoking is a major health problem in Turkey which requires attention. However, this epidemiologic information is valuable in assessing its possible effects on various systems. In our study we evaluated the possible effects of smoking on spontaneous passage rates of distal ureteral stones. Previous animal studies results have shown that nicotine increases ureteral contraction frequency [5,7].

Ureteral stones are most often encountered in the distal portion. The treatment options for stones at this location differ between interventional management and watchful waiting according to the stone dimension. For stones left for spontaneous passage medical expulsive therapy option should be kept in mind. When initiating such a treatment the consequences of obstruction on kidney functions should be known and the period of watchful waiting should be limited with 4 weeks [1].

In the guideline published by EAU in 2013, spontaneous passage rates of stones was 68% and 95% consecutively for stones below 5 mm and 4 mm independent of location [1]. However the same guideline states that these rates significantly differ according to the stone location within the ureter. Spontaneous passage rates of stones below 4 mm in the proximal, mid and distal portions of the ureter were 25%, 45% and 70% respectively. A 5 mm cut-off value was used in the joint guideline of EAU and American Urological Association (AUA) published in 2007 [8]. According to these guidelines spontaneous passage rates were 68% for stones smaller than 5 mm and interventional treatment is advised in stones greater than 5 mm independent of the location the within the ureter. However location specific spontaneous passage rates are not stated in this guideline. Location of the stone within the ureter has been evaluated by some studies and all confirm that stone passage rates are higher in the distal portion [9,10]. However, detailed evaluations and solid date with respect to stone site and stone size evaluations are scarce.

The subject of medical expulsive treatment has been analyzed in a recently published meta analysis [11]. According to this meta analysis the additional benefit of medical expulsive treatment decreased as stone diameter decreased. The fact that spontaneous expulsion rates increased as stone diameter decreased was the reason why medical expulsive treatment did not have a significant effect in smaller stones. Alpha-blocker studies have shown that stone sizes ≥5 mm demonstrated a significant benefit from medical expulsive treatment [11]. In our study the spontaneous expulsion rates of stones ≥4 mm were lower in patients with smoking habits. The rate of spontaneous expulsion was 46% in smokers and 67% in non-smokers with stones ≥4 mm. However the spontaneous expulsion rate of stones <4 mm was similar in both groups. The data from our study implies that smoking may decrease spontaneous expulsion rates of stones larger than 4 mm.

Anti-edema drugs, spasmolitics, alpha-blockers, calcium channel blockers, prostaglandin inhibitors, glycerin trinitrate and steroids have been researched as an option for medical expulsive therapy [11]. The role of the adrenergic system has been emphasized in many of these studies. The main adrenergic agonist noradrenalin has a dose dependent relationship. Noradrenalin increases the frequency of peristalsis with it s positive chronotropic effect and creates ureteral obstruction with its inotropic effect that causes contraction in the smooth muscle cells of the ureter. Due to these reasons alpha adrenergic stimulus decreases the amount of urine passed through the ureter [12]. Although, the role of the adrenergic system and ureter have extensively been evaluated similar studies about the ach receptor activity is far more less. Especially as nicotine has an effect on the ureteral ach receptors similar studies about its effect may also be carried out.

Boyarsky et al. have shown that nicotine increases the peristaltic activity of the ureter in dogs. In their study they administered nicotine by intravenous, inhaled or topical route and shown that both intravenous and inhaled nicotine, although effective at different dosages, do alter the peristalsis of the ureter [5]. Nicotine most probably exhibits this effect on the ureter over the cholinergic receptors proven to be present in the ureter also [13]. Further studies have shown that in each breath of a cigarette smoked there is 120 μg nicotine and about 50% of this is absorbed to the circulation in humans. After a single breath of a cigarette the concentration of nicotine reaches 0,15-0,25 μg/ml in the arterial blood [14]. Subsequently a person consuming one cigarette within 1 hour will have 18,3 ng/ml of nicotine in their blood. The study of Boyarsky has stroked our attention and lately the increasing attention to medical expulsive treatments has led us to evaluate the effect of smoking on spontaneous expulsion of ureteral stones.

Our study has shown that spontaneous expulsion of stones is not affected from smoking in patients with stones <4 mm. However in the group of patients with stone diameter ≥4 mm the rate of spontaneous expulsion was lower in patients with smoking habits. These results should be further confirmed with studies including larger numbers of patients.

Conclusion

Due to the small number of subjects neither a favorable nor un-favorable effect of smoking on spontaneous passage of distal ureteral stones has been shown. However, spontaneous passage rates in patients with a stone diameter of ≥4 mm was lower in smokers. These results should be further confirmed with studies including larger numbers of patients.

Competing interests
The authors declare that they have no competing interests.

Authors' contribution
AF carried out the design of the study, drafting of the manuscript and interpretation of the results. YS carried out data collection, contributed to interpretation of the results and preparation of the manuscript. ZT carried out the statistical analysis, interpretation of the results and contributed to drafting of the manuscript. FOK contributed to critical revision of the manuscript for important intellectual content. SB contributed to critical revision of the manuscript for important intellectual content. MC contributed to critical revision of the manuscript for important intellectual content. All authors read and approved the final manuscript.

Author details
[1]Department of Urology, Taksim Teaching Hospital, Istanbul, Turkey.
[2]Department of Radiology, Gaziosmanpasa Hospital, Istanbul, Turkey.
[3]Department of Urology, Trakya Medical School, Edirne, Turkey.

References

1. Turk C, Knoll T, Petrik A, Sarica K, Skolarikos A, Straub M, Seitz C, members of the European Association of Urology (EAU) Guidelines Office: *European Association of Urology Guidelineson urolithiasis.* 28th edition. Milano: EAU Annual Congress; 2013. ISBN 978-90-79754-70-0.
2. Tzortzis V, Mamoulakis C, Rioja J, Gravas S, Michel MC, De La Rosette JJMCH: **Medical expulsive therapy for distal ureteral stones.** *Drugs* 2009, **69**(6):677–692.
3. Cervenàkov I, Fillo J, Mardiak J, Kopecný M, Smirala J, Lepies P: **Speedy elimination of ureterolithiasis in lower part of ureters with the alpha 1-blocker–Tamsulosin.** *Int Urol Nephrol* 2002, **34**(1):25–29.
4. Dellabella M, Milanese G, Muzzonigro G: **Efficacy of tamsulosin in the medical management of juxtavesical ureteral stones.** *J Urol* 2003, **170**(6 Pt 1):2202–2205.
5. Boyarsky S, Labay P, Pfautz CJ: **The effect of nicotine upon ureteral peristalsis.** *South Med J* 1968, **61**(6):573–579.
6. World Health Organization: **[database on the Internet].** 2010: [cited http://data.euro.who.int/hfadb/]
7. Barastegui CA: **[Motility of the rat ureter in vitro. Responses to cholinergic drugs (author's transl)].** *Rev Esp Fisiol* 1977, **33**(1):1–4.
8. Preminger GM, Tiselius H-G, Assimos DG, Alken P, Buck AC, Gallucci M, Knoll T, Lingeman JE, Nakada SY, Pearle MS, Sarica K, Türk C, Wolf JS Jr, EAU/AUA Nephrolithiasis Guideline Panel: **2007 Guidline for the management of ureteral calculi.** *J Urol* 2007, **52**(6):1610–1631.
9. Ueno A, Kawamura T, Ogawa A, Takayasu H: **Relation of spontaneous passage of ureteral calculi to size.** *Urology* 1977, **10**(6):544–546.
10. Coll DM, Varanelli MJ, Smith RC: **Relationship of spontaneous passage of ureteral calculi to stone size and location as revealed by unenhanced helical CT.** *Am J Roentgenol* 2002, **178**(1):101–103.
11. Seitz C, Liatsikos E, Porpiglia F, Tiselius H-G, Zwergel U: **Medical therapy to facilitate the passage of stones: what is the evidence?** *Eur Urol* 2009, **56**(3):455–471.
12. Singh A, Alter HJ, Littlepage A: **A systematic review of medical therapy to facilitate passage of ureteral calculi.** *Ann Emerg Med* 2007, **50**(5):552–563.
13. Schulman CC, Duarte-Escalante O, Boyarsky S: **The ureterovesical innervation. A new concept based on a histochemical study.** *Br J Urol* 1972, **44**(6):698–712.
14. Isaac PF, Rand MJ: **Blood levels of nicotine and physiological effects after inhalation of tobacco smoke.** *Eur J Pharmacol* 1969, **8**(3):269–283.

7

A novel surgical management for male infertility secondary to midline prostatic cyst

Gong Cheng[†], Bianjiang Liu[†], Zhen Song, Aiming Xu, Ninghong Song and Zengjun Wang[*]

Abstract

Background: To summary the procedure and experience of a novel surgical management for male infertility secondary to midline prostatic cyst (MPC).

Methods: From February 2012 to February 2014, 12 patients were diagnosed with PMC by semen analysis, seminal plasma biochemical analysis, transrectal ultrasonography (TRUS), and pelvic magnetic resonance imaging (MRI). All patients underwent the transurethral unroofing of MPC using resectoscope, the dilation of ejaculatory duct, and the irrigation of seminal vesicle using seminal vesiculoscope. All patients were followed up at least 3 months after operation.

Results: Preoperative semen analyses of 12 patients showed oligoasthenozoospermia (5/12) or azoospermia (7/12), low semen volume (0–1.9 mL), and low pH level (5.5-7.0). Preoperative seminal plasma biochemical analyses showed reduced semen fructose. TURS and MRI revealed a cyst lesion located in the midline of prostatic. After 3 months follow up, the semen quality of 80% patients (4/5) with oligoasthenozoospermia improved obviously. The spermatozoa were present in the semen in 5 of 7 cases with azoospermia. In one patient, the spermatozoa occurred in the urine after ejaculation.

Conclusions: Surgical management using transurethral resectoscopy and seminal vesiculoscopy is effective, minimally invasive, and safe for male infertility secondary to MPC.

Keywords: Male infertility, Midline prostatic cyst, Transurethral resectoscopy, Seminal vesiculoscopy

Background

Male infertility affects about 8% of couples around the world [1]. Midline prostatic cyst (MPC), a rare but surgically correctable disease, is deemed to cause ejaculatory duct obstruction (EDO) which accounts for approximately 1-5% of male infertility [2]. Most MPCs are nonsymptomatic. Semen analysis, transrectal ultrasonography (TRUS) and pelvic magnetic resonance imaging (MRI) can help to diagnose MPC. For treatment, cyst puncture and simple endoscopic section are widely used. However, the efficacy is often poor. The present study shows a novel surgical management for male infertility secondary to MPC.

Methods

Approval for this study was granted by the ethics committee of Nanjing Medical University (China) and informed written consent was received from all participants.

Patients

From February 2012 to December 2013, 12 patients were recruited at Department of Urology, The First Affiliated Hospital of Nanjing Medical University. The patients were aged 18–40 years. All of them complained of infertility 2–10 years after marriage. Two cases had hematospermia. Preoperative semen analyses of 12 patients showed oligoasthenozoospermia (5/12) or azoospermia (7/12), low semen volume (0–1.9 mL), and low pH level (5.5-7.0). Preoperative seminal plasma biochemical analyses showed reduced semen fructose. TURS (Figure 1A) and MRI (Figure 1B) revealed a cyst lesion located in the midline prostate.

* Correspondence: zengjunwang@njmu.edu.cn

†Equal contributors

State Key Laboratory of Reproductive Medicine and Department of Urology, The First Affiliated Hospital of Nanjing Medical University, Nanjing 210029, China

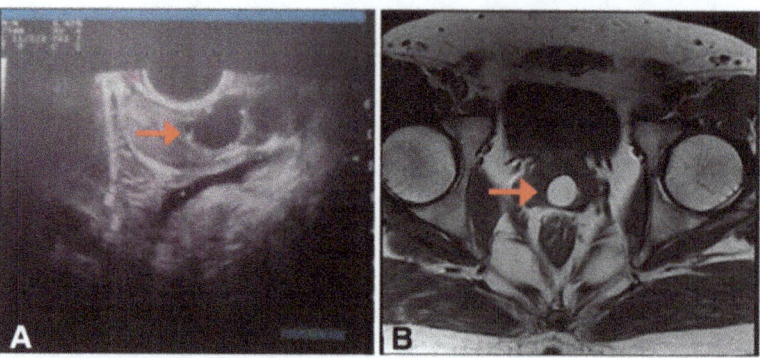

Figure 1 The representative images of MPC. A, TRUS; **B**, pelvic MRI. The arrow indicates the cystic lesion.

Procedures

The patients were placed under general anesthesia in the dorsal lithotomy position. Transurethral unroofing of MPC was performed using the F26 resectoscope. First, the resectoscope was inserted into prostatic urethra for preliminary visualization of the cyst (Figure 2A). Then the ridgy posterior wall of the urethra was resected for unroofing the MPC (Figure 2B and C). If the ejaculatory duct opening was not obvious, transurethral resection of the ejaculatory duct (TURED) was performed to make the ejaculatory duct unobstructed (Figure 2D). Lastly, the dilation of ejaculatory duct and the irrigation of seminal vesicle were performed using F7 seminal vesiculoscope according to our previous report [3]. Under the guidance of a zebra guidewire, the endoscope was inserted into the ejaculatory ducts and seminal vesicles

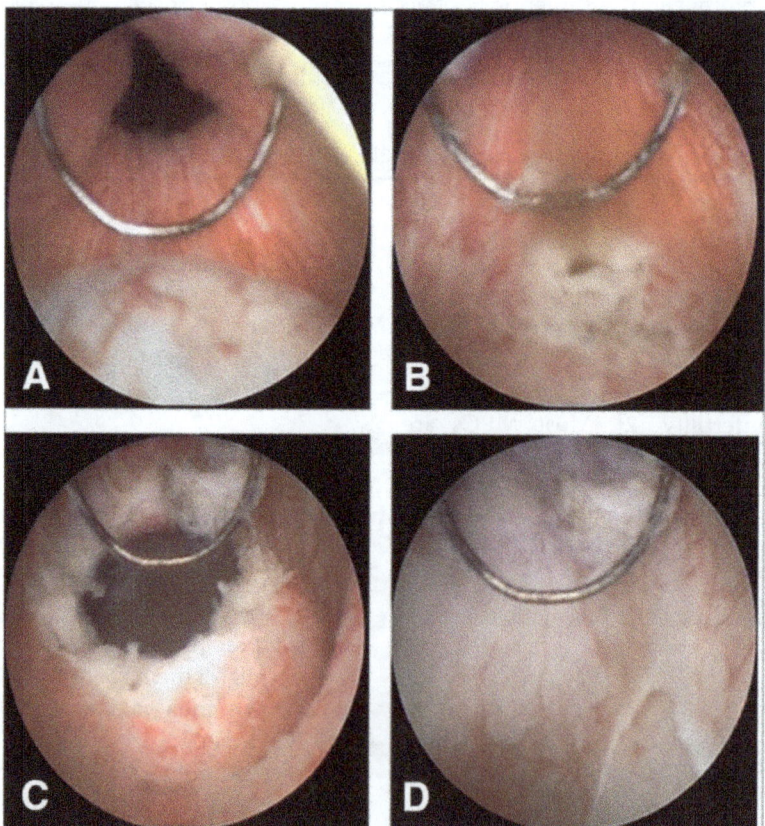

Figure 2 Transurethral unroofing of MPC. A, the cyst is visualized through the resectoscope. **B** and **C**, the ridgy posterior wall of the urethra is resected for unroofing the MPC. **D**, TURED is performed to make the ejaculatory duct unobstructed.

at the help of hand-controlled intermittent water perfusion dilation. The seminal vesicles usually contained the congestive wall, and milky, yellow or pink vesicle fluid filled with flocculent turbidity and dark blood clots (Figure 3A). In some cases, seminal vesicle stones were even found (Figure 3B). The seminal vesicles were irrigated using a levofloxacin solution (Figure 3C and D). After operation, a urethral Foley catheter was remained overnight. All patients were required to refrain from ejaculation at least two weeks and followed up at least 3 months.

Outcomes analysis

Preoperative and postoperative serum sex hormone levels were recorded. Preoperative and postoperative semen qualities were monitored using a computer-assisted semen analyzer (IVOS; Hamilton-Thorne, Beverly, MA, U.S.).

Results

All operations were completed without conversion to open surgery. There were no severe complications such as rectal injury and urethral sphincter damage. The average length of hospitalization was 3 days. Serum sex hormone levels of all patients prior to and after surgery were within the normal range. The preoperative and postoperative semen parameters were shown in Table 1. After 3 months follow up, the semen quality of 80% patients (4/5) with oligoasthenozoospermia improved obviously. The spermatozoa were present in the semen in 5 of 7 cases with azoospermia. In one patient, the spermatozoa occurred in the urine after ejaculation.

Discussion

MPC is previously thought to be Mullerian duct cyst, causing EDO and male infertility through oppressing ejaculatory duct [4]. Recent researches reveal that not all cystic lesions are located in the midline prostate originate from Mullerian duct remnant. Some cases are just the cystadenoma or the simple cyst of prostate [5]. Such cyst in the midline prostate should be termed as prostatic utricular cyst or cystic dilation of prostatic utricle, depending on whether an outlet to the urethra exists.

Despite the embryologic or histological origin, MPC is a surgically correctable disease. Many MPCs are asymptomatic, or have some non-specific symptoms such as perineal pain, hematospermia, and painful ejaculation. One of the most important and serious outcomes caused

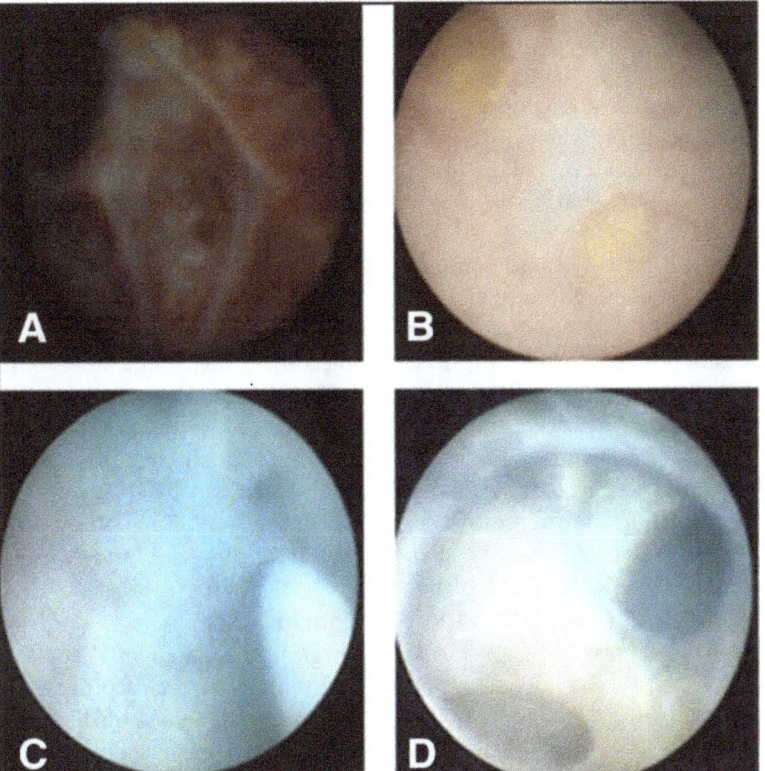

Figure 3 Transurethral irrigation of seminal vesicle. A, seminal vesiculitis contains the congestive wall, and milky, yellow or pink vesicle fluid filled with flocculent turbidity and dark blood clots. **B**, seminal vesicle stones. **C** and **D**, the seminal vesicle is washed clearly and irrigated using a levofloxacin solution.

Table 1 The preoperative and postoperative semen parameters of 12 cases

	Preoperative		Postoperative	
	Concentration (10^6/mL)	Grade a + b (%)	Concentration (10^6/mL)	Grade a + b (%)
Oligoasthenozoospermia 1	11	33.3	45	60.0
Oligoasthenozoospermia 2	6	12.7	21	48.5
Oligoasthenozoospermia 3	15	26.1	73	66.5
Oligoasthenozoospermia 4	2	12.3	4	11.1
Oligoasthenozoospermia 5	9	22.4	50	59.6
Azoospermia 1	0	0	21	62.3
Azoospermia 2	0	0	17	52.3
Azoospermia 3	0	0	0	0
Azoospermia 4	0	0	32	68.7
Azoospermia 5	0	0	10	45.5
Azoospermia 6*	0	0	0	0
Azoospermia 7	0	0	43	57.9

*The spermatozoa occurred in the urine after ejaculation.

by cystic lesion oppression is EDO and male infertility. Semen analysis of these patients often showed low semen volume and pH level, reduced semen fructose, oligoasthenozoospermia, and even azoospermia.

Vasoseminal vesiculography is the golden standard for diagnosis. Percutaneous testicular sperm aspiration (PTSA) is helpful to identify the type of MPC. However, these methods are invasive and complicated. TURS is preferred for simple and noninvasive characteristics. It can offer greater details about the relationship of prostatic, seminal vesicle, and ejaculatory duct [6]. Pelvic MRI not only clearly shows the anatomy of prostatic, seminal vesicle, and ejaculatory duct, but also helps to judge the nature of cyst fluid [7].

The treatment for MPC is still controversial. Some researchers claimed that treatment should only be performed on symptomatic or infertile patients since almost 60% of cases with MPC did not experience any cyst-related symptoms or fertility impairment [8]. Invasive procedures include transperineal or transrectal puncture and endoscopic section of the utricle meatu [9]. However, puncture therapy has a high recurrence rate while endoscopic incision faces persistent post-operative severe oligozoospermia or azoospermia [10]. We speculate that MPC may cause to seminal vesiculitis and further promote the abnormal semen quality through oppressing ejaculatory duct and causing semen stasis. Therefore, the dilation of ejaculatory duct and the irrigation of seminal vesicle using seminal vesiculoscope were performed after transurethral unroofing of the cyst in present study. A previous study achieved a better result for MPC with male infertility using transurethral endoscopic incision, in which a pregnancy rate was 30.8% (8/26) [10]. However, other reports showed a poor efficacy of unroofing of the cyst [11]. The present study is delightful with a pregnancy rate of 41.7% (5/12) and an obviously improved semen quality of 75% (9/12). One patient with azoospermia had spermatozoa in the urine after ejaculation. For the two patients of poor efficacy, seminal vesicle impairment due to long term semen stasis might cause inadequate transfer of semen quality [12]. In conclusion, our data showed that the novel surgical management is effective, minimally invasive, and safe for male infertility secondary to MPC.

The followings are our endoscopic experiences. Sometimes, it is difficult to find the opening since the ejaculatory duct is oppressed by MPC or covered by inflammatory tissues [3,13]. Increasing the velocity of water perfusion and using a zebra guidewire as the guidance are helpful to find the openings. Otherwise, vas deferens puncture and injection of methylene blue, combined with the transurethral endoscope, are helpful to observe the ejaculatory duct openings. After observing the seminal vesicle lumen carefully, appropriate therapies can be implemented. Inflammatory semen can be treated with antibiotics irrigation into seminal vesicle. Stones can be removed through holmium laser lithotripsy and forceps.

Conclusions

Surgical management using transurethral resectoscopy and seminal vesiculoscopy has good clinical outcomes for improving the semen quality. It is effective, minimally invasive, and safe for male infertility secondary to MPC.

Abbreviations

MPC: Midline prostatic cyst; EDO: Ejaculatory duct obstruction; TRUS: Transrectal ultrasonography; MRI: Magnetic resonance imaging; TURED: Transurethral resection of the ejaculatory duct.

Competing interests
The authors declare that they have no competing interests.

Authors' contributions
All authors participated in the study conception, design and coordination. CG, LB, and SZ performed the surgery and wrote the paper. XA and SN performed the data analysis. WZ designed the study. All authors read and approved the final manuscript.

Acknowledgements
This work was supported by the grants from National Natural Science Foundation of China (81270685; 81200467) and by A Project Funded by the Priority Academic Program Development of Jiangsu Higher Education Institutions (JX10231801).

References
1. Goldwasser BZ, Weinerth JL, Carson 3rd CC. Ejaculatory duct obstruction: the case for aggressive diagnosis and treatment. J Urol. 1985;134:964–6.
2. Pryor JP, Hendry WF. Ejaculatory duct obstruction in subfertile males: analysis of 87 patients. Fertil Steril. 1991;56:725–30.
3. Liu B, Li J, Li P, Zhang J, Song N, Wang Z, et al. Transurethral seminal vesiculoscopy in the diagnosis and treatment of intractable seminal vesiculitis. J Int Med Res. 2014;42:236–42.
4. Turek PJ, Magana JO, Lipshultz LI. Semen parameters before and after transurethral surgery for ejaculatory duct obstruction. J Urol. 1996;155:1291–3.
5. Yasumoto R, Kawano M, Tsujino T, Shindow K, Nishisaka N, Kishimoto T. Is a cystic lesion located at the midline of the prostatic a mullerian duct cyst? Analysis of aspirated fluid and histopathological study of the cyst wall. Eur Urol. 1997;31:187–9.
6. Wang H, Ye H, Xu C, Liu Z, Gao X, Hou J, et al. Transurethral seminal vesiculoscopy using a 6 F vesiculoscope for ejaculatory duct obstruction: initial experience. J Androl. 2012;33:637–43.
7. Moukaddam HA, Haddad MC, El-Sayyed K, Wazzan W. Diagnosis and treatment of midline prostatic cysts. Clin Imaging. 2003;27:44–6.
8. Coppens L, Bonnet P, Andrianne R, de Leval J. Adult mullerian duct or utricle cyst: clinical significance and therapeutic management of 65 cases. J Urol. 2002;167:1740–4.
9. Zhou T, Chen CL, Chen K, Wang XD, Yang J. Transrectal ultrasound-guided puncture and anhydrous alcohol sclerotherapy for Mullerian duct cyst. Zhonghua Nan Ke Xue. 2012;18:511–3.
10. Hendry WF, Pryor JP. Mullerian duct (prostatic utricle) cyst: diagnosis and treatment in subfertile males. Br J Urol. 1992;69:79–82.
11. Cornel EB, Dohle GR, Meuleman EJ. Transurethral deroofing of midline prostatic cyst for subfertile men. Hum Reprod. 1999;14:2297–300.
12. Colpi GM, Negri L, Mariani M, Balerna M. Semen anomalies due to voiding defects of the ampullo-vesicular tract. Infertility due to ampullo-vesicular voiding defects. Andrologia. 1990;22 Suppl 1:206–18.
13. Han WK, Lee SR, Rha KH, Kim JH, Yang SC. Transutricular seminal vesiculoscopy in hematospermia: technical considerations and outcomes. Urology. 2009;73:1377–82.

8

Standardised high dose versus low dose cranberry Proanthocyanidin extracts for the prevention of recurrent urinary tract infection in healthy women [PACCANN]

Babar Asma[1,2] (iD), Leblanc Vicky[2], Dudonne Stephanie[2], Desjardins Yves[2], Howell Amy[3] and Dodin Sylvie[1,2*]

Abstract

Background: Urinary tract infections (UTIs) are amongst the most common bacterial infections affecting women. Although antibiotics are the treatment of choice for UTI, cranberry derived products have been used for many years to prevent UTIs, with limited evidence as to their efficacy. Our objective is to assess the efficacy of a cranberry extract capsule standardized in A-type linkage proanthocyanidins (PACs) for the prevention of recurrent urinary tract infection.

Methods: We will perform a 1:1 randomized, controlled, double blind clinical trial in women aged 18 years or more who present ≥2 UTIs in 6 months or ≥ 3 UTIs in 12 months. One hundred and forty-eight women will be recruited and randomized in two groups to either receive an optimal dose of cranberry extract quantified and standardized in PACs (2×18.5 mg PACs per day) or a control dose (2×1 mg PACs per day). The primary outcome for the trial is the mean number of new symptomatic UTIs in women during a 6-month intervention period. Secondary outcomes are: (1) To evaluate the mean number of new symptomatic UTIs with pyuria as demonstrated by a positive leucocyte esterase test; (2) To detect the mean number of new symptomatic culture-confirmed UTIs; (3) To quantify urinary PACs metabolites in women who take a daily dose of 37 mg PACs per day compared to women who take a daily dose of 2 mg per day for 6 months; (4) To characterize women who present recurrent UTI based on known risk factors for recurrent UTI; (5) To describe the side effects of daily intake of cranberry extract containing 37 mg PACs compared to 2 mg PACs. This report provides comprehensive methodological data for this randomized controlled trial.

Discussion: The results of this trial will inform urologists, gynaecologists, family physicians and other healthcare professionals caring for healthy women with recurrent UTI, as to the benefits of daily use of an optimal dose of cranberry extract for the prevention of recurrent UTI.

Keywords: Recurrent urinary tract infection, Women's health, Proanthocyanidins, Cranberry, *Vaccinium macrocarpon*, Antioxidants, Prevention

* Correspondence: sylvie.dodin@fmed.ulaval.ca
[1]Department of Obstetrics and Gynaecology, Laval University, CHU de Québec - Université Laval, 2705, boulevard Laurier, Local A1385, Québec, Québec G1V 4G2, Canada
[2]Institute of Nutrition and Functional Foods, Laval University, 2440 Hochelaga Boulevard, Quebec City, Quebec G1V 0A6, Canada
Full list of author information is available at the end of the article

Background

Urinary tract infections (UTIs) are one of the most common bacterial infections affecting women [1, 2]. UTI preferentially affects young, sexually active women with 50–60% of women reporting at least one UTI during their lifetime [2]. Nearly 1 in 3 women will experience at least one episode of UTI requiring antibiotic therapy before the age of 24 years and a quarter of these women will present reoccurrence within 6 months [1]. Anatomical differences in male and female perineal anatomy may explain why women are more susceptible than men to the ascension of faecal bacteria in the urinary tract. More precisely, these anatomical features include a relative shortness of the urethra [3], the urethral meatus's proximity to the anus and a more humid surrounding environment comparatively to the male anatomy [4, 5]. Additional well-established risk factors include spermicide-based contraception, history of previous UTI, first UTI before 15 years of age and those with UTI history in the mother [6–10].

Recurrent UTIs (r-UTI) are defined as more than 2 episodes in the last 6 months or 3 episodes in the last year [11]. The major symptoms of UTI include dysuria, increased frequency of urine, cloudy urine and occasionally hematuria [12]. In general, uncomplicated UTIs are confined to the bladder, resolve quickly following antibiotic treatment and thus are associated with fewer severe or long-term sequelae [13]. Though viewed as a benign affliction, uncomplicated lower UTI symptoms can have considerable impacts on the patient's productivity and quality of life. A study of university women reported that patients suffering from UTI experienced 2.4 days of restricted activity, 1.2 days of lost time and 0.4 bed bound days due to their symptoms [7]. Presently, the Canadian Urological Association and Society of Obstetricians and Gynecologists of Canada recommendations for the treatment of uncomplicated r-UTI use one of three antibiotic treatment regimens: continuous antibiotic prophylaxis, post-coital antibiotic prophylaxis or self-start antibiotic therapy [11, 12]. Empirical and preventive antibiotics for the treatment of r-UTI have been established as the most cost-effective way to manage these infections. However, prescribing without confirmation of diagnosis and isolation of causal bacterial contributes to the growing problem of uropathogen resistance in primary care [14].

Cranberries have been used for numerous years to prevent UTIs. Research suggests that proanthocyanidins (PACs), a component of cranberries, inhibit the adherence of p-fimbriated *Escherichia coli* on uroepithelial cells of the bladder, preventing the adherence of bacteria to the mucosal surface of the urinary tract and thereby inhibiting bacterial proliferation [15]. A multicentre randomized clinical trial (RCT) in sexually active adult women showed that a daily dose of 36 mg PACs or more provided an optimal antibacterial effect in the urine [16]. A Cochrane systematic review published in 2012, could not definitively conclude on the efficacy of cranberry products for the prevention of r-UTI mainly because of a lack of observance to the intake of cranberry supplements in juice form and also because of varying PACs concentrations in the different clinical trials that were rarely quantified or standardized [17]. A systematic review in 2013 including trials conducted in women with r-UTI found a significantly decreased risk of UTI among women receiving cranberry-containing products compared to control (2 trials, Risk ratio (RR) = 0.53, 95%CI 0.33–0.83, I^2 = 0%) [18].

Since these reviews, several well-designed trials have evaluated the effects of daily cranberry capsules in women with r-UTI. Most notably, an RCT compared the preventive effects of a cranberry juice (UR65) containing 40 mg PACs versus placebo on the relapse of UTI in women aged 20–79 years presenting acute complicated or uncomplicated cystitis with a history of r-UTI during a six-month follow-up [19] The authors found no significant difference in the relapse rates of UTI between groups (log-rank test, $p = 0.4209$). Similarly, a double blind RCT evaluated the effects of a daily dose of 500 mg of a commercial cranberry fruit powder (2 mg PACs) compared to a placebo in 176 women who experienced at least 2 symptomatic UTI in the twelve months preceding the study [20]. In this trial, the proportion of women who experienced greater than one UTI in the cranberry powder group was significantly lower than in the placebo group during the six-month follow-up period (10.8% vs 25.8%, $p = 0.04$). Although well designed, these studies presented several methodological flaws such as the inclusion of women with complicated UTIs related to catheterization in the former as well as the use of a sub-optimal dose of cranberries in the latter.

We hypothesize that the efficacy of cranberry products for the prevention of R-UTI in women will be strongly increased by the usage of an optimal dose of cranberry extracts in capsule form (standardized to 37 mg PACs per day) and by an adequate measure of participant observance.

Methods
Study design and objectives
To assess the effects of a standardized cranberry extract in sexually active healthy women who present r-UTI, we will undertake a double blind, prospective RCT with 2 arms comparing the mean number of new UTIs during a 6-month period after consumption of a standardized cranberry extract containing 37 mg PACs (2 × 18.5 mg PACs per day) with a control dose of 2 mg PACs (2 × 1 mg PACs per day) in women presenting r-UTI. This protocol was developed in accordance with the Standard

Protocol Items: Recommendations for Interventional Trials (SPIRIT) Statement. The SPIRIT figure is illustrated in Fig. 1.

The primary objective is to evaluate, in sexually active women who present r-UTIs, the effects of a standardized cranberry extract containing 37 mg type-A linkage PACs per day, compared to a control dose of 2 mg PACs per day during a 6-month period on the incidence rate of newly symptomatic UTIs during a 6-month follow-up period. Secondary objectives are: (1) To evaluate the mean number of new symptomatic UTIs with pyuria as demonstrated by a positive leucocyte esterase test; (2) To detect the mean number of new symptomatic culture-confirmed UTIs; (3) To quantify urinary PACs metabolites in women who take a daily dose of 37 mg PACs per day compared to women who take a daily dose of 2 mg per day for 6 months; (4) To characterize women who present r-UTI based on known risk factors such as spermicidal contraception use, frequency of sexual relations, personal and familial history of UTI; (5) To describe the side effects of daily intake of cranberry extract containing 37 mg PACs compared to 2 mg PACs.

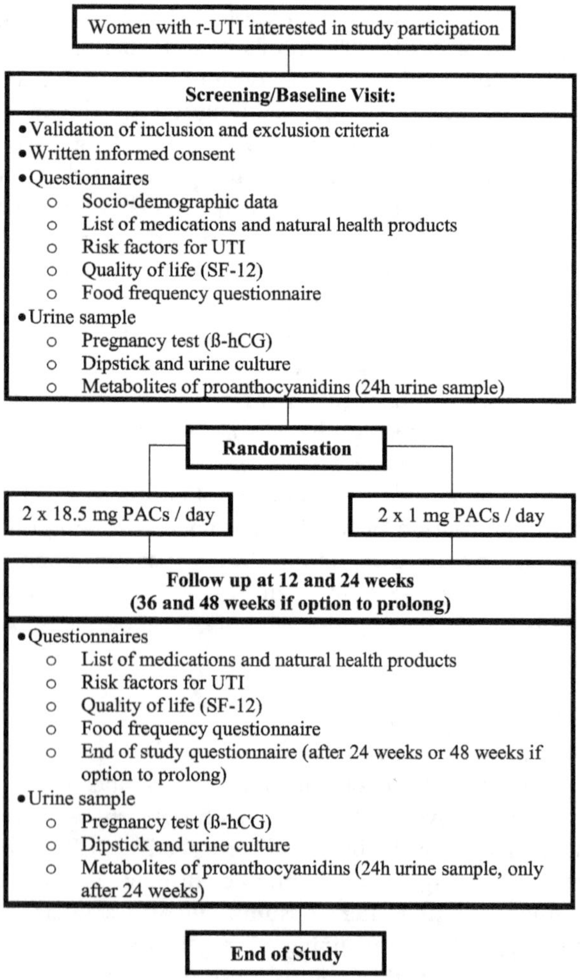

Study participants and recruitment

This clinical trial aims to enrol sexually active non-pregnant non-lactating women aged 18 years and over presenting culture-confirmed r-UTI (defined as ≥2 UTIs in the past 6 months or ≥ 3 UTIs in the past 12 months). Women will be recruited in the Laval University community in Quebec City, Canada, through list serves and local clinician referrals as well as posters in medical clinics, social media, paid advertising and word of mouth. Women wishing to participate will contact the study coordinator who will explain the research project to them and verify eligibility according to inclusion and exclusion criteria (Table 1). The risks and benefits of the study will be thoroughly discussed and the consent form will be signed at the first of three visits at the Institute on Nutrition and Functional Foods (INAF).

Potential participants will need to restrain exposure to systemic antimicrobial agents or cranberry derivatives in the two weeks preceding enrolment. Women with anatomical abnormalities of the urinary tract, a history of renal disease (renal failure, nephrolithiasis) or intestinal disease causing malabsorption (Crohn's disease, Celiac disease), or anticoagulant therapy will be excluded. Furthermore, we will exclude women with known allergy or intolerance to cranberries.

Study randomization

Concealed randomization will be generated using computer aided block randomization by blocks of 10. Eligible

Fig. 1 Study procedures and characteristics of study visits

Table 1 Admissibility criteria for the cranberry extract for prevention of recurrent urinary tract infections trial

Inclusion Criteria
Sexually active healthy women
Aged 18 years and older
Recent history of recurrent urinary tract infections (UTIs)[a]
≥ 2 UTIs in the past 6 months and/or
≥ 3 UTIs in the past 12 months
No consumption of cranberry juice, polyphenol or antioxidant supplements in the last 2 weeks
Exclusion Criteria
Pregnancy
History of anatomical urogenital anomalies, urogenital tract surgery
History of acute or chronic renal failure, nephrolithiasis
History of intestinal diseases causing malabsorption
Anticoagulant medication in the last month
Known allergy or intolerance to cranberry

[a]UTIs diagnosed by a clinician and treated with antibiotic therapy

women will be assigned 1:1 to consume a cranberry extract either formulated in high PAC content capsules (2 capsules of 18.5 mg PAC per day) or low PAC content capsules (2 capsules of 1 mg PAC per day) for 6 months. The low PAC content cranberry capsule is comparable to the majority of cranberry extract products presently approved by Health Canada [21] . The standardized capsules will be manufactured and provided by Diana Foods and will be distributed in opaque packaging in order to conceal colour variations from the research team. The PAC content of each cranberry treatment will be validated at INAF according to the standardized BL-DMAC method, using A2 procyanidin dimer as standard for the quantification [22]. All clinical investigation, laboratory analysis, data collection and assessment will be blinded to the randomization allocation.

Clinical follow-up

Each visit (0, 12 and 24 weeks) will include a short questionnaire documenting socio-demographic characteristics ($T = 0$ only), medication and natural health product intake, quality of life (SF-12) [23], risk factors for UTIs, and a validated food frequency questionnaire (FFQ) [24] modified for our study to specifically include foods containing PACs. Double data entry will be performed under the study coordinator supervision in order to promote data quality. Participants will be instructed to obtain a midstream urine sample according to standard methods suggested by the microbiological laboratory. A dipstick urinalysis using Chemstrip 9 (Roche Diagnostics USA) and a pregnancy test (ß-hCG) will be completed. Three 10 ml tubes will be placed in a – 80 °C freezer for urinary PAC metabolites measurements by ultra-high performance liquid chromatography coupled with mass spectrometry, and the urine sample for culture will be refrigerated and transported to the microbiology laboratory at the CHU de Quebec – Universite Laval within 24 h after collection.

During their participation, the women will be asked to contact the study coordinator if they present symptoms of UTI in order to schedule a visit at INAF to confirm the diagnosis by urinalysis and urine culture and to receive an appropriate antibiotic prescription based on their medical history and allergies. Women unable to present themselves at INAF will be prescribed antibiotics waiving a confirmation of their UTI. Women wishing to discontinue the consumption of capsules will be asked to present themselves at the 3 and 6-month visit in order to complete intention to treat analysis. The participants will be asked not to consume other products containing cranberry derivatives for the duration of the study and to consume their cranberry extracts 2–4 h preceding each visit. Participants will also be asked to limit intense physical activity for 24 h preceding each visit. After 24 weeks of participation, women will be provided with the option of prolonging their participation

for an additional 24 weeks, with follow-up visits at 36 and 48 weeks. This data will provide information on seasonal variations in the incidence of UTI.

Sample size and statistical analysis

Statistical analyses will be performed using SAS 9.2 (SAS Institute Inc., USA). All analyses will be based on the intention-to-treat principle before unmasking the treatment groups. The baseline characteristics of both groups will be compared using a Student's t test for continuous variables and a generalized linear model for nominal variables. The Poisson regression model, which allows us to adjust for participants that were lost to follow up, will be used to compare the incidence of UTI during the 6-month follow up period as well as side effects of the treatment. Subgroup analyses will be performed in order to evaluate the impact of cranberry capsules in pre- and post-menopausal women as well as women with certain risk factors for complicated UTI such as pelvic floor disorders and diabetes.

Based on the literature [17], we estimate that 35% of patients in the control group will present at least one UTI during the 6-month follow-up period. In total, 126 women will need to be recruited in order to detect a clinically significant difference of 25% between the 2 groups (10% of women assigned to the experimental group will have at least 1 UTI with a power of 80%). Based on our past clinical trial experience [25], we estimate that 15% of randomized participants will be lost to follow up, therefore 148 women will need to be recruited in order to have at least 126 participants who will complete the 24-week intervention.

End points

Incidence of UTI

The primary endpoint is the average number of symptomatic UTIs during the 6-month follow-up period. Individuals with acute urinary symptoms such as pollakiuria, urgency, burning, suprapubic pain, and hematuria will be assessed by study staff and will have to provide a urine sample for urinalysis. Women who present both symptom and pyuria criteria, defined as a positive leukocyte esterase dipstick result, will be diagnosed as having confirmed symptomatic UTI and prescribed appropriate antibiotic treatment. If the urine culture results are positive, the episode will be categorized as a culture-confirmed UTI. Women with symptomatic UTI during the study period will continue to take the cranberry capsules and remain in the study for the full 6 months unless they are lost to follow up or discontinue the intervention.

Urinary PAC content

At the beginning of the trial, participants will be offered the option to provide a 24-h urine collect for targeted metabolomic characterization of PAC metabolites using ultra-high-performance liquid chromatography coupled to tandem mass spectrometry, performed by a chemist blinded to treatment allocation.

Compliance and side effects

The cranberry extract capsules will be distributed at each visit and participants will be asked to bring remaining capsules the next visit in order to count remaining capsules. The participants will fill out a daily journal to record compliance, transient UTI symptoms and any adverse effects related to capsule intake. A bi-monthly email reminder will be sent to encourage participation. Each participant will receive an email reminder in the week preceding each visit. Evaluation of side effects will take place at each visit and participants will be asked to document symptoms (nausea, dyspepsia, abdominal pain, bloating and headaches) in their daily journal. In the presence of severe side effects, participants will be allowed to discontinue the intervention and remain in the study in order to preserve the intention to treat analyses.

Blinding and contamination Bias

The proportion of women who will guess their group allocation correctly will be documented with a short questionnaire at the last visit. To control for contamination bias, any antibiotic therapy during the study period will be declared to the study coordinator and PAC consumption will be measured by FFQ for the 24 h preceding each visit.

Discussion

Use of cranberry derived products in the prevention of r-UTI remains controversial, with no definitive evidence to show superiority of the cranberry compared to antibiotic therapy [17, 18]. There is some evidence that cranberry products may reduce the incidence of UTIs compared to placebo, though the most effective amount and concentration of PACs that must be consumed and the duration for the intervention are unknown [17]. To our knowledge, this study is the first large, prospective randomized clinical trial assessing the impact of a cranberry extract capsule standardized to 37 mg PAC per day compared to 2 mg PAC per day in preventing UTIs in healthy women presenting r-UTI.

Incidence of symptomatic UTI during the 6-month follow-up period was selected as the primary end-point in this trial because it is the most important, clinically relevant long-term outcome for patients. We used three classifications for UTI analyses: symptomatic UTI, dipstick-positive UTI and culture-confirmed UTI. Symptomatic UTI was diagnosed if a participant presented at least one of the following symptoms: dysuria, pollakiuria, urinary urgency, suprapubic pain or hematuria. In the presence of clinical symptoms, participants will be asked to provide a urine sample in order to perform a dipstick

test and a urine culture. Positive leucocytes or nitrites will indicate a positive dipstick test [26]. A positive urine culture will be designated by greater than 10^6 colony-forming units, according to the microbiological laboratory standards of the CHUL hospital. In our study, antibiotics will be prescribed in the presence of clinical symptoms in combination with either a positive urine dipstick test and/or positive urine culture.

Implications of findings

Many Canadian women who present r-UTI commonly use over the counter cranberries-derived products with inadequate labelling of PACs concentrations. For cranberry products with quantification of PACs, these concentrations rarely exceed 2 mg in Canada [21]. Various trials have tested the effectiveness of cranberry derived products, essentially in juice form, and their results remain discordant mainly due to the lack of standardization and low doses of PACs in tested products. Hence, the intrinsic activity of cranberry PACs, demonstrated against *Escherichia coli* in vitro, has never been optimized for the prevention of UTI. The results generated from this trial will clarify the role of cranberry extracts standardized in PACs on the decreased incidence of UTI in women presenting r-UTIs, will evaluate the differences in the incidence of UTI on the basis of different PACs concentrations and will respond to the recommendations reported in the last Cochrane meta-analysis [17].

This report provides comprehensive methods for a clinical trial on the prevention of RUTI by cranberry extract capsule intake. The strengths of this trial include the quantification and standardisation of PACs contained in the cranberry extract capsule and a randomized, double blind, controlled trial method. Our trial will add to a growing body of literature regarding cranberry extract capsule for the prevention of r-UTI in healthy women. In addition, the data set and specimen bank generated from conducting this trial will enable researchers to understand the metabolites of type-A PACs produced after prolonged consumption of cranberry capsules.

Trial status

Participant recruitment started on August 18th 2015 and was completed in March 2017. Study follow up visits will continue into Winter 2018.

Abbreviations

FFQ: Food frequency questionnaire; PAC: Proanthocyanidin; RCT: Randomized controlled trial; r-UTI: Recurrent UTI; UTI: Urinary tract infection

Acknowledgements

We thank Iseult Grenier-Ouellet and Marie-Pier Bernard-Genest for their assistance in the clinical follow-up of participants during this clinical trial at the Institute of Nutrition and Functional Foods, Laval University. The authors are very grateful to the laboratory and clinical staff and all participants in this study.

Funding
This research project was funded by the Ministry of Agriculture, Fisheries and Food of Quebec and Nutra Canada (now part of Diana Food). The funders had no role in the design and conduct of this clinical trial; the collection, management, analysis, and interpretation of data; the preparation, review, or approval of the manuscript; and the decision to submit the manuscript for publication. Nutra Canada manufactured and donated the cranberry capsules used in this study.

Availability of data and materials
All data sets will be password protected and only available to project investigators. Data sets, cleaned and blinded of any identifying participant information, as well as the full protocol, will be available after the completion of the trial on request to the contacting author.

Dissemination of results
Trial results will be accessible to health professionals and the scientific community through articles published in peer-reviewed journals and presentations at local, national and international scientific conferences in the fields of gynaecology, urology, nutraceuticals and antioxidants. Results will also be disseminated to the general public through interviews on community radio and the publication of news articles.

Authors' contributions
AB performed recruitment, clinical follow up, interpretation of data, statistical analyses and writing of the manuscript; VL. contributed to the design of this study, recruitment, clinical follow up, interpretation of data, statistical analyses and revision of the manuscript; S. Dudonne undertook supervision of the biomarker measures and review of the manuscript, AD and YD contributed to the original concept and design of this study; S. Dodin contributed to the original concept and design of this study, undertook supervision of the clinical follow-up of participants, and wrote the study grant. All authors read and approved the final manuscript.

Ethics approval and consent to participate
The protocol and consent form of this study were reviewed and approved by the institutional ethics committee of Laval University with approval number 2015–091 A-5/ 03–11-2016. Further changes to the study protocol will require ethics approval from the institutional ethics committee. The study coordinator will obtain written informed consent from all study participants. Women will be able to withdraw from the study at any time during their participation. Data will be entered electronically and original study forms will be kept locked at the study site and maintained in storage for a period of 25 years after the completion of the study. This randomized clinical trial is registered in ClinicalTrials.gov, identifier: NCT02572895.

Competing interests
The authors report no conflicts of interest. The authors alone are responsible for the content and writing of the paper.

Author details
[1]Department of Obstetrics and Gynaecology, Laval University, CHU de Québec - Université Laval, 2705, boulevard Laurier, Local A1385, Québec, Québec G1V 4G2, Canada. [2]Institute of Nutrition and Functional Foods, Laval University, 2440 Hochelaga Boulevard, Quebec City, Quebec G1V 0A6, Canada. [3]Rutgers University, 125A Lake Oswego Rd., Chatsworth, NJ 08019, USA.

References
1. Czaja CA, Hooton TM. Update on acute uncomplicated urinary tract infection in women. Postgrad Med. 2006;119(1):39–45.
2. Foxman B, Barlow R, D'Arcy H, Gillespie B, Sobel JD. Urinary tract infection: self-reported incidence and associated costs. Ann Epidemiol. 2000;10(8):509–15.
3. Hickling DR, Sun TT, Wu XR. Anatomy and physiology of the urinary tract: relation to host defense and microbial infection. Microbiol Spectr. 2015;3(4)
4. Yamamoto S, Tsukamoto T, Terai A, Kurazono H, Takeda Y, Yoshida O. Genetic evidence supporting the fecal-perineal-urethral hypothesis in cystitis caused by Escherichia coli. J Urol. 1997;157(3):1127–9.
5. Hooton TM. Pathogenesis of urinary tract infections: an update. J antimicrobial chemotherapy. 2000;46(Suppl A):1–7.
6. Strom BL, Collins M, West SL, Kreisberg J, Weller S. Sexual activity, contraceptive use, and other risk factors for symptomatic and asymptomatic bacteriuria. A case-control study. Ann Intern Med. 1987;107(6):816–23.
7. Foxman B, Frerichs RR. Epidemiology of urinary tract infection: I. Diaphragm use and sexual intercourse. Am J Public Health. 1985;75(11):1308–13.
8. McDonald AM, Knight RC, Campbell MK, Entwistle VA, Grant AM, Cook JA, Elbourne DR, Francis D, Garcia J, Roberts I, et al. What influences recruitment to randomised controlled trials? A review of trials funded by two UK funding agencies. Trials. 2006;7:9.
9. Foxman B, Frerichs RR. Epidemiology of urinary tract infection: II. Diet, clothing, and urination habits. Am J Public Health. 1985;75(11):1314–7.
10. Scholes D, Hawn TR, Roberts PL, Li SS, Stapleton AE, Zhao LP, Stamm WE, Hooton TM. Family history and risk of recurrent cystitis and pyelonephritis in women. J Urol. 2010;184(2):564–9.
11. Epp A, Larochelle A, Lovatsis D, Walter JE, Easton W, Farrell SA, Girouard L, Gupta C, Harvey MA, Robert M, et al. Recurrent urinary tract infection. J Obstet Gynaecol Can. 2010;32(11):1082–101.
12. Dason S, Dason JT, Kapoor A. Guidelines for the diagnosis and management of recurrent urinary tract infection in women. Can Urol Assoc J. 2011;5(5):316–22.
13. Little P, Merriman R, Turner S, Rumsby K, Warner G, Lowes JA, Smith H, Hawke C, Leydon G, Mullee M, et al. Presentation, pattern, and natural course of severe symptoms, and role of antibiotics and antibiotic resistance among patients presenting with suspected uncomplicated urinary tract infection in primary care: observational study. BMJ (Clinical research ed). 2010;b5633:340.
14. Giesen LG, Cousins G, Dimitrov BD, van de Laar FA, Fahey T. Predicting acute uncomplicated urinary tract infection in women: a systematic review of the diagnostic accuracy of symptoms and signs. BMC Fam Pract. 2010;11:78.
15. Gupta K, Chou MY, Howell A, Wobbe C, Grady R, Stapleton AE. Cranberry products inhibit adherence of p-fimbriated Escherichia coli to primary cultured bladder and vaginal epithelial cells. J Urol. 2007;177(6):2357–60.
16. Howell AB, Botto H, Combescure C, Blanc-Potard AB, Gausa L, Matsumoto T, Tenke P, Sotto A, Lavigne JP. Dosage effect on uropathogenic Escherichia coli anti-adhesion activity in urine following consumption of cranberry powder standardized for proanthocyanidin content: a multicentric randomized double blind study. BMC Infect Dis. 2010;10:94.
17. Jepson RG, Williams G, Craig JC. Cranberries for preventing urinary tract infections. Cochrane Database Syst Rev. 2012;10:CD001321.
18. Wang CH, Fang CC, Chen NC, Liu SS, Yu PH, Wu TY, Chen WT, Lee CC, Chen SC. Cranberry-containing products for prevention of urinary tract infections in susceptible populations: a systematic review and meta-analysis of randomized controlled trials. Arch Intern Med. 2012;172(13):988–96.
19. Takahashi S, Hamasuna R, Yasuda M, Arakawa S, Tanaka K, Ishikawa K, Kiyota H, Hayami H, Yamamoto S, Kubo T, et al. A randomized clinical trial to evaluate the preventive effect of cranberry juice (UR65) for patients with recurrent urinary tract infection. J Infection Chemotherapy : official journal of the Japan Society of Chemotherapy. 2013;19(1):112–7.
20. Fromentin E, Vostalova J, Vidlar A, Galandakova A, Vrbkova J, Ulrichova J, Student V, Simanek V. A randomized, double-blind, placebo-controlled clinical trial to investigate the efficacy of cranberry fruit powder (Pacran) in the prevention of recurrent urinary tract infection in women. FASEB J. 2014;28
21. Licensed Natural Health Products Database [https://www.canada.ca/en/health-canada/services/drugs-health-products/natural-non-prescription/applications-submissions/product-licensing/licensed-natural-health-products-database.html].
22. Prior RL, Fan E, Ji H, Howell A, Nio C, Payne MJ, Reed J. Multi-laboratory validation of a standard method for quantifying proanthocyanidins in cranberry powders. J Sci Food Agric. 2010;90(9):1473–8.
23. Jenkinson C, Layte R, Jenkinson D, Lawrence K, Petersen S, Paice C, Stradling J. A shorter form health survey: can the SF-12 replicate results from the SF-36 in longitudinal studies? J Public Health Med. 1997;19(2):179–86.
24. Goulet J, Nadeau G, Lapointe A, Lamarche B, Lemieux S. Validity and reproducibility of an interviewer-administered food frequency questionnaire for healthy French-Canadian men and women. Nutr J. 2004;3:13.

25. Mogollon JA, Bujold E, Lemieux S, Bourdages M, Blanchet C, Bazinet L, Couillard C, Noel M, Dodin S. Blood pressure and endothelial function in healthy, pregnant women after acute and daily consumption of flavanol-rich chocolate: a pilot, randomized controlled trial. Nutr J. 2013;12:41.
26. Deville WL, Yzermans JC, van Duijn NP, Bezemer PD, van der Windt DA, Bouter LM. The urine dipstick test useful to rule out infections. A meta-analysis of the accuracy. BMC Urol. 2004;4:4.

9

Reliability of pelvic floor muscle strength assessment in healthy continent women

Dulcegleika VB Sartori[1], Monica O Gameiro[2], Hamilto A Yamamoto[1], Paulo R Kawano[1], Rodrigo Guerra[1], Carlos R Padovani[3] and João L Amaro[1,4*]

Abstract

Background: The aim of this study was to compare pelvic floor muscle (PFM) strength using transvaginal digital palpation in healthy continent women in different age groups, and to compare the inter- and intra-rater reliability of examiners performing anterior and posterior vaginal assessments.

Methods: We prospectively studied 150 healthy multiparous women. They were distributed into four different groups, according to age range: G1 (n = 37), 30–40 years-old; G2 (n = 39), 41–50 years-old; G3 (n = 39), 51–60 years-old; and G4 (n = 35), older than 60 years-old. PFM strength was evaluated using transvaginal digital palpation in the anterior and posterior areas, by 3 different examiners, and graded using a 5-point Amaro's scale.

Results: There was no statistical difference among the different age ranges, for each grade of PFM strength. There was good intra-rater concordance between anterior and posterior PFM assessment, being 64.7%, 63.3%, and 66.7% for examiners A, B, and C, respectively. The intra-rater concordance level was good for each examiner. However, the inter-rater reliability for two examiners varied from moderate to good.

Conclusions: Age has no effect on PFM strength profiles, in multiparous continent women. There is good concordance between anterior and posterior vaginal PFM strength assessments, but only moderate to good inter-rater reliability of the measurements between two examiners.

Keywords: Gynecological examination, Parity, Pelvic floor, Urinary Incontinence, Reproducibility of results

Background

Urinary incontinence (UI) in women is common and prevalence increases with age [1,2]. Damage to the pelvic floor muscle (PFM) can decrease the muscle strength and consequently could result in urinary and fecal incontinence [2]. It has been demonstrated that the weakness of the PFM is significantly higher in incontinent women [3,4] and also that this weakness is worse in women with urge urinary incontinence [5]. According to the International Classifications of Impairments, Disabilities and Handicaps (ICIDH), a nonfunctioning PFM occurs when there is a reduction in force generation and incorrect timing or coordination of muscle contraction [6].

The PFM function can be evaluated using vaginal palpation, visual observation, electromyography, ultrasound, and magnetic resonance imaging [6]. The vaginal palpation is currently used by most physical therapists to assess PFM contraction. However, there has been no systematic research to determine the best method of vaginal palpation to evaluate the pelvic floor contraction [6], and different score systems have been described.

The Brink score [7] and the Laycock PERFECT assessment scheme [8] are commonly used to evaluate PFM function [9]. Some authors have reported that the best reliability is obtained by a digital examination (Brink Score) followed by perineometer evaluation and then by vaginal cone tests in incontinent elderly women [10]. Despite this, other authors have shown poor inter-rater reliability using a modified Oxford scale to assess PFM function [11,12]. A simplified non-validated scale for PFM assessment was proposed by Amaro [13]. On the other hand, some authors have observed that PFM contractions at 50% intensity, in

* Correspondence: jamaro@fmb.unesp.br
[1]Department of Urology, Medical School of Botucatu, São Paulo State University, Botucatu, Brazil
[4]Department of Urology, School of Medicine, São Paulo State University (UNESP), Campus de Rubião Júnior, s/n, 18618-970 Botucatu, SP, Brazil
Full list of author information is available at the end of the article

asymptomatic subjects, actually had a gradient of pressure, which increases in the anterior and posterior directions of the vagina, and which is greater than in incontinent patients [4]. This indicates that there is an antero-posterior vaginal pressure profile (VPP) along the vagina, and therefore highlights the importance of assessing PFM strength both at the anterior and posterior regions of the vagina, instead of evaluating it at any random position [4].

It would be interesting to determine the baseline and distribution of force along the vagina of healthy continent women. Despite the number of different studies on the reliability of PFM evaluation, there is no consensus

about the most valid and reliable method. Additionally, knowledge about normal PFM evolution with aging is limited.

The aim of this study was to evaluate PFM strength using transvaginal digital palpation (TDP) in healthy multiparous continent women, in different age groups, and to compare anterior and posterior vaginal assessment, establishing examiners' inter and intra-rater reliability.

Methods

We prospectively studied 150 healthy multiparous women with an average age of 50 years. All patients were informed

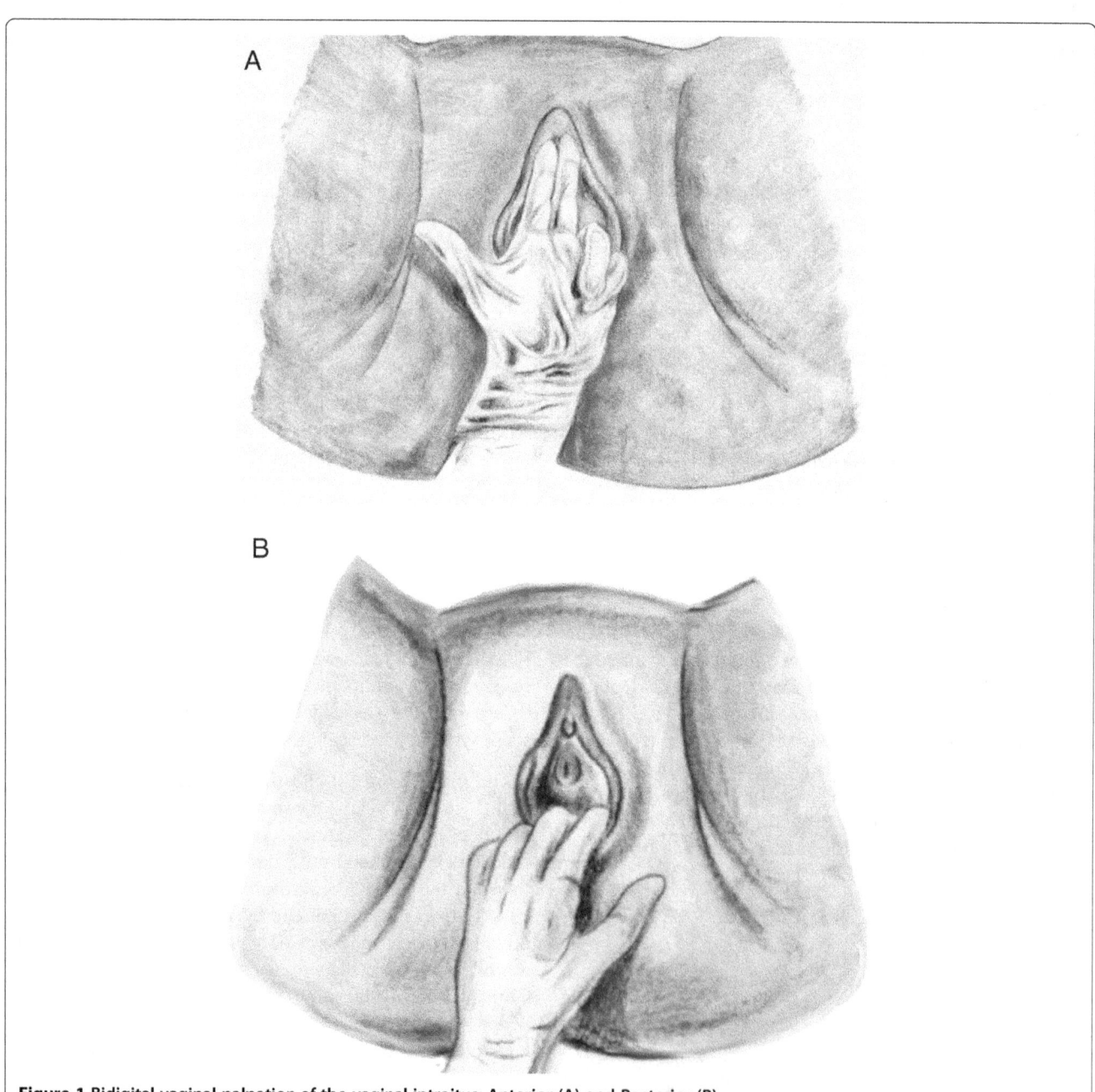

Figure 1 Bidigital vaginal palpation of the vaginal introitus: Anterior (A) and Posterior (B).

about the procedures and study objectives and provided written consent, as approved by the Ethical Committee in Research of Universidade do Sagrado Coração - USC (protocol number: 61/07). Exclusion criteria were UI and/or lower urinary tract symptoms, neurological diseases, previous pelvic surgeries, diabetes mellitus, smoking, and cognitive problems.

The participants were distributed into four different groups according to age range: G1 (n = 37), 30–40 years-old; G2 (n = 39), 41–50 years-old; G3 (n = 39), 51–60 years-old; and G4 (n = 35), older than 60 years-old. Demographic data, such as age, number of deliveries, body mass index (BMI), and physical and sexual activity, were all obtained using a clinical questionnaire. BMI was calculated and classified according to World Health Organization [14] guidelines.

PFM strength assessments were performed using TDP. The subjects lay in a supine position with a pillow under their heads, with their knees straight and legs abducted. The examiners used their second and third fingers for examination, extended and fully inserted into the vagina, but avoiding any excessive discomfort. The participants were then instructed to contract the pelvic floor muscles against the examiner's fingers and hold this contraction as long as possible. Contractions at either anterior and posterior regions of the vagina were assessed sequentially, with the same method (Figure 1A and B). Muscle strength was graded using the 4-point Amaro´s Scale: 0 = no contraction, 1 = mild muscular contraction, sustained for less than 3 seconds (s), 2 = moderate muscular contraction, sustained for less than 5 s, and 3 = Normal muscular contraction, sustained for more than 5 s. This classification was tested but not validated [13]. Three experienced physical therapists (more than 1 year since graduation) conducted this study (A, B, and C). They sequentially graded each participant's PFM strength, both at anterior and posterior vaginal regions, separately from each other. The palpation test was performed in random order of examiner, and the results of each evaluation were kept in sealed envelopes, blinded to the other examiners, in order to avoid influencing their evaluations.

Statistical analysis

Sample size was calculated for a significance level of 10% and test power of 95%. The characteristics of our health service were also taken into account. We invited three of each four women seen consecutively to enroll. According to these results and considering the range between percentages of answers as the casual error, the minimum of 150 women was established, proportionally distributed in four different age groups.

Data were analyzed using SPSS® software (IBM Corp., Armonk, New York, USA). When the data followed a Gaussian or normal distribution, analysis of variance was used. When the data were not normally distributed, the nonparametric Spearman coefficient and Kruskal–Wallis test were used [15]. A confidence interval of 95% was considered for the proportion of intra-examiner concordance [15]. The Cronbach alpha was used for inter-examiner reliability of PFM strength scores, using TDP in the anterior and posterior areas [16]. The kappa test was used for inter- and intra-rater concordance of PFM strength, using TDP in the anterior and posterior areas [15]. Differences were considered statistically significant when $p < 0.05$.

Results

The median ages were 35, 45, 54, and 67 years in the G1, G2, G3, and G4 age groups, respectively. There was a statistically significant difference between groups in age, BMI, number of pregnancies and vaginal delivery, as shown in Table 1. Of the 150 women, 69.3% reported sexual activity and in 40.7% reported regular physical activity, defined as occurring at least three times a week. There was a positive linear relationship between age and BMI ($r = 0.188$, $p = 0.0212$). There was a positive linear relationship between age and number of pregnancies

Table 1 Demographic characteristic

Variables	GROUPS				Statistical analysis
	G1	G2	G3	G4	
	(n = 37)	(n = 39)	(n = 39)	(n = 35)	
Age[1]	35.0 (30.0; 40.0)	45.0 (41.0; 50.0)	54.0 (50.0; 59.0)	67.0 (61.0; 86.0)#	p < 0.001
Body Mass Index[2]	24.9 (4.1)	26.5 (4.9)	25.7 (4.0)	28.0 (3.5)##	p = 0.015
Number of pregnancies[1]	3.0 (2.0; 7.0)	3.0 (2.0; 5.0)	3.0 (2.0; 8.0)	4.0 (2.0; 14.0)##	p = 0.015
Vaginal deliveries[1]	1.0 (0.0; 7.0)	1.0 (0.0; 3.0)	1.0 (0.0; 6.0)	2.0 (0.0; 8.0)###	p = 0.016

[1]Median (minimum value; maximum value).
[2]Mean (standard deviation).
#($p < 0.001$) G4 xG3 xG2 xG1.
##($p < 0.05$)G4 x G1.
###($p < 0.05$) G4 x (G2,G3).

Table 2 Descriptive measures of ages according with grade of PFM strength using TDP assessment on anterior and posterior areas

Grade Of Pfm strength*	(n)	Anterior (age)[1]	(n)	Posterior (age)[1]	p value
0	(5)	42 (33; 52)	(4)	38 (30; 43)	p = 0.190
1	(49)	48 (30; 73)	(36)	51 (30; 73)	p = 0.578
2	(71)	51 (30; 86)	(64)	48 (30; 86)	p = 0.611
3	(25)	49 (30; 72)	(46)	51 (30; 72)	p = 0.896
p value	(150)	p = 0.408	(150)	p = 0.123	

*Amaro's classification [13].
[1]Median (minimum value; maximum value).

(r = 0.265, p = 0.0010), and between age and vaginal deliveries (r = 0.258, p = 0.0014).

Considering the subjects graded as having mild contraction (Amaro grade 1), using TDP in both the anterior and posterior areas, there was a positive linear relationship between BMI and vaginal deliveries (r = 0.418, p = 0.013 and r = 0.302, p = 0.037, respectively). We observed no linear relationship between these factors in grades 2 and 3 of the PFM strength evaluation. There was no statistically significant difference in the different grades of PFM strength, in neither the anterior nor posterior areas, in relation to age (Table 2). There was good intra-rater concordance between anterior and posterior PFM assessments, being 64.7%, 63.3%, and 66.7% for examiners A, B, and C, respectively (Tables 3 and 4). The inter-rater concordance level was moderate to good, with kappa tests in the range of 0.523–0.736, between two examiners (Table 5).

Discussion

BMI was higher in the older age range, compared with younger women, and there was a progressive increase in BMI with aging. Other authors have also observed an increase in weight with aging and this factor could be correlated with menopause [17,18]. Different studies have demonstrated the presence of PFM dysfunction related to aging, parity, and vaginal deliveries [19,20]. Interestingly, in our series of continent women, despite the higher BMI and the higher number of pregnancies and

Table 3 Intra- rater concordance between anterior and posterior transvaginal digital palpation (TDP) assessment and their respective confidence interval considering each examiner according Amaro's Scale [13]

Examiners	Concordance	Confidence interval	
		Lowerbound	Upperbound
A	97/150 (64.7%)	57.0%	72.4%
B	95/150 (63.3%)	55.6%	71.0%
C	100/150 (66.7%)	59.2%	74.2%

Table 4 Intra-rater concordance between anterior and posterior transvaginal digital palpation (TDP) assessment considering each examiner

Examiner	Transvaginal Digital Palpation (TDP)
A	0.71*
B	0.67*
C	0.74*

*CONCORDANCE LEVEL (Kappa Test): 0–0.20: weak; 0.21-0.40: regular; 0.41-0.60: moderate; 0.61-0.80: good; >0.81: excellent.

vaginal deliveries in older women, there was no statistically significant difference in PFM strength in the different age ranges, showing that the aging process in continent women generally did not influence PFM strength. There was a positive linear relationship between PFM weakness, BMI, and vaginal deliveries though, and considering this, probably the interaction of these factors may have contributed to the decrease in PFM strength encountered in some of these continent women.

The International Continence Society (ICS) has defined by consensus, the diagnosis and treatment of pelvic floor dysfunctions [21]. They standardized the terminology of pelvic floor muscle function and acknowledged that assessing it by vaginal digital palpation is easy to perform, but emphasized that quantification of PFM contraction is problematic [21,22]. In our study, we used a scale of four grades, varying from 0 to 3, as described by Amaro et al. [13], with the objective to facilitate the understanding and reproducibility in clinical practice. However, different authors do not consider digital palpation of the vagina as a sensitive and reproducible method for the assessment of PFM function [11,23,24]. On the other hand, others have reported that this would be the best qualitative method to assess the contraction and muscular strength of PFM [11,25,26].

In our study, there was no correlation between muscle weakness and age. This finding is in agreement with the literature where the physiological aging "per se" in continent women does not correlate with decrease of PFM strength [27]. However, in incontinent women the PFM strength was significantly lower than continents and worsens during the aging process [3,28].

Table 5 Concordance level considering each two examiners in transvaginal digital palpation (TDP) assessment of PFM on anterior and posterior areas (Amaro's classification) [13]

Examiners	Transvaginal Digital Palpation (TDP)	
	Anterior	Posterior
AxB	0.591*	0.571*
AxC	0.682*	0.736*
BxC	0.685*	0.523*

*CONCORDANCE LEVEL (Kappa Test): 0–0.20: weak; 0.21-0.40: regular; 0.41-0.60: moderate; 0.61-0.80: good; >0.81: excellent.

Our results are consistent with the literature that reports the difficulty of assessing PFM function by vaginal digital palpation, due to variability of its anatomy. This assessment still depends on the skill and experience of examiners. The examiners who participated in our study had 4–5 years of work experience after graduation and, despite that, there were some different interpretations of PFM contraction degree. Our find are in agreement with the literature, that shows reproducibility of the TDP method, with some restrictions [26,28-30]. Slieker-ten Hove et al. [31], conducted a reproducibility study with 4 different examiners by TDP, demonstrating high intra-observer rates of reproducibility, and low inter-examiner rates. According to the authors, the classifications used in the studies may not have enough accuracy to properly distinguish between individuals.

Morin et al. [30] reported that it is not possible to establish any correlation between TDP and objective methods of evaluation, such as dynamometer or perineometer. In another study of our group, we also observed that the correlation with objective methods of evaluation of PFM and its reproducibility are questionable [3,13].

The intra-rater reliability refers to the concordance of each anterior and posterior TDP assessment of pelvic floor contractions, for each subject and for each examiner. Our results objectively revealed a good level of concordance, indicating that the TDP assessment is accurate for evaluating the pelvic floor muscular strength in either position. However, when we take in consideration the inter-rater reliability between each two examiners, the concordance varied between moderate to good. Inter-rater reliability refers to the concordance of PFM grading on the same subject, by different examiners. This fact is in agreement with the findings of other authors that have highlighted the differential profile of vaginal pressure distributed along the vaginal canal [4], and that this is a subjective evaluation, dependent of examiners' training [32]. Consequently, the accuracy of this assessment test depends on the skill and experience of the examining physical therapist.

Different measurement tools assess different aspects of PFM function, and it is important to look at them as complementary in a thorough PFM evaluation, not mutually exclusive. Further studies are necessary to evaluate the concordance between tests using different classifications and their inter-rater reliability.

Conclusions

Age does not affect PFM strength profiles, in continent women. There is a good relationship between anterior and posterior vaginal PFM strength assessments, but only moderate to good inter-rater reliability of the measurements.

Brief summary

This work intends to evaluate transvaginal palpation, as a clinical method to assess baseline strength of the pelvic floor, in multiparous continent women.

Abbreviations
UI: Urinary incontinence; PFM: Pelvic floor muscle; ICIDH: International Classifications of Impairments, Disabilities and Handicaps; TDP: Transvaginal digital palpation; BMI: Body mass index; s: Seconds (s); ICS: International Continence Society.

Competing interest
The authors declare that they have no competing interests.

Authors' contributions
DVBS: Data collection, management and analysis; manuscript writing. MOG: Protocol development; data analysis. HY: Manuscript review. PRK: Manuscript review and editing. RG: Manuscript review and editing. CRP: Other (statistical analysis). JLA: Protocol development; data analysis; review of manuscript. All authors read and approved the final manuscript.

Acknowledgements
We would like to thank the Universidade do Sagrado Coração - USC by the support and all researchers and patients involved in the study for their dedication to the project, which has made the present work possible.

Author details
[1]Department of Urology, Medical School of Botucatu, São Paulo State University, Botucatu, Brazil. [2]Coordinator of Pelvic Floor Rehabilitation Service, Medical School of Botucat, São Paulo State University, Botucatu, Brazil. [3]Department of Biostatistics, Medical School of Botucatu, São Paulo State University, Botucatu, Brazil. [4]Department of Urology, School of Medicine, São Paulo State University (UNESP), Campus de Rubião Júnior, s/n, 18618-970 Botucatu, SP, Brazil.

References
1. Brown JS, Seeley DG, Fong J, Black DM, Ensrud KE, Grady D. Urinary incontinence in older women: who is at risk? Study Osteoporotic Fractures Research Group. Obstet Gynecol. 1996;87:715.
2. Amaro JL, Macharelil CA, Yamamoto H, Kawano PR, Padovani CR, Agostinho AD. Prevalence and risk factors for urinary and fecal incontinence in Brazilian women. Int Braz J Urol. 2009;35:592–8.
3. Amaro JL, Moreira EC, De Oliveira OGM, Padovani CR. Pelvic floor muscle evaluation in incontinent patients. Int Urogynecol J Pelvic Floor Dysfunct. 2005;16:352–4.
4. Shishido K, Peng Q, Jones R, Omata S, Constantinou CE. Influence of pelvic floor muscle contraction on the profile of vaginal closure pressure in continent and stress urinary incontinent women. J Urol. 2008;179:1917–22.
5. Gameiro MO, Moreira EC, Ferrari RS, Kawano PR, Padovani CR, Amaro JL. A comparative analysis of pelvic floor muscle strength in women with stress and urge urinary incontinence. Int Braz J Urol. 2012;38:661–6.
6. Bo K, Sherburn M. Evaluation of female pelvic-floor muscle function and strength. Phys Ther. 2005;85:269–82.
7. Brink CA, Sampselle CM, Wells TJ, Diokno AC, Gillis GL. A digital test for pelvic muscle strength in older women with urinary incontinence. Nurs Res. 1989;38:196–9.
8. Incontinence LJ. Pelvic floor re-education. Nursing. 1991;4:15–7.
9. Slieker-ten Hove MC, Pool-Goudzwaard AL, Eijkemans MJ, Steegers-Theunissen RP, Burger CW, Vierhout ME. Face validity and reliability of the first digital assessment scheme of pelvic floor muscle function conform the new standardized terminology of the International Continence Society. Neurourol Urodyn. 2009;28:295.
10. Kerschan-Schindl K, Uher E, Wiesinger G, Kaider A, Ebenbichler G, Nicolakis P, et al. Reliability of pelvic floor muscle strength measurement in elderly incontinent women. Neurourol Urodyn. 2002;21:42–7.

11. Bo K, Finckenhagen HB. Vaginal palpation of pelvic floor muscle strength: inter-test reproducibility and comparison between palpation and vaginal squeeze pressure. Acta Obstet Gynecol Scand. 2001;80:883.

12. Ferreira CH, Barbosa PB, de Oliveira SF, Antônio FI, Franco MM, Bø K. Inter-rater reliability study of the modified Oxsford Grading scale and the Peritron manometer. Physiotherapy. 2011;97:132–8.

13. Amaro JL, Oliveira Gameiro MO, Padovani CR. Treatment of urinary stress incontinence by intravaginal electrical stimulation and pelvic floor physiotherapy. Int Urogynecol J Pelvic Floor Dysfunct. 2003;14:204–8.

14. World Health Organization [homepage on the Internet]. BMI Classification. 2006. Geneva: WHO [cited 2008 nov1 12]. Available from: www.who.int/bmi.

15. Norman GR, Streiner DL. Biostatistics: the bare essentials. 3rd ed. St. Louis: Mosby Year Book; 2008. p. 393.

16. Cronbach LJ. Coefficient alpha and the internal structure of tests. Psychometrika. 1951;16:297–334.

17. Panatopoulos G, Raison J, Ruiz JC, Guy-Grand B, Basdevant A. Weight gain at the time of menopause. Hum Reprod. 1997;12:126–33.

18. Lins APM, Sichieri R, Coutinho WF, Ramos EG, Peixoto MVM, Fonseca VM. Healthy eating, schooling and being overweight among low-income women.Cien Saude Colet. 2013;18:357–66.

19. Kearney R, Miller JM, Ashton-Miller JA, De Lancey JO. Obstetric factors associated with levatorani muscle injury after vaginal birth. Obstet Gynecol. 2006;107:144–9.

20. Nygaard I, Barber MD, Burgio KL, Kenton K, Meikle S, Schaffer J. Prevalence of symptomatic pelvic floor disorders in US women. JAMA. 2008;300:1311–6.

21. Abrams P, Cardozo L, Fall M, Griffiths D, Rosier P, Ulmsten U, et al. The standardization of terminology of lower urinary tract function: report from the standardization sub-committee of International Continence Society. NeurourolUrodyn. 2002;21:167–78.

22. Messelink B, Benson T, Berghmans B, Bø K, Corcos J, Fowler C, et al. Standardization of Terminology of Pelvic Floor muscle function and dysfunction: report from the pelvic floor clinical assessment group of the International Continence Society. NeurourolUrodyn. 2005;24:374–80.

23. Worth A, Dougerty M, Mokey P. Development and testing of the circunvaginal muscles rating scale. Nurs Res. 1986;35:166–8.

24. Brink CA, Wells TJ, Sampselle CM, Faillie ER, Mayer R. A digital test for pelvic muscle strengh in women with urinary incontinence. Nurs Res. 1994;43:352–6.

25. Laycock J, Jerwood D. Pelvic floor muscle assessment: The PERFECT Scheme. Physiotherapy. 2001;87:631–42.

26. Thompson LV, O'Sullivan PB, Briffa NK, Neumann P. Assessment of voluntary pelvic floor muscle contraction in continent and incontinent women using transperineal ultrasound, manual muscle testing and vaginal squeeze pressure measurements. Int Urogynecol J Pelvic Floor Dysfunc. 2006;17:624–30.

27. FitzGerald MP, Burgio KL, Borello-France DF, Menefee SA, Schaffer J, Kraus S, et al. Pelvic-floor strength in women with incontinence as assessed by the brink scale. Phys Ther. 2007;87:1316–24.

28. Bø K, Finckenhagen HB. Is there any difference in measurement of pelvic floor muscle strength in supine and standing position. Acta ObstetGynecol Scand. 2003;82:1120–4.

29. Frawley H, Galea M, Phillips B, Sherburn M, Bø K. Effect of test position on pelvic floor muscle assessment. Int Urogynecol J. 2006;17:365–71.

30. Morin M, Dumoulin C, Bourbonnais D, Gravel D, Lemieux MC. Pelvic floor maximal strength using vaginal digital assessment compared to dynamometric measurements. Neurourol Urodynamics. 2004;23:336–41.

31. Slieker-ten Hove MC, Pool-Goudzwaard AL, Eijkemans MJ, Steegers-Theunissen RP, Burger CW, Vierhout ME. Face validity and reliability of the first digital assessment scheme of pelvic floor muscle function conform the new standardized terminology of the International Continence Society. Neurourol Urodyn. 2009;28:295–300.

32. McArdle WD, Katch FI, Katch VL. Fisiologia do exercícioEnergia, nutrição e desempenho do corpo humano. 5th ed. Rio de Janeiro: Guanabara Koogan; 2008. cap. 31:p.902-3.

10

The MAPP research network: a novel study of urologic chronic pelvic pain syndromes

J Quentin Clemens[1]*, Chris Mullins[2], John W Kusek[2], Ziya Kirkali[2], Emeran A Mayer[3], Larissa V Rodríguez[3], David J Klumpp[4], Anthony J Schaeffer[4], Karl J Kreder[5], Dedra Buchwald[6], Gerald L Andriole[7], M Scott Lucia[8], J Richard Landis[9], Daniel J Clauw[10] and The MAPP Research Network Study Group

Abstract

Urologic chronic pelvic pain syndrome (UCPPS) may be defined to include interstitial cystitis/bladder pain syndrome (IC/BPS) and chronic prostatitis/chronic pelvic pain syndrome (CP/CPPS). The hallmark symptom of UCPPS is chronic pain in the pelvis, urogenital floor, or external genitalia often accompanied by lower urinary tract symptoms. Despite numerous past basic and clinical research studies there is no broadly identifiable organ-specific pathology or understanding of etiology or risk factors for UCPPS, and diagnosis relies primarily on patient reported symptoms. In addition, there are no generally effective therapies. Recent findings have, however, revealed associations between UCPPS and "centralized" chronic pain disorders, suggesting UCPPS may represent a local manifestation of more widespread pathology in some patients. Here, we describe a new and novel effort initiated by the National Institute of Diabetes and Digestive and Kidney Diseases (NIDDK) of the U.S. National Institutes of Health (NIH) to address the many long standing questions regarding UCPPS, the Multidisciplinary Approach to the Study of Chronic Pelvic Pain (MAPP) Research Network. The MAPP Network approaches UCPPS in a systemic manner, in which the interplay between the genitourinary system and other physiological systems is emphasized. The network's study design expands beyond previous research, which has primarily focused on urologic organs and tissues, to utilize integrated approaches to define patient phenotypes, identify clinically-relevant subgroups, and better understand treated natural history and pathophysiology. Thus, the MAPP Network provides an unprecedented, multi-layered characterization of UCPPS. Knowledge gained is expected to provide important insights into underlying pathophysiology, a foundation for better segmenting patients for future clinical trials, and ultimately translation into improved clinical management. In addition, the MAPP Network's integrated multi-disciplinary research approach may serve as a model for studies of urologic and non-urologic disorders that have proven refractory to past basic and clinical study.

Keywords: Urological chronic pelvic pain syndromes, Interstitial cystitis, Chronic prostatitis, Translational research, Multi-disciplinary

Background

Urologic chronic pelvic pain syndrome (UCPPS) encompasses two highly prevalent non-malignant urologic disorders, interstitial cystitis/bladder pain syndrome (IC/BPS) and chronic prostatitis/chronic pelvic pain syndrome (CP/CPPS). UCPPS is primarily characterized by chronic and often debilitating pain in the pelvic region and/or genitalia and typically a spectrum of defects in bladder and lower urinary tract function [1,2].

Numerous studies have been conducted over the past two decades to define the pathophysiology and natural history of UCPPS and to examine the efficacy of therapies. Many of those studies were supported by the National Institute of Diabetes and Digestive and Kidney Diseases (NIDDK) of the U.S. National Institutes of Health (NIH). The first NIDDK-sponsored pelvic pain clinical research network, the Interstitial Cystitis Database study (ICDB) was initiated in 1991 [3]. This five-year prospective cohort

* Correspondence: qclemens@med.umich.edu
[1]Department of Urology, University of Michigan, Ann Arbor, MI, USA
Full list of author information is available at the end of the article

study collected data on more than 600 persons and characterized them across demographic and clinical characteristics, including bladder biopsy [4]. The Interstitial Cystitis Clinical Trials Group (ICCTG) was subsequently established to conduct randomized clinical trials beginning in 1996 [5-9]. In 2003, this group became the Interstitial Cystitis Collaborative Research Network (ICCRN) and carried out additional randomized clinical trials [10-12]. In 1998, the Chronic Prostatitis Cohort (CPC) study began to prospectively collect patient data to systematically examine the demographics, clinical characteristics and natural history of CP/CPPS [13]. The NIDDK subsequently initiated the Chronic Prostatitis Collaborative Research Network (CPCRN) which performed clinical trials for CP/CPPS [14-17]. Results from these clinical research studies failed to identify definitive risk factors or generally effective treatments, with the exception of a single study suggesting that myofascial physical therapy might be effective in IC/BPS [18]. The NIDDK-supported Boston Area Community Health (BACH) Survey [19-21] and the RAND IC Epidemiology (RICE) Study [22,23] provided estimates on the prevalence of IC-related symptoms for both men and women, as well as an expanded understanding of symptom morbidity. In addition to these clinical and epidemiological studies, many basic research efforts were developed to describe pathophysiology at the cellular level, including *in vivo* studies of model systems. However, no consensus agreement has been achieved on an underlying etiology for UCPPS, though co-occurrence of UCPPS with other chronic non-urologic pain syndromes has been revealed [24-30].

In light of the limitations of previous studies and results showing potential associations between UCPPS and other chronic pain conditions, the NIDDK proposes that the traditional bladder and prostate centered focus of UCPPS research be broadened to a systemic view of disease in which the interplay between the genitourinary system and other physiological systems (e.g., the central nervous system), is highlighted. In addition, it is suggested that studies of UCPPS would benefit from incorporating broad approaches involving a diversity of urologic and non-urologic disciplines to promote a more comprehensive characterization of patient phenotype.

These concepts, as well as recommendations solicited from the scientific community [31], prompted the NIDDK to initiate a new research program for the study of UCPPS, the Multidisciplinary Approach to the Study of Chronic Pelvic Pain (MAPP) Research Network. Since its inception in 2008, the MAPP Research Network has adopted a highly collaborative and integrated research strategy that incorporates new and novel approaches conducted by investigators representing traditional urologic disciplines and broad non-urologic expertise, including experts in pain research, neurobiology and neuroimaging, infectious disease, biomarker discovery, animal modeling,

epidemiology, psychology, immunology, among many others. The overarching goal of the MAPP Research Network is to provide findings useful for designing future clinical trials and ultimately to improve clinical management for UCPPS patients. Importantly, the design and goals of the MAPP Network are complementary to other large phenotyping efforts for non-urologic pain conditions being conducted, such as the OPPERA study [32].

The MAPP Research Network includes six Discovery Sites and several specialized sub-sites that conduct multiple, collaborative Trans-MAPP (i.e., across sites) studies, as well as a number of single-site studies, and two specialized Cores (see Acknowledgement for complete listing of MAPP Network Sites and affiliated personnel). The Data Coordination Core (DCC) serves as the central site for data acquisition and storage; provides bio-statistical analyses for all studies; and promotes network-wide quality assurance. The DCC also provides administrative support, including development and maintenance of a public website (http://www.mappnetwork.org/). The Tissue Analysis and Technology Core (TATC) monitors biosample collection and provides sample banking, annotation, and distribution services.

The MAPP Research Network is currently conducting complementary basic, translational, and clinical science studies to investigate questions of significant clinical relevance and adopts the view that UCPPS potentially involves significant systemic contributions. The primary scientific protocol is a prospective observational study of the treated natural history UCPPS, the Trans-MAPP Epidemiology/Phenotyping (EP) Study. A full description of the central Trans-MAPP EP Study and the complement of urologic and non-urologic measures employed are described in the companion report by Landis et al. [33]. In addition to the extensive phenotyping, the Trans-MAPP EP Study also provide a source of highly characterized participants for further phenotyping through other integrated network protocols. Assembled network working groups develop and conduct complementary Trans-MAPP studies that broadly address potential contributions of various physiological systems and hypotheses of underlying etiology, pathophysiology, risk, and relationships between UCPPS and commonly associated non-urologic syndromes. These include structural and functional assessments of the central nervous system; efforts to uncover potential contributions of infectious agents to etiology; discovery efforts to identify new biological markers; extensive characterizations of symptom variation (e.g., flares); and efforts to develop new and more informative patient reported outcome measures. The network is also engaged in collaborative research to establish and assess animal models validated for the presence of clinically-relevant phenotypes, thus allowing for improved translation between animal and human studies. The MAPP study will provide comprehensive, state-of-the-art phenotyping data which will set the standard for future UCPPS research. Results from the MAPP study can be integrated with other, more clinically focused phenotyping efforts (such as the UPOINT system [34,35]) to better define the 'minimal data set' required to provide optimal patient care for UCPPS patients.

Within the MAPP Research Network all clinical Trans-MAPP protocols and site-specific efforts, which primarily serve to pilot test ideas complementary to the collaborative protocols, are highly integrated through their use of shared patients and controls evaluated through standard phenotyping; common biological samples; and a standardized data collection, storage, and analysis strategy. In addition, neuroimaging study parameters are standardized across sites and scan data is centrally managed by the University of California at Los Angeles (UCLA) Center for Neurobiology of Stress (painrepository.org), in close collaboration with UCLA-Laboratory of Neuroimaging (LONI), which has extensive experience in the collection, storage and analysis of large multi-site MRI data sets (loni.usc.edu). In this way diverse findings across protocols may be integrated to allow a detailed characterization of a single UCPPS patient or patient sub-groups. Importantly, these efforts are also generating a unique national resource of highly detailed longitudinal clinical and epidemiological data associated with data from additional, integrated phenotyping studies and linked biological samples, for future use by the wider research community through the NIDDK Data and Sample Repositories (http://www3.niddk.nih.gov/researchprograms/repositories/).

Conclusions

UCPPS research is clearly at a cross-road in which the traditional basic and clinical scientific strategies are being re-evaluated in light of evolving ideas of UCPPS and recognition of the limitations of previous study designs. The MAPP Research Network was created to address these challenges. Advances from network efforts are expected to provide a more comprehensive understanding of UCPPS pathophysiology, identify clinically relevant patient subgroups, inform the design of future clinical trials, and ultimately improve clinical care. The unique organization and approach of the MAPP Network may also provide a blueprint for multi-site, multi-disciplinary research in the broader pain field, as well as for those disciplines addressing other disorders with ill-defined pathophysiology.

Appendix: MAPP Research Network Study Group
MAPP Network Executive Committee
J. Quentin Clemens, MD, FACS, MSci,
Network Chair, 2013-Philip Hanno, MD

Ziya Kirkali, MD
John W. Kusek, PhD
J. Richard Landis, PhD
M. Scott Lucia, MD
Chris Mullins, PhD
Michel A. Pontari, MD

Northwestern University Discovery Site
David J. Klumpp, PhD, Co-Director
Anthony J. Schaeffer, MD, Co-Director
Apkar (Vania) Apkarian, PhD
David Cella, PhD
Melissa A. Farmer, PhD
Colleen Fitzgerald, MD
Richard Gershon, PhD
James W. Griffith, PhD
Charles J. Heckman II, PhD
Mingchen Jiang, PhD
Laurie Keefer, PhD
Darlene S. Marko, RN, BSN, CCRC
Jean Michniewicz
Todd Parrish, PhD
Frank Tu, MD, MPH

University of California, Los Angeles Discovery Site and PAIN Neuroimaging Core
Emeran A. Mayer, MD, Co-Director
Larissa V. Rodríguez, MD, Co-Director
Jeffry Alger, PhD
Cody P. Ashe-McNalley
Ben Ellingson, PhD
Nuwanthi Heendeniya
Lisa Kilpatrick, PhD
Jason Kutch, PhD
Jennifer S. Labus, PhD
Bruce D. Naliboff, PhD
Fornessa Randal
Suzanne R. Smith, RN, NP

University of Iowa Discovery Site
Karl J. Kreder, MD, MBA, Director
Catherine S. Bradley, MD, MSCE
Mary Eno, RN, RA II
Kris Greiner, BA
Yi Luo, PhD, MD
Susan K. Lutgendorf, PhD
Michael A. O'Donnell, MD
Barbara Ziegler, BA

University of Michigan Discovery Site
Daniel J. Clauw, MD, Co-Director;
Network Chair, 2008-2013
J. Quentin Clemens, MD, FACS, MSci,
Co-Director; Network Chair, 2013-

Suzie As-Sanie, MD
Sandra Berry, MA
Megan E. Halvorson, BS, CCRP
Richard Harris, PhD
Steve Harte, PhD
Eric Ichesco, BS
Ann Oldendorf, MD
Katherine A. Scott, RN, BSN
David A. Williams, PhD

University of Washington, Seattle Discovery Site
Dedra Buchwald, MD, Director
Niloofar Afari, PhD, Univ. Of California, San Diego
John Krieger, MD
Jane Miller, MD
Stephanie Richey, BS
Susan O. Ross, RN, MN
Roberta Spiro, MS
TJ Sundsvold, MPH
Eric Strachan, PhD
Claire C. Yang, MD

Washington University, St. Louis Discovery Site
Gerald L. Andriole, MD, Co-Director
H. Henry Lai, MD, Co-Director
Rebecca L. Bristol, BA, BS, Coordinator
Graham Colditz, MD, DrPH
Georg Deutsch, PhD, Univ. of Alabama at Birmingham
Vivien C. Gardner, RN, BSN, Coordinator
Robert W. Gereau IV, PhD
Jeffrey P Henderson, MD, PhD
Barry A. Hong, PhD, FAACP
Thomas M. Hooton, MD, Univ of Miami
Timothy J. Ness, MD, PhD, Univ. of Alabama at Birmingham
Carol S. North, MD, MPE, Univ. Texas Southwestern
Theresa M. Spitznagle, PT, DPT, WCS
Siobhan Sutcliffe, PhD, ScM, MHS

University of Pennsylvania Data Coordinating Core (DCC)
J. Richard Landis, PhD, Core Director
Ted Barrell, BA
Philip Hanno, MD
Xiaoling Hou, MS
Tamara Howard, MPH
Michel A. Pontari, MD
Nancy Robinson, PhD
Alisa Stephens, PhD
Yanli Wang, MS

University of Colorado Denver Tissue Analysis & Technology Core (TATC)
M. Scott Lucia, MD, Core Director
Adrie van Bokhoven, PhD

Andrea A. Osypuk, BS
Robert Dayton, Jr
Karen R. Jonscher, PhD
Holly T. Sullivan, BS
R. Storey Wilson, MS

Additional Sites: Drexel University College of Medicine
Garth D.Ehrlich, PhD

Harvard Medical School/Boston Children's Hospital
Marsha A. Moses, PhD, Director
Andrew C. Briscoe
David Briscoe, MD
Adam Curatolo, BA
John Froehlich, PhD
Richard S. Lee, MD
Monisha Sachdev, BS
Keith R. Solomon, PhD
Hanno Steen, PhD

Stanford University
Sean Mackey, MD, PhD, Director
Epifanio Bagarinao, PhD
Lauren C. Foster, BA
Emily Hubbard, BA
Kevin A. Johnson, PhD, RN
Katherine T. Martucci, PhD
Rebecca L. McCue, BA
Rachel R. Moericke, MA
Aneesha Nilakantan, BA
Noorulain Noor, BS

Queens University
J. Curtis Nickel, MD, FRCSC, Director

National Institutes of Diabetes and Digestive and Kidney Diseases (NIDDK), National Institutes of Health (NIH)
Chris Mullins, PhD
John W. Kusek, PhD
Ziya Kirkali, MD
Tamara G. Bavendam, MD

Abbreviations
BACH: Boston area community health survey; BPS: Bladder pain syndrome; CFS: Chronic fatigue syndrome; CNS: Central nervous system; CPC: Chronic prostatitis cohort; CP/CPPS: Chronic prostatitis/chronic pelvic pain syndrome; DCC: Data coordinating core; DNA: Deoxyribonucleic acid; EEP: External experts panel; FM: Fibromyalgia; IBS: Irritable bowel syndrome; IC/BPS: Interstitial cystitis/bladder pain syndrome; ICCRN: Interstitial cystitis collaborative research network; ICCTG: The interstitial cystitis clinical trials group; ICDB: Interstitial cystitis database study; LONI: Laboratory of neuroimaging; MAPP: Multidisciplinary approach to the study of chronic pelvic pain; MRI/fMRI: Magnetic resonance imaging/functional magnetic resonance imaging; NIDDK: The national institute of diabetes, digestive, and kidney diseases; NUAS: Non-urologic associated syndromes; PPT: Pressure pain threshold; RICE: RAND IC epidemiology study; TATC: Tissue analysis and technology core; Trans-MAPP EP: Trans-MAPP epidemiology and phenotyping study; UCLA: University of california at Los

Angeles; UCPPS: Urological chronic pelvic pain syndromes; VB1, VB2: Voided bladder 1, 2.

Competing interests
JQ Clemens, C Mullins, JW Kusek, Z Kirkali, EA Mayer, LV Rodriguez, AJ Schaeffer, D Buchwald, and JR Landis declare no competing interests. DJ Klumpp declares ownership and equity interests in ProbioTx Inc, and Gold Coast Therapeutics Inc. KJ Kreder is a Consultant for Medtronic, Astellas, Symptelligence, and Tengion. GL Andriole is a Consultant for Augmenix, Bayer, Genomic Health, GlaxoSmithKline and Myriad Genetics and has received research grants from Johnson & Johnson, Medivation and Wilex. MS Lucia declares ownership of 3D Biopsy and has consulted for Myriad Genetics and Bayer Healthcare. DJ Clauw has received grants from Pfizer, Cerephex, Lilly, Merck, Nuvo and Furest, and Consulting Fees and Honoraria from Pfizer, Cerephex, Lilly, Merck, Nuvo, Furest, Tonix, Purdue, Therauance, and Johnson & Johnson.

Authors' contributions
JQC wrote the initial draft manuscript. All authors read and approved the final manuscript.

Acknowledgements
The MAPP Research Network acknowledges support through NIH grants: U01 DK82315, U01 DK82316, U01 DK82325, U01 DK82333, U01 DK82342, U01 DK82344, U01 DK82345, and U01 DK82370. The NIDDK and MAPP Network investigators wish to thank the Interstitial Cystitis Association (ICA) and the Prostatitis Foundation (PF) for their assistance in study participant recruitment and other network efforts.
We thank the participants and staff from the following sites that participated in the study: Northwestern University; University of California, Los Angeles; University of Iowa; Washington University, St. Louis; University of Washington, Seattle; University of Michigan; University of Pennsylvania (Data Coordinating Core); University of Colorado Denver (Tissue Analysis & Technology Core); Stanford University; NIDDK.
This article outlines independent research commissioned by the National Institute for Health (NIH). The views expressed in this article are those of the author(s) and are not necessarily those of the NIH, the NIDDK, or the Department of Health and Human Services (DHHS).

Author details
[1]Department of Urology, University of Michigan, Ann Arbor, MI, USA. [2]National Institute of Diabetes and Digestive and Kidney Diseases, National Institutes of Health, Bethesda, MD, USA. [3]Division of Digestive Diseases, University of California, Los Angeles, CA, USA. [4]Department of Urology, Northwestern University, Chicago, IL, USA. [5]Department of Urology, University of Iowa, Iowa City, IA, USA. [6]Departments of Epidemiology and Medicine, University of Washington, Seattle, WA, USA. [7]Division of Urologic Surgery, Department of Surgery, Washington University School of Medicine, St Louis, MO, USA. [8]Department of Pathology, University of Colorado Anschutz Medical Campus, Aurora, CO, USA. [9]Department of Biostatistics and Epidemiology, University of Pennsylvania Perelman School of Medicine, Philadelphia, PA, USA. [10]Departments of Anesthesiology and Medicine, University of Michigan, Ann Arbor, MI, USA.

References
1. Bogart LM, Berry SH, Clemens JQ: Symptoms of interstitial cystitis, painful bladder syndrome and similar diseases in women: a systematic review. J Urol 2007, 177(2):450–456.
2. Clemens JQ, Markossian TW, Meenan RT, O'Keeffe Rosetti MC, Calhoun EA: Overlap of voiding symptoms, storage symptoms and pain in men and women. J Urol 2007, 178(4 Pt 1):1354–8. discussion 1358.
3. Simon LJ, Landis JR, Erickson DR, Nyberg LM: The interstitial cystitis data base study: concepts and preliminary baseline descriptive statistics. Urology 1997, 49(5A Suppl):64–75.
4. Propert KJ, Schaeffer AJ, Brensinger CM, Kusek JW, Nyberg LM, Landis JR: A prospective study of interstitial cystitis: results of longitudinal followup of the interstitial cystitis data base cohort: the interstitial cystitis data base study group. J Urol 2000, 163(5):1434–1439.
5. Sant GR, Propert KJ, Hanno PM, Burks D, Culkin D, Diokno AC, Hardy C, Landis JR, Mayer R, Madigan R, Messing EM, Peters K, Theoharides TC, Warren J, Wein AJ, Steers W, Kusek JW, Nyberg LM, Interstitial Cystitis Clinical Trials Group: A pilot clinical trial of oral pentosan polysulfate and oral hydroxyzine in patients with interstitial cystitis. J Urol 2003, 170(3):810–815.
6. Mayer R, Propert KJ, Peters KM, Payne CK, Zhang Y, Burks D, Culkin DJ, Diokno A, Hanno P, Landis JR, Madigan R, Messing EM, Nickel JC, Sant GR, Warren J, Wein AJ, Kusek JW, Nyberg LM, Foster HE, Interstitial Cystitis Clinical Trials Group: A randomized controlled trial of intravesical bacillus calmette-guerin for treatment refractory interstitial cystitis. J Urol 2005, 173(4):1186–1191.
7. Propert KJ, Mayer RD, Wang Y, Sant GR, Hanno PM, Peters KM, Kusek JW, Interstitial Cystitis Clinical Trials Group: Responsiveness of symptom scales for interstitial cystitis. Urology 2006, 67(1):55–59.
8. Propert KJ, Mayer R, Nickel JC, Payne CK, Peters KM, Teal V, Burks D, Kusek JW, Nyberg LM, Foster HE, Interstitial Cystitis Clinical Trials Group: Did patients with interstitial cystitis who failed to respond to initial treatment with bacillus calmette-guerin or placebo in a randomized clinical trial benefit from a second course of open label bacillus calmette-guerin? J Urol 2007, 178(3 Pt 1):886–890.
9. Propert KJ, Mayer R, Nickel JC, Payne CK, Peters KM, Teal V, Burks D, Kusek JW, Nyberg LM, Foster HE, Interstitial Cystitis Clinical Trials Group: Followup of patients with interstitial cystitis responsive to treatment with intravesical bacillus Calmette-Guerin or placebo. J Urol 2008, 179(2):552–555.
10. Foster HE Jr, Hanno PM, Nickel JC, Payne CK, Mayer RD, Burks DA, Yang CC, Chai TC, Kreder KJ, Peters KM, Lukacz ES, Fitzgerald MP, Cen L, Landis JR, Propert KJ, Yang W, Kusek JW, Nyberg LM, Interstitial Cystitis Collaborative Research Network: Effect of amitriptyline on symptoms in treatment naive patients with interstitial cystitis/painful bladder syndrome. J Urol 2010, 183(5):1853–1858.
11. Yang CC, Burks DA, Propert KJ, Mayer RD, Peters KM, Nickel JC, Payne CK, FitzGerald MP, Hanno PM, Chai TC, Kreder KJ, Lukacz ES, Foster HE, Cen L, Landis JR, Kusek JW, Nyberg LM, Interstitial Cystitis Collaborative Research Network: Early termination of a trial of mycophenolate mofetil for treatment of interstitial cystitis/painful bladder syndrome: lessons learned. J Urol 2011, 185(3):901–906.
12. FitzGerald MP, Payne CK, Lukacz ES, Yang CC, Peters KM, Chai TC, Nickel JC, Hanno PM, Kreder KJ, Burks DA, Mayer R, Kotarinos R, Fortman C, Allen TM, Fraser L, Mason-Cover M, Furey C, Odabachian L, Sanfield A, Chu J, Huestis K, Tata GE, Dugan N, Sheth H, Bewyer K, Anaeme A, Newton K, Featherstone W, Halle-Podell R, Cen L, Landis JR, Propert KJ, Foster HE Jr, Kusek JW, Nyberg LM, Interstitial Cystitis Collaborative Research Network: Randomized multicenter clinical trial of myofascial physical therapy in women with interstitial cystitis/painful bladder syndrome and pelvic floor tenderness. J Urol 2012, 187(6):2113–2118.
13. Schaeffer AJ, Landis JR, Knauss JS, Propert KJ, Alexander RB, Litwin MS, Nickel JC, O'Leary MP, Nadler RB, Pontari MA, Shoskes DA, Zeitlin SI, Fowler JE Jr, Mazurick CA, Kishel L, Kusek JW, Nyberg LM, Chronic Prostatitis Collaborative Research Network Group: Demographic and clinical characteristics of men with chronic prostatitis: the National Institutes of Health chronic prostatitis cohort study. J Urol 2002, 168(2):593–598.
14. Alexander RB, Propert KJ, Schaeffer AJ, Landis JR, Nickel JC, O'Leary MP, Pontari MA, McNaughton-Collins M, Shoskes DA, Comiter CV, Datta NS, Fowler JE Jr, Nadler RB, Zeitlin SI, Knauss JS, Wang Y, Kusek JW, Nyberg LM Jr, Litwin MS, Chronic Prostatitis Collaborative Research Network: Ciprofloxacin or tamsulosin in men with chronic prostatitis/chronic pelvic pain syndrome: a randomized, double-blind trial. Ann Intern Med 2004, 141(8):581–589.
15. Nickel JC, Krieger JN, McNaughton-Collins M, Anderson RU, Pontari M, Shoskes DA, Litwin MS, Alexander RB, White PC, Berger R, Nadler R, O'Leary M, Liong ML, Zeitlin S, Chuai S, Landis JR, Kusek JW, Nyberg LM, Schaeffer AJ, Chronic Prostatitis Collaborative Research Network: Alfuzosin and symptoms of chronic prostatitis-chronic pelvic pain syndrome. N Engl J Med 2008, 359(25):2663–2673.
16. Nickel JC, Alexander RB, Anderson R, Berger R, Comiter CV, Datta NS, Fowler JE, Krieger JN, Landis JR, Litwin MS, McNaughton-Collins M, O'Leary MP, Pontari MA, Schaeffer AJ, Shoskes DA, White P, Kusek J, Nyberg L, Chronic Prostatitis Collaborative Research Network Study Group: Category III chronic prostatitis/chronic pelvic pain syndrome: insights from the National Institutes of Health Chronic Prostatitis Collaborative Research Network studies. Curr Urol Rep 2008, 9(4):320–327.

17. Pontari MA, Krieger JN, Litwin MS, White PC, Anderson RU, McNaughton-Collins M, Nickel JC, Shoskes DA, Alexander RB, O'Leary M, Zeitlin S, Chuai S, Landis JR, Cen L, Propert KJ, Kusek JW, Nyberg LM Jr, Schaeffer AJ, Chronic Prostatitis Collaborative Research Network-2: **Pregabalin for the treatment of men with chronic prostatitis/chronic pelvic pain syndrome: a randomized controlled trial.** *Arch Intern Med* 2010, **170**(17):1586–1593.

18. FitzGerald MP, Anderson RU, Potts J, Payne CK, Peters KM, Clemens JQ, Kotarinos R, Fraser L, Cosby A, Fortman C, Neville C, Badillo S, Odabachian L, Sanfield A, O'Dougherty B, Halle-Podell R, Cen L, Chuai S, Landis JR, Mickelberg K, Barrell T, Kusek JW, Nyberg LM: **Randomized multicenter feasibility trial of myofascial physical therapy for the treatment of urological chronic pelvic pain syndromes.** *J Urol* 2013, **189**(1):S75–S85.

19. Clemens JQ, Link CL, Eggers PW, Kusek JW, Nyberg LM Jr, McKinlay JB, BACH Survey Investigators: **Prevalence of painful bladder symptoms and effect on quality of life in black, Hispanic and white men and women.** *J Urol* 2007, **177**(4):1390–1394.

20. Link CL, Pulliam SJ, Hanno PM, Hall SA, Eggers PW, Kusek JW, McKinlay JB: **Prevalence and psychosocial correlates of symptoms suggestive of painful bladder syndrome: results from the Boston area community health survey.** *J Urol* 2008, **180**(2):599–606.

21. Barry MJ, Link CL, McNaughton-Collins MF, McKinlay JB, Boston Area Community Health (BACH) Investigators: **Overlap of different urological symptom complexes in a racially and ethnically diverse, community-based population of men and women.** *BJU Int* 2008, **101**(1):45–51.

22. Berry SH, Elliott MN, Suttorp M, Bogart LM, Stoto MA, Eggers P, Nyberg L, Clemens JQ: **Prevalence of symptoms of bladder pain syndrome/interstitial cystitis among adult females in the United States.** *J Urol* 2011, **186**(2):540–544.

23. Suskind AM, Berry SH, Ewing BA, Elliott MN, Suttorp MJ, Clemens JQ: **The prevalence and overlap of interstitial cystitis/bladder pain syndrome and chronic prostatitis/chronic pelvic pain syndrome in men: results of the RAND Interstitial Cystitis Epidemiology male study.** *J Urol* 2013, **189**(1):141–145.

24. Warren JW, Wesselmann U, Morozov V, Langenberg PW: **Numbers and types of nonbladder syndromes as risk factors for interstitial cystitis/painful bladder syndrome.** *Urology* 2011, **77**(2):313–319.

25. Warren JW, Howard FM, Cross RK, Good JL, Weissman MM, Wesselmann U, Langenberg P, Greenberg P, Clauw DJ: **Antecedent nonbladder syndromes in case–control study of interstitial cystitis/painful bladder syndrome.** *Urology* 2009, **73**(1):52–57.

26. Clauw DJ, Schmidt M, Radulovic D, Singer A, Katz P, Bresette J: **The relationship between fibromyalgia and interstitial cystitis.** *J Psychiatr Res* 1997, **31**(1):125–131.

27. Heitkemper M, Jarrett M: **Overlapping conditions in women with irritable bowel syndrome.** *Urol Nurs* 2005, **25**(1):25–30. quiz 31.

28. Aaron LA, Herrell R, Ashton S, Belcourt M, Schmaling K, Goldberg J, Buchwald D: **Comorbid clinical conditions in chronic fatigue: a co-twin control study.** *J Gen Intern Med* 2001, **16**(1):24–31.

29. Clemens JQ, Meenan RT, O'Keeffe Rosetti MC, Kimes TA, Calhoun EA: **Case–control study of medical comorbidities in women with interstitial cystitis.** *J Urol* 2008, **179**(6):2222–2225.

30. Rodriguez MA, Afari N, Buchwald DS, National Institute of Diabetes and Digestive and Kidney Diseases Working Group on Urological Chronic Pelvic Pain: **Evidence for overlap between urological and nonurological unexplained clinical conditions.** *J Urol* 2009, **182**(5):2123–2131.

31. Nickel JC: **The multidisciplinary approach to defining the urologic chronic pelvic pain syndromes: report from a National Institutes of Health workshop, December 13–14, 2007, Baltimore.** *MD Rev Urol* 2008, **10**(2):157–159.

32. Fillingim RB, Ohrbach R, Greenspan JD, Knott C, Dubner R, Bair E, Baraian C, Slade GD, Maixner W: **Potential psychosocial risk factors for chronic TMD: descriptive data and empirically identified domains from the OPPERA case–control study.** *J Pain* 2011, **12**(11 Suppl):T46–60.

33. Landis JR, Williams DA, Lucia MS, Clauw DJ, Naliboff BD, Robinson NA, van Bokhoven A, Sutcliffe S, Schaeffer AJ, Rodriguez LV, Mayer EA, Lai HH, Krieger JN, Kreder KJ, Afari N, Andriole GL, Bradley CS, Griffith JW, Klumpp DJ, Hong BA, Lutgendorf SK, Buchwald D, Yang CC, Mackey S, Pontari MA, Hanno P, Kusek JW, Mullins C, Clemens JQ, The MAPP Research Network Study Group: *The MAPP research network: design, patient characterization, and operations*; Accepted to BMC Urology on 23 July 2014.

34. Shoskes DA, Nickel JC, Dolinga R, Prots D: **Clinical phenotyping of patients with chronic prostatitis/chronic pelvic pain syndrome and correlation with symptom severity.** *Urology* 2009, **73**(3):538–42. discussion 542–3.

35. Nickel JC, Shoskes D, Irvine-Bird K: **Clinical phenotyping of women with interstitial cystitis/painful bladder syndrome: a key to classification and potentially improved management.** *J Urol* 2009, **182**(1):155–160.

11

Effects of surgeon variability on oncologic and functional outcomes in a population-based setting

Sigrid Carlsson[1,2*], Anders Berglund[3], Daniel Sjoberg[4], Ali Khatami[2], Johan Stranne[2], Svante Bergdahl[2], Pär Lodding[2], Gunnar Aus[5], Andrew Vickers[4] and Jonas Hugosson[2]

Abstract

Background: Oncologic and functional outcomes after radical prostatectomy (RP) can vary between surgeons to a greater extent than is expected by chance. We sought to examine the effects of surgeon variation on functional and oncologic outcomes for patients undergoing RP for prostate cancer in a European center.

Methods: The study comprised 1,280 men who underwent open retropubic RP performed by one of nine surgeons at an academic institution in Sweden between 2001 and 2008. Potency and continence outcomes were measured preoperatively and 18 months postoperatively by patient-administered questionnaires. Biochemical recurrence (BCR) was defined as a prostate-specific antigen (PSA) value > 0.2 ng/mL with at least one confirmatory rise. Multivariable random effect models were used to evaluate heterogeneity between surgeons, adjusting for case mix (age, PSA, pathological stage and grade), year of surgery, and surgical experience.

Results: Of 679 men potent at baseline, 647 provided data at 18 months with 122 (19%) reporting potency. We found no evidence for heterogeneity of potency outcomes between surgeons (P = 1). The continence rate for patients at 18 months was 85%, with 836 of the 979 patients who provided data reporting continence. There was statistically significant heterogeneity between surgeons (P = 0.001). We did not find evidence of an association between surgeons' adjusted probabilities of functional recovery and 5-year probability of freedom from BCR.

Conclusions: Our data support previous studies regarding a large heterogeneity among surgeons in continence outcomes for patients undergoing RP. This indicates that some patients are receiving sub-optimal care. Quality assurance measures involving performance feedback, should be considered. When surgeons are aware of their outcomes, they can improve them to provide better care to patients.

Keywords: Prostate cancer, Radical prostatectomy, Erectile function, Urinary function

Background

Radical prostatectomy (RP) with curative intent is the most common treatment for men with localized prostate cancer [1]. A prospective, randomized Swedish trial demonstrated that surgery provides a survival benefit in men with mainly clinically diagnosed, palpable tumors when compared to watchful waiting [2]. However, surgical treatment is associated with long-term morbidity, mainly erectile dysfunction (ED) and urinary incontinence, which affect a patient's quality of life (QoL) substantially [3,4].

Previous studies performed in high-volume referral centers in the United States (US) have shown that both oncologic [5] and functional outcomes [6,7] after RP vary between surgeons to a greater extent than is expected by chance. In the present validation study, we sought to explore whether such heterogeneity exists in long-term functional and oncologic outcomes among surgeons in a European center who operate in a population-based academic setting. Another rationale for the present study is that there is limited data on

* Correspondence: carlssos@mskcc.org
[1]Urology Service at the Department of Surgery, Memorial Sloan-Kettering Cancer Center, 307 E. 63rd St, 2nd floor, New York, NY 10065, USA
[2]Department of Urology, Sahlgrenska Academy at the University of Göteborg, Göteborg, Sweden
Full list of author information is available at the end of the article

variability in patient-reported outcomes (PRO). Therefore, the present study provides a unique opportunity to explore any variability in outcomes as assessed by validated PRO instruments.

Methods

The original database consisted of 1,447 men who were scheduled for open retropubic RP at Sahlgrenska University Hospital in Göteborg, Sweden, during the study period 2001–2008, when standardized data recording into a quality assurance database was performed.

The quality control program was approved by the Ethical Committee at Göteborg University in 2001. Patients were mailed questionnaires, a cover letter with information regarding the quality assurance program, and a statement of voluntary participation in the study.

Of the 58 patients excluded, 38 were enrolled in another clinical RP trial (LAPPRO) [8], 4 underwent surgery outside the university hospital, 7 did not undergo surgery (with 4 switching to radiotherapy and 3 receiving hormonal therapy), and 9 did not undergo surgery but may have had surgery elsewhere for unknown reasons (moved or loss-to-follow-up). This left 1,389 patients in the cohort. Surgery dates ranged from Jan 2, 2001 through July 16, 2008.

Biochemical recurrence (BCR) post-prostatectomy was defined as a prostate-specific antigen (PSA) value > 0.2 ng/mL with at least one confirmatory rise. Measurements were obtained from medical charts.

Of 1,389 patients, an additional 109 were excluded from analysis since they were never administered any questionnaires, leaving 1,280 patients available for analysis of functional outcomes. Patients responded to questionnaires regarding continence and potency on 4 occasions, approximately 2 weeks preoperatively and at 6, 18, and 36 months after surgery.

Patients were administered questionnaires assessing urinary continence using pads [9]. Continence was defined as no leakage or occasional leakage associated with physical activity requiring sporadic use of pads (score 0–1 on a 0–4 point scale, where 2–4 implies incontinence with regular use of pads).

Erectile function was assessed by the standardized International Index of Erection Function questionnaire IIEF-5 [10]. The IIEF-5 score consists of 5 items with 6 responses. The total score is the sum of the 5 items and ranges from 5–25, the higher the score the better potency. For patients missing responses for an item, the sum of the remaining items was used. Potency was defined as an IIEF-5 score of ≥ 17, which corresponds to Rosen et al.'s categorization of mild ED (17–21) and no ED (22–25) [10]. This also makes our study comparable to functional outcomes reported in an earlier study by Vickers et al. where postoperative potency was defined

as 1 = normal, full erections and 2 = full, but diminished erections [6].

Missing data on potency status (potent/impotent) and continence (incontinent/continent) at 18 months were imputed following an algorithm assuming that few men regain and then lose function as well as that recovery of function can occur beyond 18 months. If a patient was missing a questionnaire at 18 months but reported potency at 6 months, he was assumed to be potent at 18 months. Comparably, a patient reporting impotence at 6 and 36 months was considered impotent at 18 months. A similar approach was used for the continence endpoint.

Patients reporting use of alprostadil injections for erectile aid were categorized as impotent (3 men preoperatively, 222 men at 18 months, and 198 men at 36 months). Men reporting use of PDE5-inhibitors were included in the analysis.

Statistics

Data on a total of 25 individual surgeons working at the hospital during the study period were included in the database. We analyzed patient-reported functional outcomes for 9 surgeons who performed ≥ 20 surgeries during the study period. Data for these surgeons were entered both as random and fixed effects.

Logistic regression models were adjusted for age at surgery, PSA at diagnosis, pathologic stage (pT0, pT2, pT3), pathologic Gleason score (≤ 6, 7, ≥ 8), year of surgery, and surgical experience. We defined surgical experience as a variable that took into account both the surgeon's prior experience, i.e., number of RPs before 2001, and the annual number of prostatectomies performed during the study period [6]. To statistically test for heterogeneity, a random effect following an inverse Gaussian distribution was included in the model.

The logistic regression model used to predict the probability of potency at 18 months was restricted to men who were potent preoperatively and also adjusted for the IIEF-5 score as a continuous variable. The model for continence at 18 months was restricted to men who were continent preoperatively. Since there have been changes in patient characteristics as well as operative technique, we also included year of surgery as a covariate. Nerve sparing status was not included in the model since it is a surgical decision. Take the case of two surgeons, one of whom only spared nerves if the cancer was very low risk and accordingly resected far from the neurovascular bundles, the other of whom only resected nerves for advanced disease. Overall, the former surgeon would have far lower potency rates, but adjusting for nerve sparing would lead to higher apparent rates.

A log-logistic distributed parametric regression survival model was used to model BCR rates following adjustment for the same covariates as for functional outcomes. To statistically test for heterogeneity, a shared frailty survival model was fitted.

For each surgeon studied, forest plots were created for the adjusted predicted probability of potency and continence, respectively, using the mean value for the covariates from the fixed regression model with a 95% confidence interval.

A scatter plot was created for adjusted rates of continence and potency with the size of each surgeon's data point proportional to the number of RPs (prior experience and during the study period) performed by each surgeon. Spearman's rank correlation was applied to test the correlation between surgeons' adjusted probabilities of potency and continence at 18 months as well as BCR.

Statistical analyses were performed using Stata v. 12.0 (Stata Corp, College Station, TX, USA).

Results

Table 1 shows clinical characteristics for all 1,280 men who underwent RP. The median age at surgery was 64 years. Crude functional outcome rates per surgeon along with prior experience and the number of cases operated upon during the study period are shown in Table 2. Nine surgeons performed ≥ 20 surgeries during the study period, with a maximum of 248 cases. The prior experience of these surgeons ranged between 0 and 360 cases (Table 2).

Regarding functional outcomes, a total of 1,039 men responded to the IIEF-5 questionnaire, with 679 reporting being potent preoperatively (65%). Data were available for 647 (95%) patients at 18 months with 122 (19%) reporting potency (without alprostadil).

Crude potency rates at 18 months were higher for men who underwent bilateral nerve-sparing RP (31.8%) and for those < 60 years of age (45.7%) (data not shown).

Of the 1,078 patients who responded preoperatively to the continence question, 25 were considered incontinent

Table 1 Clinical characteristics for all patients who underwent radical prostatectomy

		All patients N = 1,280	
Age at surgery, median years (IQR)		64	(60,67)
PSA at diagnosis, median (IQR) ng/mL (Missing n=3)		6.3	(4.5,9.8)
Follow-up for biochemical recurrence, median years (IQR)		5.28	(3.59-6.83)
		n	(%)
Pathological Gleason score (Missing n=2)	≤ 6	593	(46.5)
	7	624	(48.9)
	≥ 8	59	(4.6)
	No tumor found	2	-
Nerve-sparing surgery (Missing n=3)	No	625	(48.9)
	Unilateral	196	(15.3)
	Bilateral	456	(35.7)
Surgical margins (Missing n=5)	Positive	333	(26.1)
	Negative	942	(73.9)
Seminal vesicle invasion (Missing n=16)	Yes	109	(8.6)
	No	1155	(91.4)
Pathological stage (Missing n=7)	pT0	2	(0.2)
	pT2	906	(71.2)
	pT3	365	(28.7)
Preoperative erectile function (Missing n=241)	Potent	679	(65.4)
	Impotent	360	(34.7)
Postoperative erectile function at 18 months (Missing n=633)	Potent	122	(18.9)
	Impotent	525	(81.1)
Preoperative urinary function (Missing n=202)	Continent	1053	(97.7)
	Incontinent	25	(2.3)
Postoperative urinary function at 18 months (Missing n=301)	Continent	836	(85.4)
	Incontinent	143	(14.6)

PSA = prostate-specific antigen, IQR = Inter Quartile Range.

Table 2 Unadjusted functional outcome rates per surgeon (among preoperatively potent and continent men) in relation to prior experience and number of cases performed during study period

Surgeon number	Prior experience, number of RPs performed before study period (n)	Number of cases during study period (n)	Potent at 18 months, n (%)	Impotent at 18 months, n (%)	Missing potency information at 18 months, n (%)	Continent at 18 months, n (%)	Incontinent at 18 months, n (%)	Missing continence information at 18 months, n (%)
1	32	94	4 (9.1)	38 (86.4)	2 (4.5)	56 (78.9)	14 (19.7)	1 (1.4)
2	120	248	20 (15.9)	98 (77.8)	8 (6.3)	171 (86.8)	15 (7.6)	11 (5.6)
3	2	104	12 (20.0)	45 (75.0)	3 (5.0)	69 (76.7)	14 (15.6)	7 (7.8)
4	360	156	20 (24.1)	59 (71.1)	4 (4.8)	115 (84.6)	14 (10.3)	7 (5.1)
5	13	239	25 (19.4)	98 (76.0)	6 (4.7)	157 (83.1)	18 (9.5)	14 (7.4)
6	115	138	16 (19.3)	64 (77.1)	3 (3.6)	80 (66.1)	27 (22.3)	14 (11.6)
7	67	97	9 (16.1)	46 (82.1)	1 (1.8)	69 (82.1)	11 (13.1)	4 (4.8)
8	2	75	7 (20.6)	25 (73.5)	2 (5.9)	43 (71.7)	12 (20.0)	5 (8.3)
9	0	49	4 (13.8)	22 (75.9)	3 (10.3)	21 (58.3)	10 (27.8)	5 (13.9)

RPs = radical prostatectomies.

(2%). Of the 979 (91%) patients responding at 18 months, 836 were continent (85%). The degrees of incontinence at 18 months among preoperatively continent men were as follows: never urinary leakage (39.0%), sometimes urinary leakage when coughing, sneezing or performing physical exercise with sporadic use of pads (46.4%), regular use of pads but they are not always wet (9.4%), regular use of pads that are wet (3.3%), and constant urinary leakage (1.7%).

Between-surgeon variation in functional outcomes is shown in the forest plots for potency in Figure 1A and continence in Figure 1B. For potency at 18 months, we found no evidence for heterogeneity between surgeons (random effects variance = 0.0002, P = 1). For continence at 18 months, there was a statistically significant

heterogeneity between surgeons, (random effects variance = 0.0318; 95% CI 0.0125 – 0.1649, P = 0.001) with continence rates varying from 70 to 93% between surgeons. For BCR at a mean follow-up of 5.12 years (SD 0.07), heterogeneity between surgeons was not observed (random effects variance = 0.0133, P = 0.484) (Figure 1C).

The correlation between surgeons' adjusted probabilities of potency and continence was not statistically significant (Spearman's rho −0.20, P = 0.61) (Figure 2A).

Postoperatively, the 5-year probability of freedom from BCR adjusted for case mix was 86%. We observed a weak and non-significant association between surgeons' adjusted probabilities of functional recovery (i.e., both potent and continent) and 5-year probability of freedom from BCR (P = 0.9) (Figure 2B). The present findings

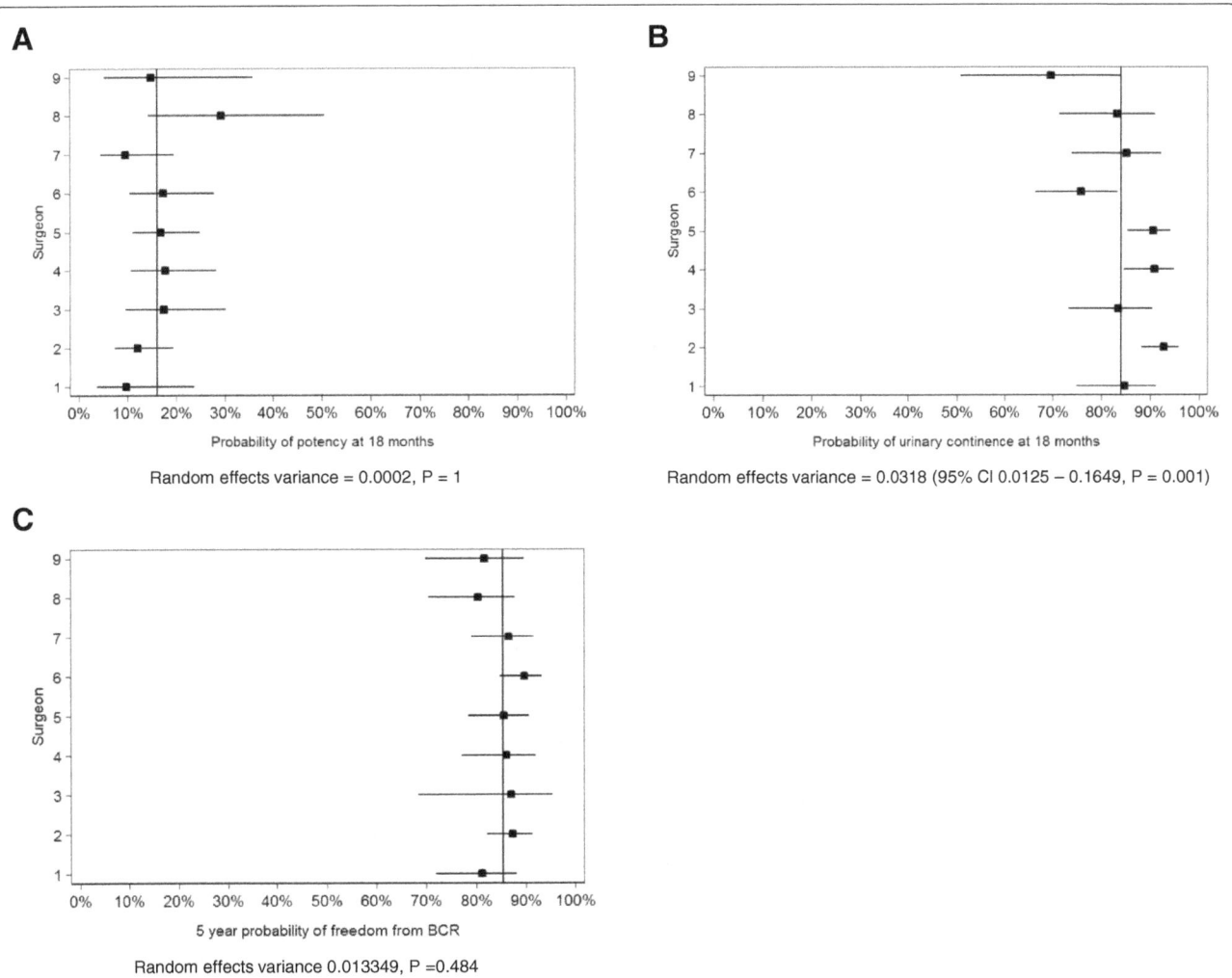

Figure 1 Forest plots for the probability of functional and oncologic outcomes by surgeon. A. Probability of potency at 18 months postoperatively. **B**. Probability of continence at 18 months postoperatively. **C**. 5-year probability of freedom from biochemical-free recurrence. Proportions (squared dots) and 95% confidence intervals (horizontal lines) are adjusted for patients with the mean level of the covariates: age at surgery, PSA at diagnosis, pathological stage, pathologic Gleason score, year of surgery and surgical experience. The vertical line represents the mean adjusted probability for all surgeons. Potency was defined as an IIEF-5 total score ≥ 17, with alprostadil-users defined as impotent. Continence was defined as urinary control with no leakage or sporadic use of pads due to leakage associated with physical activity.

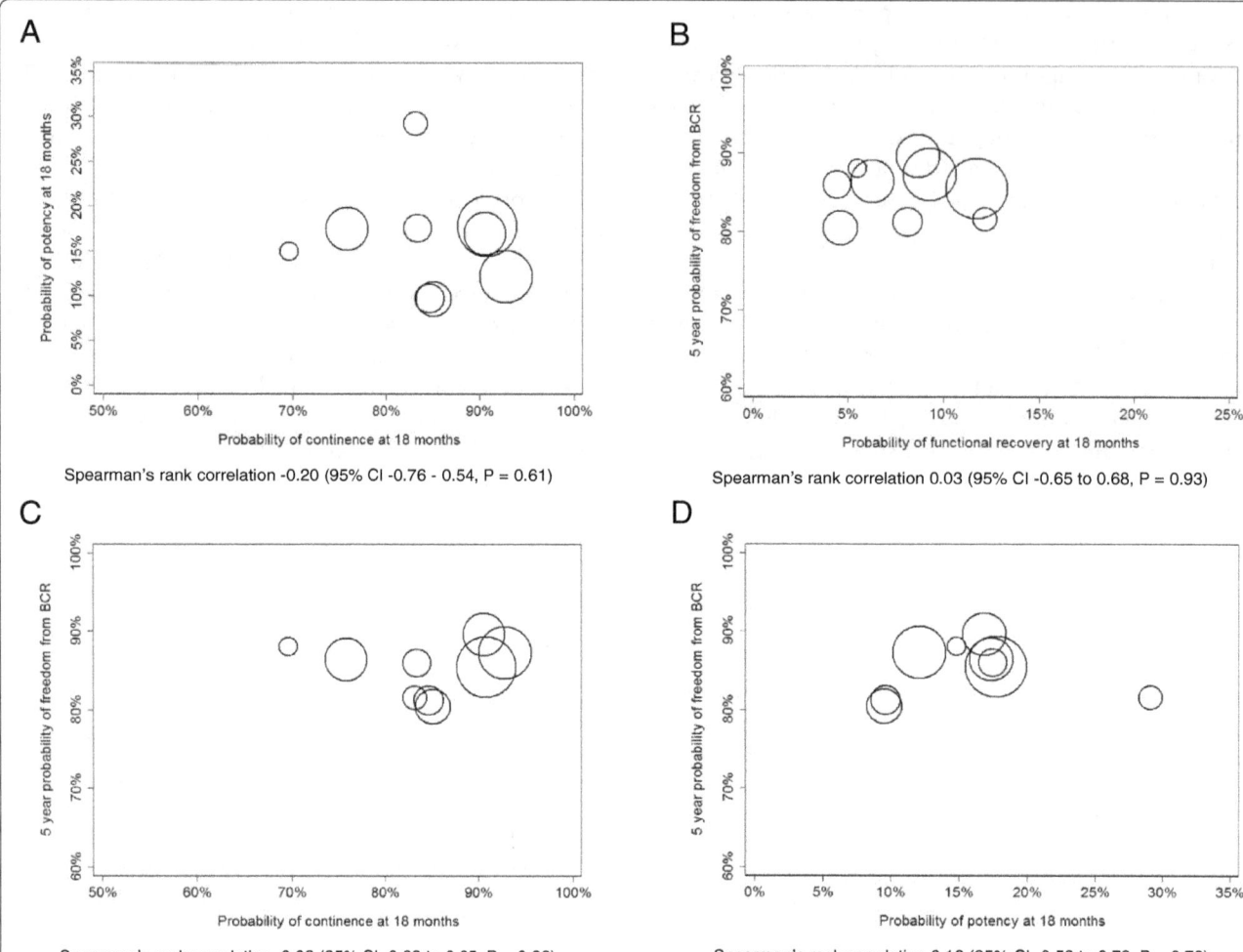

Figure 2 Scatter plots. A. Adjusted probability of continence and potency at 18 months postoperatively. **B**. Adjusted probability of functional recovery and 5-year probability of freedom from biochemical recurrence at 18 months postoperatively. **C**. Adjusted probability of continence and 5-year probability of freedom from biochemical recurrence at 18 months postoperatively. **D**. Adjusted probability of potency and 5-year probability of freedom from biochemical recurrence at 18 months postoperatively. Each circle represents a single surgeon and the size is proportionate to the surgeon's prior experience and the number of radical prostatectomies that surgeon performed during the study period.

were not altered when the correlation between functional recovery and BCR was assessed separately; continence and potency, respectively (Figure 2C and 2D).

Discussion

In the present validation study, we explored whether heterogeneity in long-term functional outcomes in a European academic center is comparable to that previously reported in a very high-volume referral center in the US [6]. Our data confirms prior studies on the existence of surgeon heterogeneity for continence, but not for potency [5-7].

Continence rates were similar when comparing our present study to the Vickers et al. study in which 1,910 patients were treated with RP by 1 of 11 surgeons between 1997 and 2007 at a high-volume US referral center [6], with a rate of 85% at 18 months vs. 83% at 12 months,

respectively. However, potency rates were lower in the present study, with a rate of 19% at 18 months compared to 43% at 12 months in Vickers et al. Overall, the rate of impotence at 18 months postoperatively was high in the present study, with less than two-thirds of patients being potent preoperatively. The lower rate of potency is most plausibly explained by the fact that the men in this study were considerably older, with a median age of 64 years, as compared to the median age of 58 years in the Vickers et al. study. Another possible explanation is that the study cohort was derived from a population-based sample in an area where active surveillance is frequently used, implying that only the most aggressive tumors are treated; this likely results in more advanced tumor features leading to more radical surgery with wider resection and lower potency rates. This is exemplified in that only one third of patients underwent a bilateral nerve-sparing procedure. Additionally, center-specific differences in indication for nerve-sparing procedures may explain these results.

A major strength of the current study is that potency and continence outcomes were assessed from patient-administered questionnaires in contrast to the study by Vickers et al., where the same outcomes were evaluated by the treating surgeon. PROs provide an assessment of functional outcomes from the patient's perspective. Therefore, collecting data from the patient may protect against bias due to patients minimizing symptoms when they are asked by the treating physician directly. Published rates of impotence after RP based on physician reports may be underestimates, since patients may not report this side effect accurately and completely to their doctor [11].

Furthermore, the patient-reported potency rate in the present study is in line with other population-based series on unselected patients in the literature [11-15]. In the Scandinavian Prostate Cancer Group Study 4 (SPCG-4) trial, the prevalence of ED 12 years after RP was 84% [3].

We found no evidence of heterogeneity in potency by surgeon. Our failure to replicate a prior finding of heterogeneity for potency outcomes [6] may be related to a floor effect of low overall rates as well as limited power (9 surgeons). Other possible explanations are that potency post-operatively is more a question of inherent patient factors or also dependent upon the individual decision of the surgeon and patient to elect for a nerve-sparing procedure.

For continence outcomes at 18 months, we found evidence of significant heterogeneity between surgeons. The difference was quite remarkable (7%–30% incontinence rates). This finding is in line with a previous US study. Using the SEER-Medicare database (patients ≥ 65 years old); Begg et al. found that case mix-adjusted incontinence rates 1 year after RP were lower in very high-volume hospitals than in low-volume hospitals. They also studied, in detail, long-term incontinence in patients for 159 surgeons in the 2 highest-volume categories (20–32 RPs per surgeon and 33–121 RPs per surgeon during the study period) and noted significant surgeon-to-surgeon variations in outcome [7].

Urinary incontinence and impotence after RP have a major impact on QoL [4] and these side effects, especially in the long-term, are one of the major drawbacks of PSA screening [16]. In the present study the average incontinence rate was 15%, which is very similar to the 17% reported by Vickers et al. [6]. The large variation between surgeons suggests a need for formal quality assurance programs and performance feedback systems. Surgeons need to know their results so that they can evaluate and find ways to improve them [17].

Previous studies have shown heterogeneity between surgeons regarding not only functional outcomes but also risk for BCR and clinical recurrence [5,6,18]. In particular,

Vickers et al. found that functional preservation did not come at the expense of cancer control [6]. Indeed, there was a positive correlation between oncologic and functional outcomes, suggesting that both are markers of surgical quality. We were not able to replicate this finding, possibly due to a floor effect for potency.

Conclusion

RP is associated with long-term side effects such as incontinence and ED. In this study we replicated prior findings that individual surgeon technique is related to the risk of permanent incontinence; we were unable to replicate findings relating surgical technique to erectile dysfunction and oncologic outcome. Quality assurance measures involving performance feedback should be considered. When surgeons are aware of their outcomes, they can improve them to provide better care to patients.

Abbreviations
BCR: Biochemical recurrence; ED: Erectile dysfunction; PSA: Prostate-specific antigen; RP: Radical prostatectomy; PRO: Patient-reported outcomes; QoL: Quality of life; IIEF-5: International index of erectile function 5 questionnaire; SPCG-4: Scandinavian prostate cancer group study 4.

Competing interest
None of the authors have any competing interest to declare.

Authors' contributions
AV, JH and SC conceived the study concept and design. The data acquisition was performed by JH and SC. AV supervised the statistical methods and analyses. AB and DS carried out the statistical analyses and plotted the figures. SC and AV drafted the manuscript. SC, JH and AV obtained funding. AK, VH, SB, PL, GA and JH performed the radical prostatectomies in the study. All authors interpreted the data and critically revised the manuscript for important intellectual content. All authors read and approved the final manuscript.

Acknowledgements
We thank study nurse Maria Nyberg for extensive medical charts review. We sincerely thank Joyce Tsoi for her assistance with editing this manuscript. S.C. is supported by funding from the Swedish Society for Medical Research, the Swedish Cancer Society, the Sweden America Foundation and the Swedish Council for Working Life and Social Research. Further support was received from NIH grant P50-CA92629, the Sidney Kimmel Center for Prostate and Urologic Cancers; David H. Koch through the Prostate Cancer Foundation.

Author details
[1]Urology Service at the Department of Surgery, Memorial Sloan-Kettering Cancer Center, 307 E. 63rd St, 2nd floor, New York, NY 10065, USA. [2]Department of Urology, Sahlgrenska Academy at the University of Göteborg, Göteborg, Sweden. [3]Department of Surgical Sciences, Uppsala University, Uppsala University Hospital, Uppsala, Sweden. [4]Department of Epidemiology and Biostatistics, Memorial Sloan-Kettering Cancer Center, New York, USA. [5]Department of Urology, Carlanderska hospital, Göteborg, Sweden.

References
1. Cooperberg MR, Broering JM, Carroll PR: Time trends and local variation in primary treatment of localized prostate cancer. *J Clin Oncol* 2010, 28(7):1117–1123.
2. Bill-Axelson A, Holmberg L, Ruutu M, Garmo H, Stark JR, Busch C, Nordling S, Häggman M, Andersson SO, Bratell S, Spångberg A, Palmgren J, Steineck

G, Adami HO, Johansson JE: SPCG-4 Investigators: radical prostatectomy versus watchful waiting in early prostate cancer. *New Engl J Med* 2011, **364**(18):1708–1717.

3. Johansson E, Steineck G, Holmberg L, Johansson JE, Nyberg T, Ruutu M, Bill-Axelson A, SPCG-4 Investigators: Long-term quality-of-life outcomes after radical prostatectomy or watchful waiting: the Scandinavian Prostate Cancer Group-4 randomised trial. *Lancet Oncol* 2011, **12**(9):891–899.

4. Sanda MG, Dunn RL, Michalski J, Sandler HM, Northouse L, Hembroff L, Lin X, Greenfield TK, Litwin MS, Saigal CS, Mahadevan A, Klein E, Kibel A, Pisters LL, Kuban D, Kaplan I, Wood D, Ciezki J, Shah N, Wei JT: Quality of life and satisfaction with outcome among prostate-cancer survivors. *New Engl J Med* 2008, **358**(12):1250–1261.

5. Bianco FJ Jr, Vickers AJ, Cronin AM, Klein EA, Eastham JA, Pontes JE, Scardino PT: Variations among experienced surgeons in cancer control after open radical prostatectomy. *J Urol* 2010, **183**(3):977–982.

6. Vickers A, Savage C, Bianco F, Mulhall J, Sandhu J, Guillonneau B, Cronin A, Scardino P: Cancer control and functional outcomes after radical prostatectomy as markers of surgical quality: analysis of heterogeneity between surgeons at a single cancer center. *Eur Urol* 2011, **59**(3):317–322.

7. Begg CB, Riedel ER, Bach PB, Kattan MW, Schrag D, Warren JL, Scardino PT: Variations in morbidity after radical prostatectomy. *New Engl J Med* 2002, **346**(15):1138–1144.

8. Thorsteinsdottir T, Stranne J, Carlsson S, Anderberg B, Bjorholt I, Damber JE, Hugosson J, Wilderäng U, Wiklund P, Steineck G, Haglind E: LAPPRO: a prospective multicentre comparative study of robot-assisted laparoscopic and retropubic radical prostatectomy for prostate cancer. *Scand J Urol Nephrol* 2011, **45**(2):102–112.

9. Wallerstedt A, Carlsson S, Nilsson AE, Johansson E, Nyberg T, Steineck G, Wiklund NP: Pad use and patient reported bother from urinary leakage after radical prostatectomy. *J Urol* 2012, **187**(1):196–200.

10. Rosen RC, Cappelleri JC, Smith MD, Lipsky J, Pena BM: Development and evaluation of an abridged, 5-item version of the International Index of Erectile Function (IIEF-5) as a diagnostic tool for erectile dysfunction. *Int J Impot Res* 1999, **11**(6):319–326.

11. Talcott JA, Rieker P, Propert KJ, Clark JA, Wishnow KI, Loughlin KR, Richie JP, Kantoff PW: Patient-reported impotence and incontinence after nerve-sparing radical prostatectomy. *J Natl Cancer Inst* 1997, **89**(15):1117–1123.

12. Steineck G, Helgesen F, Adolfsson J, Dickman PW, Johansson JE, Norlén BJ, Holmberg L, Scandinavian Prostatic Cancer Group Study Number 4: Quality of life after radical prostatectomy or watchful waiting. *New Engl J Med* 2002, **347**(11):790–796.

13. Madalinska JB, Essink-Bot ML, de Koning HJ, Kirkels WJ, van der Maas PJ, Schröder FH: Health-related quality-of-life effects of radical prostatectomy and primary radiotherapy for screen-detected or clinically diagnosed localized prostate cancer. *J Clin Oncol* 2001, **19**(6):1619–1628.

14. Potosky AL, Legler J, Albertsen PC, Stanford JL, Gilliland FD, Hamilton AS, Eley JW, Stephenson RA, Harlan LC: Health outcomes after prostatectomy or radiotherapy for prostate cancer: results from the prostate cancer outcomes study. *JNCI* 2000, **92**(19):1582–1592.

15. Stanford JL, Feng Z, Hamilton AS, Gilliland FD, Stephenson RA, Eley JW, Albertsen PC, Harlan LC, Potosky AL: Urinary and sexual function after radical prostatectomy for clinically localized prostate cancer: the prostate cancer outcomes study. *JAMA* 2000, **283**(3):354–360.

16. Heijnsdijk EA, Wever EM, Auvinen A, Hugosson J, Ciatto S, Nelen V, Kwiatkowski M, Villers A, Páez A, Moss SM, Zappa M, Tammela TL, Mäkinen T, Carlsson S, Korfage IJ, Essink-Bot ML, Otto SJ, Draisma G, Bangma CH, Roobol MJ, Schröder FH, de Koning HJ: Quality-of-life effects of prostate-specific antigen screening. *New Engl J Med* 2012, **367**(7):595–605.

17. Vickers AJ, Sjoberg D, Basch E, Sculli F, Shouery M, Laudone V, Touijer K, Eastham J, Scardino PT: How do you know if you are any good? A surgeon performance feedback system for the outcomes of radical prostatectomy. *Eur Urol* 2012, **61**(2):284–289.

18. Vickers AJ, Bianco FJ, Gonen M, Cronin AM, Eastham JA, Schrag D, Klein EA, Reuther AM, Kattan MW, Pontes JE, Scardino PT: Effects of pathologic stage on the learning curve for radical prostatectomy: evidence that recurrence in organ-confined cancer is largely related to inadequate surgical technique. *Eur Urol* 2008, **53**(5):960–966.

12

Long-term experience of hyperbaric oxygen therapy for refractory radio- or chemotherapy-induced haemorrhagic cystitis

Stephan Degener[1]*, Alexander Pohle[2], Hartmut Strelow[3], Michael J Mathers[4], Jürgen Zumbé[2], Stephan Roth[1] and Alexander S Brandt[1]

Abstract

Background: Radiotherapy and cyclophosphamide-induced haemorrhagic cystitis are rare but severe complications occurring in 3–6% of patients. Hyperbaric oxygen treatment (HBOT) has been demonstrated to be an effective treatment for haematuria not responding to conventional management. Only very few data exist for long-term follow-up after HBOT.

Methods: We retrospectively reviewed 15 patients referred for HBOT for haemorrhagic cystitis (HC). HBOT was performed for 130 min/day at a pressure of 2.4 atmospheres. We evaluated patient demographics, type of radio- and chemotherapy and characteristics of haematuria. The effect of HBOT was defined as complete or partial resolution of hematuria according to the RTOG/EORTC grade and Gray score.

Results: A total of 15 patients (12 after radiotherapy, two after chemotherapy and one patient with a combination of both) were treated with a median of 34 HBO treatments. Radiotherapy patients received primary, adjuvant, salvage and HDR radiotherapy (60 – 78 Gy) for prostate, colon or cervical cancer. The patient with combination therapy and both of the chemotherapy patients were treated with cyclophosphamide. First episodes of haematuria occurred at a median of 48 months after completion of initial therapy. The first HBOT was performed at a median of 11 months after the first episode of hematuria. After a median of a 68-month follow-up after HBOT, 80% experienced a complete resolution and two patients suffered a singular new minor haematuria (p < 0.00001). A salvage-cystectomy was necessary in one patient. No adverse effects were documented.

Conclusions: Our experience indicate that HBOT is a safe and effective therapeutic option for treatment-resistant radiogenic and chemotherapy-induced haemorrhagic cystitis. For a better evaluation prospective clinical trials are required.

Keywords: Haemorrhagic cystitis, Radiotherapy, Cyclophosphamide, Hyperbaric oxygenation

Background

Radiotherapy-induced haemorrhagic cystitis (RHC) after pelvic radiation therapy is a rare but known long-term complication which develops in 3–6.5% of patients. RHC can occur from 6 months to 20 years after radiation therapy [1-3]. Chemotherapy-induced haemorrhagic cystitis (CHC) can also cause chemotherapy-limiting haematuria (cyclophosphamide or others oxazaphosphorines) [4-7]. Since the introduction of Mesna (2-mercaptoethanesulfonic acid), a thiol compound, for uroprotection the incidence of CHC has decreased to less than 5% [5]. Despite the underlying cause, HC is a relevant impairment of the patients' quality of life with often multiple and mostly emergency admissions to hospitals.

As for other severe haematurias, bladder irrigation is the primary treatment for HC. Different systemic or intravesical agents such as hyaluronic acid, aminocaproic acid, formalin or prostaglandins have been used, however with limited success [8]. As a consequence, bladder fulguration is repeatedly used as a therapeutic option to

---
* Correspondence: stephan.degener@helios-kliniken.de
[1]Department of Urology, HELIOS Medical Center Wuppertal, University of Witten/Herdecke, Heusnerstrasse 40, 42283 Wuppertal, Germany
Full list of author information is available at the end of the article

stop bleeding and blood is transfused when indicated. In the most severe cases selective embolization of the hypogastric arteries or salvage cystectomy with urinary diversion may be necessary [9].

Hyperbaric oxygen therapy (HBOT) is a promising but still extreme rarely-used therapeutic option for patients in whom the standard management has failed. By increasing the tissue oxygen level by up to 15-fold, HBOT promotes capillary angiogenesis which also increases the regeneration of damaged urothelium. Studies report success rates of 73 to 96% [1,3,10-13]. We present here our results of HBOT for the treatment of RHC and CHC.

Methods

We retrospectively reviewed all 23 patients treated with HBOT for haemorrhagic cystitis between 01/2002 and 10/2014 in two urological departments. In 15 patients a complete follow-up was achievable. Patient demographics were recorded, as was for RHC the total radiation dosage and the type of radiation therapy. Follow-up was ensured by outpatient contacts in the clinic and by cooperating ambulatories. Each patient gave informed consent and the study was approved by the institutional review committee of Witten/Herdecke University.

Evaluation of hematuria

Initially, all patients underwent permanent bladder irrigation and evacuation of blood clots. Urine cultures were set up before irrigation to detect infectious haematuria. When urine cleared after bladder irrigation patients underwent a cystoscopy or, in cases of heavy bleeding, a transurethral resection / fulguration to rule out an urothelial carcinoma (including carcinoma in situ). Additionally, the upper urinary tract was evaluated to exclude it as a source of bleeding.

The onset of the first relevant haematuria and the maximum severity of all haematuria episodes were evaluated. The grading of haematuria was determined from the RTOG/EORTC grade for RHC, and the Gray score for CHC [14,15] (Table 1). The difference in haematuria grade before and after treatment was analyzed by using a paired t-test. Statistical significance was selected as a value of $p < 0.05$.

Hyperbaric oxygen therapy

Hyperbaric oxygen therapy was initiated when conventional therapy options remained unsuccessful and when no contraindication for HBOT was given (assessment with otoscopy, spirometry and ECG). We evaluated the time between the first haemorrhagic episode and the beginning of HBOT, the number of HBOTs and all HBOT-related data (Table 2).

All patients were treated in the same HBOT centre where HBOT was performed in a treatment chamber with a capacity of up to 12 patients (Haux Starmed, HAUX-LIFE-SUPPORT GmbH, Karlsbad-Ittersbach, Germany) (Figure 1) under continued monitoring. The therapy scheme TS240-90 [16] is composed of 3x30 minute periods of pure oxygen (at a pressure of 2.4 atmospheres). The episodes of pure oxygen were interrupted by 10 minutes with normal air (21% (v/v) oxygen) to reduce oxygen toxicity (Figure 2). The increase of the partial pressure of oxygen (pO_2) was measured percutaneously. HBOT was performed five days a week. After each HBOT session the grade of haematuria was evaluated and patients were checked for barotraumas.

The effect of HBOT was defined as complete (no further macro-haematuria until completion of follow-up) or partial resolution of haematuria (defined as a lower RTOG/EORTC or Gray score than before HBOT).

Results

In 15 patients (12 males, 3 females) undergoing HBOT for therapy-resistant haemorrhagic cystitis between 2002 and 2014 a complete retrospective follow-up was achieved. Additionally, two patients suffered from haemorrhagic proctitis. At the beginning of HBOT the age ranged from 22 to 86 years (mean age 71). At the end of follow-up the age ranged from 33 to 90 years (mean age 76 y).

Radiotherapy was performed owing to prostate (10 patients, 67%), colon or cervical cancer (1 patient each, 7%). One patient underwent combined radio-chemotherapy owing to retroperitoneal synovial sarcoma (with Ifosfamide,

Table 1 Classification scores for radiotherapy and chemotherapy induced haemorrhagic cystitis: RTOG/ EORTC and Gray scores (modified from [14] and [15])

Classification scores for chronic radio- and chemotherapy induced haemorrhagic cystitis					
Radiotherapy	RTOG/ EORTC scale	Grade 1	Grade 2	Grade 3	Grade 4
		Microscopic haematuria, requiring no medication; Minor telangiectasia	Moderate haematuria requiring medication; Moderate telangiectasia	Severe haematuria; Severe telangiectasia	Necrosis; Severe haemorrhagic cystitis
Chemotherapy	Gray score	Grade 0	Grade 1	Grade 2	Grade 3
		Normal, no haematuria	Mild haematuria with telangiectasia or dilatation of the bladder vessels	Severe haematuria with mucosal haematomas	Severe haematuria with intravesical clots

Table 2 Clinical characteristics of patients and details of CHC and RHC and HBO treatment

Sex	Age/ Therapy	Age/ End of Follow-up	Diagnosis	Treatment	HBO Indication Indikation	End of Therapy	Time till Haematuria [m]	RTOG/ Gray before HBOT	Admissions to Hospital	Number blood transfusions	Duration till HBO [m]	HBO Treatments	Follow Up [m]	Events/ Follow-up	RTOG/ Gray after HBO
M	68	70	PCA	adj	RC	08/2008	34	3	5	0	4	40	33	no relapse	0
M	82	86	PCA	prim	RC	07/2004	54	3	3	0	15	24	53	no relapse	0
M	73	81	PCA	HDR	RC	08/2002	11	4	4	2	33	24	100	1x haematuria 2007	3
W	71	83	CCA	adj	RC	07/1997	30	3	3	0	28	128	142	no relapse	0
M	80	86	PCA	prim	RC	07/1998	5	4	2	2	110	40	78	no relapse	0
M	71	76	PCA	adj	RC	01/1999	76	4	2	1	36	35	28	no relapse, †2010	0
W	86	90	UCA	adj	RC	01/1990	234	4	3	2	0	6	29	no relapse, †2012	0
M	80	83	PCA	adj	RC	01/2000	124	4	3	3	1	51	16	SRC 2010, †2012	4
M	65	72	PCA	adj	RC	03/2000	50	4	3	1	30	26	94	no relapse	0
M	61	63	PCA	sal	RC	02/2010	20	4	3	4	7	20	133	no relapse	0
M	22	33	RPSS	comb	RC/CC	01/1999	43	4	2	12	11	34	28	no relapse	0
M	73	78	PCA	sal	RC/RP	07/2007	14	3	2	2	1	48	68	no relapse	0
M	65	71	PCA	adj	RC/RP	07/2003	48	4	3	2	3	20	49	no relapse, †2011	0
W	49	56	LE	prim	CC	01/1974	362	3	4	0	40	40	86	1x haematuria 2008	3
M	39	49	WG	prim	CC	01/1993	120	4	3	1	4	17	136	no relapse	0

†=deceased.

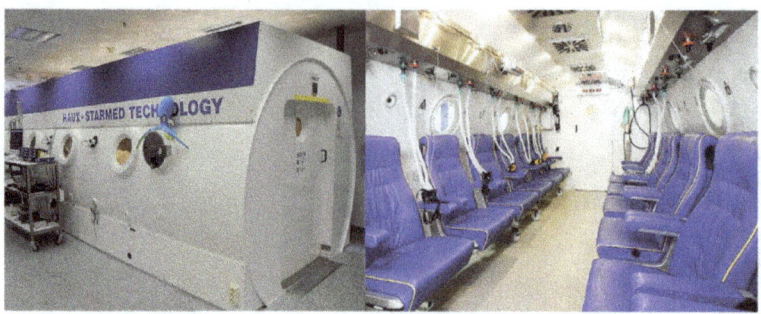

Figure 1 Exterior and interior view on the pressure chamber for max. 12 persons.

ISF) and two patients (13%) were treated with cyclophosphamide for Wegener's granulomatosis or Lupus erythematosus.

In 7 patients (47%) radiotherapy was performed as an adjuvant because of prostate, colon or cervical cancer (60–64 Gy). Primary and salvage radiation was applied to two patients (13%) for prostate cancer (66 and 70 Gy) and one patient (7%) was treated with HDR brachytherapy (78 Gy) for prostate cancer. The radiation dose of the patient with retroperitoneal synovial sarcoma was 66 Gy.

The first episodes of haematuria occurred between 5 and 362 months (median 48 months) after the beginning of radiation or chemotherapy. A median of three (2 – 5) admissions to the hospital and up to seven outpatient treatments were necessary. According to the RTOG/EORTC score haemorrhagic complication Grade 4 occurred in nine patients (60%) and Grade 3 in four (27%). Patients with CHC had haemorrhagic complication Grade 3 or 4 respectively (Gray score). Blood transfusions (between 1 and 12 units) were necessary in 11 patients (73%).

In all patients urothelial malignancy was excluded by histology. At least one bladder fulguration was performed in every case in order to stop the bleeding but no patient received any intravesical instillation therapy.

When HC was resistant to conventional therapy (without instillation therapy) HBOT was initiated, in a median of eleven months (0 – 110) after the first episode of haematuria. Between 6 and 128 HBOT sessions (mean 34) were necessary to achieve a total resolution of haematuria. In all

HBOT sessions the partial pressure of oxygen measured percutaneously was increased to 1250–1480 mmHg.

Follow-up ranged from 16 to 142 months (mean 68). In 12 patients (80%) a total resolution of the HC could be achieved without any further haematuria. In two patients (13%) bladder irrigation had to be re-performed once for a singular recurrence of haematuria (RTOG/EORTC Grade 3). Changes in RTOG/EORTC scores were statistically significant (p < 0.00001).

In one case a salvage cystectomy with urinary diversion (ileum conduit) was necessary owing to a fulminant bleeding episode. The overall success rate was 93%. The radiogenic proctitis completely recovered in both cases. No side effects were noted in any patient.

Discussion

Radiation and cyclophosphamide-induced HC is a severe and potentially life threatening complication. Management can be highly challenging with well-known urological treatment options. It is to be expected that the number of radiation therapies will increase during the next decades [17]. In parallel a rise in complications and side effects, such as RHC, can be expected. The results of this study suggest that HBOT is a promising option in therapy-resistant HC with a success rate of more than 90%.

In both CHC and RHC the acute reaction on urothelial damage is an inflammatory response causing oedema, ulceration, neovascularisation and haemorrhagic necrosis. This is usually limited to the treatment period.

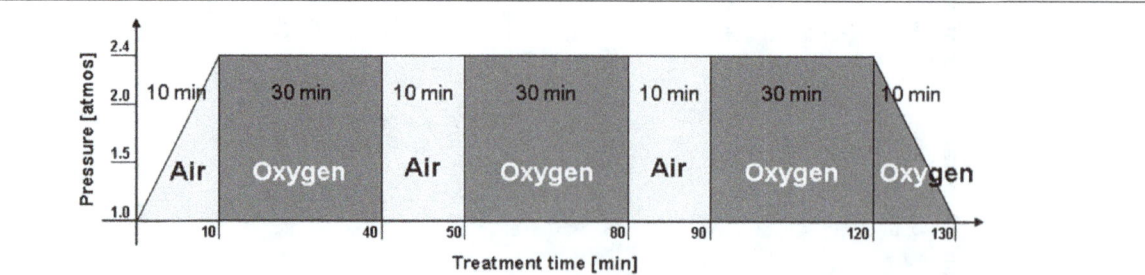

Figure 2 Diagram of the therapy scheme TS 240–90. "Air" is defined as normal ambient air with 21% (v/v) oxygen. "Oxygen" is defined as the application of 100% (v/v) oxygen. The pressure [atmosphere] is plotted on the y-axis, the treatment time [min] on the x-axis (adopted from [24]).

In CHC urotoxicity is caused directly by the renal excretion of acrolein, metabolites of oxazaphosphorine alkylated drugs. There is no clear dose-related relationship. Since the 1970s the prophylactic application of Mesna has been used as a standard protocol for prevention of haemorrhagic complications. It neutralises acrolein and its toxic effects to the urothelium. The incidence of CHC is reduced from about 68% to about 5% [5].

In RHC urothelial damage is caused by radiolysis of water. The concentration of activated free oxygen radicals increases; as these are highly reactive, they cause cell membrane injury by lipid peroxidation, which induces immediate cell death. Additionally, direct (by radiation energy) and indirect (by oxygen radicals) DNA damage causes replication failures resulting in delayed cell death [8]. This damage is dose-related.

This acute reaction can escalate into a chronic endarteritis which seems to be the determining pathology of late-onset RHC and has been described as the "three-H model": the progressive endarteritis and vascular rarefaction (**hypovascular**) results in critical ischaemia (**hypoxia**) with a reduction in oxygen concentration of up to 70-80%. Ischaemia of the mucosal tissue can lead to necrosis and sloughed off cells because of impaired healing capacity. A compensatory teleangiectasia develops and causes (persistent) haematuria. Finally, fibrotic repair processes can lead to impaired bladder capacity (**hypocellular**) [3,11]. This process can still become relevant up to 20 years after radiation therapy [2]. In our study haematuria occurred in a median of 41 months after completion of radiation therapy. This is within the range of previously described periods of 35–48 months [1,2,8,10].

Tissue oxygen supply occurs primarily via diffusion from the capillaries by significantly increasing the physically dissolved oxygen in the plasma (100% O_2 pressure of 1.4 atmosphere). HBOT improves the local and regional tissue oxygen supply. Our results demonstrate a drastically increased pO_2 in the tissue from 1250 to 1480 mmHg from percutaneous measurements. By increasing pO_2, macrophages, fibroblasts and granulocytes may resume their normal function and mediate repair processes. In addition, HBOT directly induces neo-angiogenesis, whereby 80% of the normal capillary density can be achieved. Furthermore HBOT causes anti-oedematous vasoconstriction without secondary ischaemic hypoxia [18-20].

Hyperbaric oxygen in patients with severe RHC or CHC not responding to conventional urological treatment is an extremely rare and not yet standardised treatment option.

In RHC different research groups and we have reported success rates between 75 and 96% in both prospective and retrospective study designs [10,13,19,21-23]. In contrast to our study, other cohorts have varied between 13–60 patients with only short follow-up periods of 12–30 months.

We could demonstrate a success rate of 90% even after a median long-term follow-up period of 68 months, confirming the excellent long-term results reported by Nakada et al. whose success rate was 75-88% [12].

Only a few cases patients with CHC have been reported. One of the larger series with six CHC patients reported a 100% success rate after 11 to 36 months of follow-up (although they noted that in one patient haematuria recurred after three months) [24]. In other reported case reports a complete loss of haematuria occurred after a follow-up period of 11–36 months [7,24-26].

The main advantage of this therapy is that there are no severe side-effects. The most common adverse effects of HBOT are middle ear or sinus barotraumas requiring myringotomy in up to 5% [27]. Reversible myopia has also been described as a dose-dependent HBOT side effect [27]. Our study, as many other reports, did not show any adverse effects of HBTO.

So far variable success of HBOT has been discussed without any clear results, mainly because of the small sample size in most series.

In RHC the total radiation dose seems to have an influence on HBOT success: generally, complications such as RHC begin at a total dosage of 45–55 Gy and increase significantly at a cumulative dose of ≥60 Gy (≥5% with late effects) [28]. Nakada et al. showed a significantly better HBOT success in patients exposed to lower radiation doses (62Gy vs. 76Gy, p < 0.001). In addition del Pizzo et al. reported relatively poor HBOT long-term success rates (27% after 5 years) in patients with high dosage radiotherapy (75Gy) [29]. In the present study most of the patients received a cumulative dose between 60 – 66Gy. One patient with high dose therapy (78 Gy) suffered one unique relapse of haematuria.

Some authors discuss that there might be an influence of the number of HBOT sessions on the therapeutic success in RHC. Most of the studies applied between 30 and 40 treatment sessions [13,19,21,29] which is comparable to our data with a median of 34 treatments. The significantly higher number of HBOTs (62) may be the reason for the excellent long-term success in Nakada's study compared with a study with a success rate of 64% after only 14 HBOTs [30]. The few existing data suggest that fewer HBOTs are sufficient in CHC patients. The reported series of six CHC cases required a median of 27 HBOTs, other published cases between 14 and 40 treatments [7,24-26].

The period of time between the onset of haematuria and the beginning of HBOT is discussed as another success factor for RHC. In some studies, patients with a shorter pre-treatment interval (6–8 months) showed significantly better results on HBOT (p <0.001) [12,13]. We could not demonstrate any relationship between the time to beginning of HBOT and its success. This is most probably because, as CHC is the more acute event, HBOT was started at a mean of 47 days after the onset of symptoms. However, intervals of up to four months between first admission and the beginning of HBOT have been described [24].

Finally the influence of patient age is controversially discussed. Some studies suggest that younger patients (≤70 years) have higher success rates. Other studies, as well as ours, have not found any correlation between age and HBOT success. Furthermore, in CHC patients a complete remission of haematuria is reported in cases aged from 15 to 82 years [1,12,13,24-26].

The costs amount to approximately €200 per HBOT session. Accordingly, the median costs per patient in this study were €6,800 (34 HBOT sessions). The costs are comparable to a cost-analysis case study from Australia which showed HBOT to provide major health cost savings [31].

Our study, as many others, is certainly limited by the small study population and the retrospective design. Furthermore different treatment protocols reduce the comparability of treatment outcomes. Prospective trials would be desirable for further evaluation but the first planned prospective and randomized study (initiated by the Baromedical Research Foundation) was cancelled because of poor recruitment (NCT00134628). Nevertheless, we believe that our results show the long-term efficiency and safety of this therapy option in patients suffering from radiation- and cyclophosphamide-induced haemorrhagic cystitis.

Conclusions

Our data suggest that hyperbaric oxygen therapy is a safe and simple therapy option with a long-term success rate of approximately 90% with hardly any side-effects. Therefore HBOT should be considered more often in cases of severe haemorrhagic cystitis induced by radiation and/or cyclophosphamide.

Abbreviations

HC: Hemorrhagic Cystitis; HBOT: Hyperbaric Oxygen Treatment; RHC: Radiotherapy-induced Hemorrhagic Cystitis; CHC: Chemotherapy-induced Hemorrhagic Cystitis; RTOG: Radio Therapy Oncology Group; EORTC: European Organisation for Research and Treatment of Cancer; ECG: Electrocardiography; PCA: Prostate Cancer; CCA: Colon Cancer; UCA: Uterine / Cervical Cancer; RPSS: Retroperitoneal Synovial Sarcoma; LE: Lupus Erythematosus; WG: Wegener's Granulomatosis; Adj: Adjuvant Radiation; Prim: Primary Radiotherapy; HDR: High-Dose Rate; Sal: Salvage Radiotherapy; Comb: Combined Chemoradiation; RC: Radiotherapy-induced Cystitis; RP: Radiotherapy-induced Proctitis; CC: Chemotherapy – induced Cystitis; SRC: Salvage Cystectomy.

Competing interests

The authors declare that they have no competing interests.

Authors' contributions

S.D. and A.S.B. have made conception, design and analysis of data. S.D., A.P., H.S. and M.J.M. have made acquisition of data. J.Z. and S.R. reviewed the manuscript critically. All authors approved the final version of the manuscript.

Author details

[1]Department of Urology, HELIOS Medical Center Wuppertal, University of Witten/Herdecke, Heusnerstrasse 40, 42283 Wuppertal, Germany. [2]Department of Urology, Medical Center Leverkusen, Am Gesundheitspark 11, 51375 Leverkusen, Germany. [3]Institute of Hyperbaric Oxygen (HBO), University Hospital Düsseldorf, Moorenstrasse 5, 40225 Düsseldorf, Germany. [4]Urological Ambulatory PandaMED, Alleestrasse 105-107, 42853 Remscheid, Germany.

References

1. Corman JM, McClure D, Pritchett R, Kozlowski P, Hampson NB. Treatment of radiation induced hemorrhagic cystitis with hyperbaric oxygen. J Urol. 2003;169(6):2200–2.
2. Levenback C, Eifel PJ, Burke TW, Morris M, Gershenson DM. Hemorrhagic cystitis following radiotherapy for stage Ib cancer of the cervix. Gynecol Oncol. 1994;55(2):206–10.
3. Mendenhall WM, Henderson RH, Costa JA, Hoppe BS, Dagan R, Bryant CM, Nichols RC, Williams CR, Harris SE, Mendenhall NP: Hemorrhagic Radiation Cystitis. American journal of clinical oncology 2013. [Epub ahead of print].
4. Lima MV, Ferreira FV, Macedo FY, De Castro Brito GA, Ribeiro RA. Histological changes in bladders of patients submitted to ifosfamide chemotherapy even with mesna prophylaxis. Cancer Chemother Pharmacol. 2007;59(5):643–50.
5. Korkmaz A, Oter S, Deveci S, Goksoy C, Bilgic H. Prevention of further cyclophosphamide induced hemorrhagic cystitis by hyperbaric oxygen and mesna in guinea pigs. J Urol. 2001;166(3):1119–23.
6. Kalayoglu-Besisik S, Abdul-Rahman IS, Erer B, Yenerel MN, Oguz FS, Tunc M, et al. Outcome after hyperbaric oxygen treatment for cyclophosphamide-induced refractory hemorrhagic cystitis. J Urol. 2003;170(3):922.
7. Hughes MJ, Davis FM, Mark SD, Spearing RL. Hyperbaric oxygen for cyclophosphamide-induced cystitis. Br J Haematol. 2002;119(2):575.
8. Smit SG, Heyns CF. Management of radiation cystitis. Nat Rev Urol. 2010;7(4):206–14.
9. Linder BJ, Tarrell RF, Boorjian SA. Cystectomy for refractory hemorrhagic cystitis: contemporary etiology, presentation and outcomes. J Urol. 2014;192(6):1687–92.
10. Bevers RF, Bakker DJ, Kurth KH. Hyperbaric oxygen treatment for haemorrhagic radiation cystitis. Lancet. 1995;346(8978):803–5.
11. Crew JP, Jephcott CR, Reynard JM. Radiation-induced haemorrhagic cystitis. Eur Urol. 2001;40(2):111–23.
12. Nakada T, Nakada H, Yoshida Y, Nakashima Y, Banya Y, Fujihira T, Karasawa K: Hyperbaric Oxygen Therapy for Radiation Cystitis in Patients with Prostate Cancer: A Long-Term Follow-Up Study. Urologia internationalis. 2012;89(2):208–14.
13. Chong KT, Hampson NB, Corman JM. Early hyperbaric oxygen therapy improves outcome for radiation-induced hemorrhagic cystitis. Urology. 2005;65(4):649–53.
14. Peeters ST, Heemsbergen WD, Van Putten WL, Slot A, Tabak H, Mens JW, et al. Acute and late complications after radiotherapy for prostate cancer: results of a multicenter randomized trial comparing 68 Gy to 78 Gy. Int J Radiat Oncol Biol Phys. 2005;61(4):1019–34.
15. Gray KJ, Engelmann UH, Johnson EH, Fishman IJ. Evaluation of misoprostol cytoprotection of the bladder with cyclophosphamide (Cytoxan) therapy. J Urol. 1986;136(2):497–500.
16. Marx RE, Johnson RP. Problem wounds in oral and maxillofacial surgery: The role of hyperbaric oxygen. In: Davis JC, Hunt TK, editors. Problem Wounds: The Role of Oxygen edn. New York: Elsevir Science Publishing; 1988. p. 65–123.
17. Frodin JE, Jonsson E, Moller T, Werko L. Radiotherapy in Sweden–a study of present use in relation to the literature and an estimate of future trends. Acta Oncol. 1996;35(8):967–79.
18. Anderson LH, Wilson B, Herring RF, Mehm WJ. Influence of intermittent hyperoxia on hypoxic fibroblasts. J Hyperbaric Med. 1992;7:103–14.
19. Weiss JP, Mattei DM, Neville EC, Hanno PM. Primary treatment of radiation-induced hemorrhagic cystitis with hyperbaric oxygen: 10-year experience. J Urol. 1994;151(6):1514–7.
20. Muhonen A, Haaparanta M, Gronroos T, Bergman J, Knuuti J, Hinkka S, et al. Osteoblastic activity and neoangiogenesis in distracted bone of irradiated rabbit mandible with or without hyperbaric oxygen treatment. Int J Oral Maxillofac Surg. 2004;33(2):173–8.
21. Oscarsson N, Arnell P, Lodding P, Ricksten SE, Seeman-Lodding H. Hyperbaric oxygen treatment in radiation-induced cystitis and proctitis: a prospective

cohort study on patient-perceived quality of recovery. Int J Radiat Oncol Biol Phys. 2013;87(4):670–5.

22. Degener S, Strelow H, Pohle A, Lazica DA, Windolf J, Zumbe J, et al. Hyperbaric oxygen in the treatment of hemorrhagic radiogenic cystitis after prostate cancer. Der Urologe Ausg A. 2012;51(12):1735–40.

23. Yoshida T, Kawashima A, Ujike T, Uemura M, Nishimura K, Miyoshi S. Hyperbaric oxygen therapy for radiation-induced hemorrhagic cystitis. International journal of urology : official journal of the Japanese Urological Association. 2008;15(7):639–41.

24. Davis M, MacDonald H, Sames C, Nand K. Severe cyclophosphamide-induced haemorrhagic cystitis treated with hyperbaric oxygen. The New Zealand medical journal. 2011;124(1340):48–54.

25. Shameem IA, Shimabukuro T, Shirataki S, Yamamoto N, Maekawa T, Naito K. Hyperbaric oxygen therapy for control of intractable cyclophosphamide-induced hemorrhagic cystitis. Eur Urol. 1992;22(3):263–4.

26. Yazawa H, Nakada T, Sasagawa I, Miura M, Kubota Y. Hyperbaric oxygenation therapy for cyclophosphamide-induced haemorrhagic cystitis. Int Urol Nephrol. 1995;27(4):381–5.

27. Tahir AR, Westhuyzen J, Dass J, Collins MK, Webb R, Hewitt S, et al. Hyperbaric oxygen therapy for chronic radiation-induced tissue injuries: Australasia's largest study. Asia Pac J Clin Oncol. 2015;11(1):68–77.

28. Roswit B, Malsky SJ, Reid CB. Severe radiation injuries of the stomach, small intestine, colon and rectum. Am J Roentgenol Radium Ther Nucl Med. 1972;114(3):460–75.

29. Del Pizzo JJ, Chew BH, Jacobs SC, Sklar GN. Treatment of radiation induced hemorrhagic cystitis with hyperbaric oxygen: long-term followup. J Urol. 1998;160(3 Pt 1):731–3.

30. Mathews R, Rajan N, Josefson L, Camporesi E, Makhuli Z. Hyperbaric oxygen therapy for radiation induced hemorrhagic cystitis. J Urol. 1999;161(2):435–7.

31. Smart D, Wallington M. A cost-analysis case study of radiation cystitis treatment including hyperbaric oxygen therapy. Diving and hyperbaric medicine. 2012;42(2):92–7.

13

The MAPP research network: design, patient characterization and operations

J Richard Landis[1], David A Williams[2], M Scott Lucia[3], Daniel J Clauw[2], Bruce D Naliboff[4], Nancy A Robinson[1], Adrie van Bokhoven[3], Siobhan Sutcliffe[5], Anthony J Schaeffer[6], Larissa V Rodriguez[7], Emeran A Mayer[8], H Henry Lai[9], John N Krieger[10], Karl J Kreder[11], Niloofar Afari[12], Gerald L Andriole[9], Catherine S Bradley[13], James W Griffith[14], David J Klumpp[6], Barry A Hong[15], Susan K Lutgendorf[13], Dedra Buchwald[16], Claire C Yang[10], Sean Mackey[17], Michel A Pontari[18], Philip Hanno[19], John W Kusek[20], Chris Mullins[20], J Quentin Clemens[21]* and The MAPP Research Network Study Group

Abstract

Background: The "Multidisciplinary Approach to the Study of Chronic Pelvic Pain" (MAPP) Research Network was established by the NIDDK to better understand the pathophysiology of urologic chronic pelvic pain syndromes (UCPPS), to inform future clinical trials and improve clinical care. The evolution, organization, and scientific scope of the MAPP Research Network, and the unique approach of the network's central study and common data elements are described.

Methods: The primary scientific protocol for the Trans-MAPP Epidemiology/Phenotyping (EP) Study comprises a multi-site, longitudinal observational study, including bi-weekly internet-based symptom assessments, following a comprehensive in-clinic deep-phenotyping array of urological symptoms, non-urological symptoms and psychosocial factors to evaluate men and women with UCPPS. Healthy controls, matched on sex and age, as well as "positive" controls meeting the non-urologic associated syndromes (NUAS) criteria for one or more of the target conditions of Fibromyalgia (FM), Chronic Fatigue Syndrome (CFS) or Irritable Bowel Syndrome (IBS), were also evaluated. Additional, complementary studies addressing diverse hypotheses are integrated into the Trans-MAPP EP Study to provide a systemic characterization of study participants, including biomarker discovery studies of infectious agents, quantitative sensory testing, and structural and resting state neuroimaging and functional neurobiology studies. A highly novel effort to develop and assess clinically relevant animal models of UCPPS was also undertaken to allow improved translation between clinical and mechanistic studies. Recruitment into the central study occurred at six Discovery Sites in the United States, resulting in a total of 1,039 enrolled participants, exceeding the original targets. The biospecimen collection rate at baseline visits reached nearly 100%, and 279 participants underwent common neuroimaging through a standardized protocol. An extended follow-up study for 161 of the UCPPS participants is ongoing.

Discussion: The MAPP Research Network represents a novel, comprehensive approach to the study of UCPPS, as well as other concomitant NUAS. Findings are expected to provide significant advances in understanding UCPPS pathophysiology that will ultimately inform future clinical trials and lead to improvements in patient care. Furthermore, the structure and methodologies developed by the MAPP Network provide the foundation upon which future studies of other urologic or non-urologic disorders can be based.

(Continued on next page)

* Correspondence: qclemens@med.umich.edu
[21]Department of Urology, Division of Neurourology and Pelvic Reconstructive Surgery, University of Michigan, Ann Arbor, MI, USA
Full list of author information is available at the end of the article

(Continued from previous page)

Keywords: Urologic chronic pelvic pain syndromes, Interstitial cystitis, Chronic prostatitis, Urine biomarkers, Plasma biomarkers, Non-urologic associated syndromes, Quantitative sensory testing (QST), Neuroimaging

Background

Interstitial cystitis/bladder pain syndrome (IC/BPS) and chronic prostatitis/chronic pelvic pain syndrome (CP/CPPS) are defined by the hallmark symptom of chronic pain in the region of the pelvis, urogenital floor, or external genitalia, often accompanied by urinary symptoms, such as urinary urgency or frequency [1,2]. The bladder has historically been thought to be the origin of IC/BPS symptoms; whereas the prostate gland has traditionally been believed to be the source of CP/CPPS symptoms. However, this viewpoint has come under recent challenge, in large part from the observation that many IC/BPS and CP/CPPS patients exhibiting symptoms do not have identifiable pathology in these organs [3-5].

The impact and burden of IC/BPS and CP/CPPS are substantial. Patients suffer considerable morbidity resulting in a significant decrease in quality of life for both the patient and his/her partner due to the physical and psychological impact of the condition. In fact, the quality of life of IC patients has been characterized as being worse than that of patients undergoing dialysis [6]. In the U.S., the prevalence of IC/BPS symptoms has been estimated to be 2.7% in women [7]; whereas the prevalence for analogous symptoms is estimated to be 1.3% in men [8]. Prevalence estimates for CP/CPPS in men vary between 1.8 – 6.4%, depending upon case definitions and screening methods [9,10].

Traditionally, the diagnosis of IC required cystoscopy and pathological findings, although more typically IC/BPS is defined from patient reported symptoms, due to the lack of consistent pathological findings, defined disease phenotypes or biological markers. Similarly, patient symptoms are used to define CP/CPPS. Each of these separate syndromes, however, may in fact represent a group of related conditions that manifest in a similar manner, but have differing etiologies. Based primarily on their somewhat similar symptom profiles [2], IC/BPS and CP/CPPS are here collectively termed urologic chronic pelvic pain syndromes (UCPPS) (see Table 1 for research definitions used in the MAPP Research Network). As noted in the only published phenotyping system, referred to as UPOINT [11,12], UCPPS patients have significant symptoms across the urinary, psychosocial, organ specific, infection, neurological/systemic and tenderness domains, confirming the heterogenous nature of these syndromes.

Despite intensive study over the past decade, clinical trials have failed to identify effective therapies, and basic science studies have failed to identify specific pathophysiology for these conditions (for a review of previous research efforts see companion Commentary by Clemens, et al) [13]. Intriguing new clues into the pathophysiology of UCPPS have come from several epidemiological studies revealing shared pathophysiology between UCPPS and other conditions having chronic pain as a cardinal or prominent symptom (e.g., fibromyalgia, irritable bowel syndrome, endometriosis, chronic fatigue syndrome, and vulvodynia) [14-20]. Some of these chronic pain conditions were previously thought to be due to "peripheral" etiologies (i.e., damage or inflammation in the region of the body where the individual was experiencing pain) but are now known to have prominent central nervous system (CNS) contributions (i.e. centralized pain). In light of this new understanding, even the names of some of these

Table 1 Terminology used in the MAPP Research Network to described disorders under study

Term	MAPP Network Research Definition
Urologic chronic pelvic pain syndrome (UCPPS)	General term to describe idiopathic chronic pelvic pain of urologic origin in men or women. In MAPP Network studies, this includes men and women with IC/BPS, or men with CP/CPPS (see below).
Interstitial cystitis/bladder pain syndrome (IC/BPS)	Chronic unpleasant sensation (pain, pressure, discomfort) perceived to be related to the urinary bladder, associated with lower urinary tract symptoms, in the absence of infection or other identifiable causes.
Chronic prostatitis/chronic pelvic pain syndrome (CP/CPPS)	Chronic idiopathic pelvic pain or discomfort in males, commonly in the perineum, suprapubic region, penis, or testicles, which is often exacerbated by ejaculation or urination.
Non-Urologic Associated Syndromes (NUAS)	General term used to describe symptom-based non-urologic syndromes which co-occur with UCPPS at a rate greater than observed in the general population. Within the MAPP Network, initial efforts have focused on studying specific NUAS (fibromyalgia, irritable bowel syndrome, chronic fatigue syndrome), though other examples exist (e.g. vulvodynia, temporomandibular joint disorder, and migraine headaches, among others).

conditions have changed, reflecting the fact that peripheral inflammation is not the primary cause of symptoms (e.g., fibrositis became fibromyalgia, spastic colitis became irritable bowel syndrome). In a similar manner, it has been suggested that IC be renamed Bladder Pain Syndrome (BPS), based on the fact that the majority of patients do not have identifiable inflammation or even pathology in the bladder [21]. Collectively, these findings suggest the merits of exploring common underlying CNS pathophysiology (i.e., pain centralization or augmentation) [22-24] rather than continuing the search for a uniform malfunction of a single end organ [23].

In recognition of these emerging insights and the limitations of previous basic research and clinical studies, the NIDDK established the "Multidisciplinary Approach to the Study of Chronic Pelvic Pain" (MAPP) Research Network to better understand the etiology and treated natural history of UCPPS. This network holds the promise of advancing UCPPS treatment through the identification of clinically relevant patient subgroups potentially requiring distinct interventions [13]. By moving beyond traditional bladder- and prostate-focused investigations toward an innovative multidisciplinary research strategy, the MAPP Research Network is able to more fully investigate the relationship between UCPPS and non-urologic associated syndromes (NUAS), and better define urologic and more systemic contributions to the pathophysiology of these disabling syndromes.

This manuscript describes the approach to clinical phenotyping developed in the MAPP Research Network, with a focus on its central epidemiological study. This integrated research design is highly unique in its evaluation of visceral pain and lower urinary tract symptoms associated with UCPPS, and represents the largest and most detailed characterization of UCPPS to date.

Methods/design
Scientific focus
The MAPP Research Network conducts complementary basic, translational, and clinical science studies to investigate questions of clinical relevance, motivated by the view that UCPPS involves substantial central systemic mechanisms. Studies have been designed to advance our understanding of the underlying pathophysiology and etiology, treated natural history, "flare" etiology, risk factors associated with biologic, genetic, and behavioral factors, and the discovery of comprehensive characterizations of patient phenotypes. Another key objective has been to address the relationships between UCPPS and commonly associated non-urologic syndromes (Table 1). The MAPP Network also supports translational studies using UCPPS animal models founded on key clinical criteria and leading hypotheses of UCPPS etiology.

MAPP network organization
The MAPP Research Network consists of six discovery sites (Los Angeles, CA; Chicago, IL; St. Louis, MO; Iowa City, IA, Seattle, WA, and Ann Arbor, MI); several satellite sites (Miami, FL; Birmingham, AL; Palo Alto, CA; Boston, MA; Kingston, Ontario, Canada (CA); a data coordinating core (DCC) in Philadelphia, PA; a tissue analysis and technology core (TATC) in Aurora, CO; a neuro-imaging scan repository and reading center (Los Angeles, CA); an external experts panel (EEP); and NIDDK project scientists (Figure 1).

MAPP network core functions
The DCC provides biostatistical design and analysis leadership for all studies, serves as the central site for electronic protocol and data management system development, web-based deployment of data capture tools, data acquisition and storage, and promotes network-wide quality assurance across all protocol-specific domains of data. The DCC also provides administrative and project coordination support, including development and maintenance of a public website (http://www.mappnetwork.org/). The TATC provides a central location for bio-specimen processing, storage, and analysis of blood, urine, and DNA samples. The TATC established and implemented standards for specimen collection, identification, and handling to promote consistent specimen collection procedures. DCC and TATC personnel conducted centralized coordinator training before initiating patient enrollment, with follow-up refresher training at periodic Steering Committee meetings. Standardized modular barcoded collection kits with specimen annotation forms for blood, urine, and cheek swab DNA were designed for use at all recruitment sites. The data-sharing model allows sites to enter material requests, specimen collection and shipment information through the DCC portal, with replication in real-time between both DCC and TATC databases (Figure 2). Sites request kits via the DCC portal, following which the TATC sends a shipment of unlinked specimen kits, uniquely identified with a barcode system, to the site, which are individually linked through the DCC portal to a MAPP participant at the time of biospecimen collection. Blood specimens are shipped on the day of collection to the TATC for next day delivery; whereas cheek swab and urine specimens are temporary stored at the collection sites and batch-shipped to the TATC. At-home specimen collection is facilitated by participants, using barcoded collection materials and pre-labeled shipping containers for direct shipping to the TATC. Centralized processing at the TATC ensures standardized processing using best practice standards [25]. Derivative specimen aliquots are barcoded without participant identifying information, allowing for blinded discovery and validation projects. A rigorous

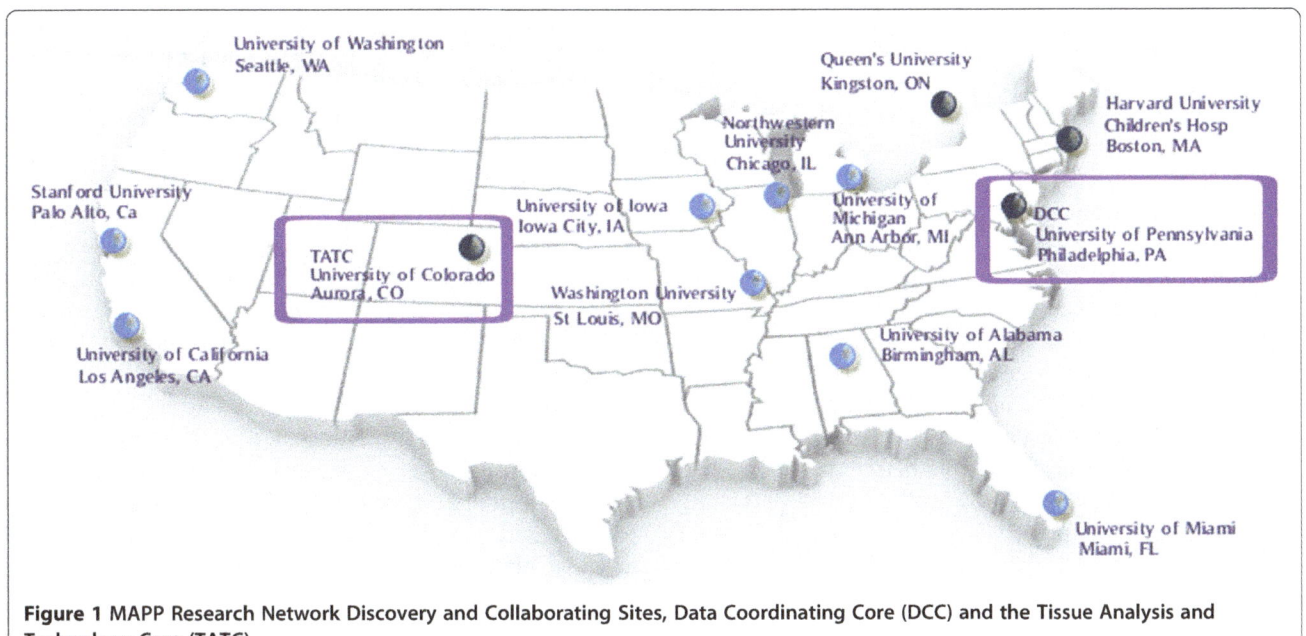

Figure 1 MAPP Research Network Discovery and Collaborating Sites, Data Coordinating Core (DCC) and the Tissue Analysis and Technology Core (TATC).

series of identity management procedures were implemented between the DCC and TATC to ensure unambiguous links between specimen and participant data. Discovery sites submit specimen requests for research projects to the DCC. Sharing of real-time specimen inventory and annotation data between the TATC and DCC database allows full control by the DCC to match specimens with the required clinical data, and select specimens at the aliquot tube level. After selection by the DCC, a specimen distribution request is transferred to the TATC, triggering shipment to the discovery site. Real-time updates allow the DCC to monitor progress of distribution projects.

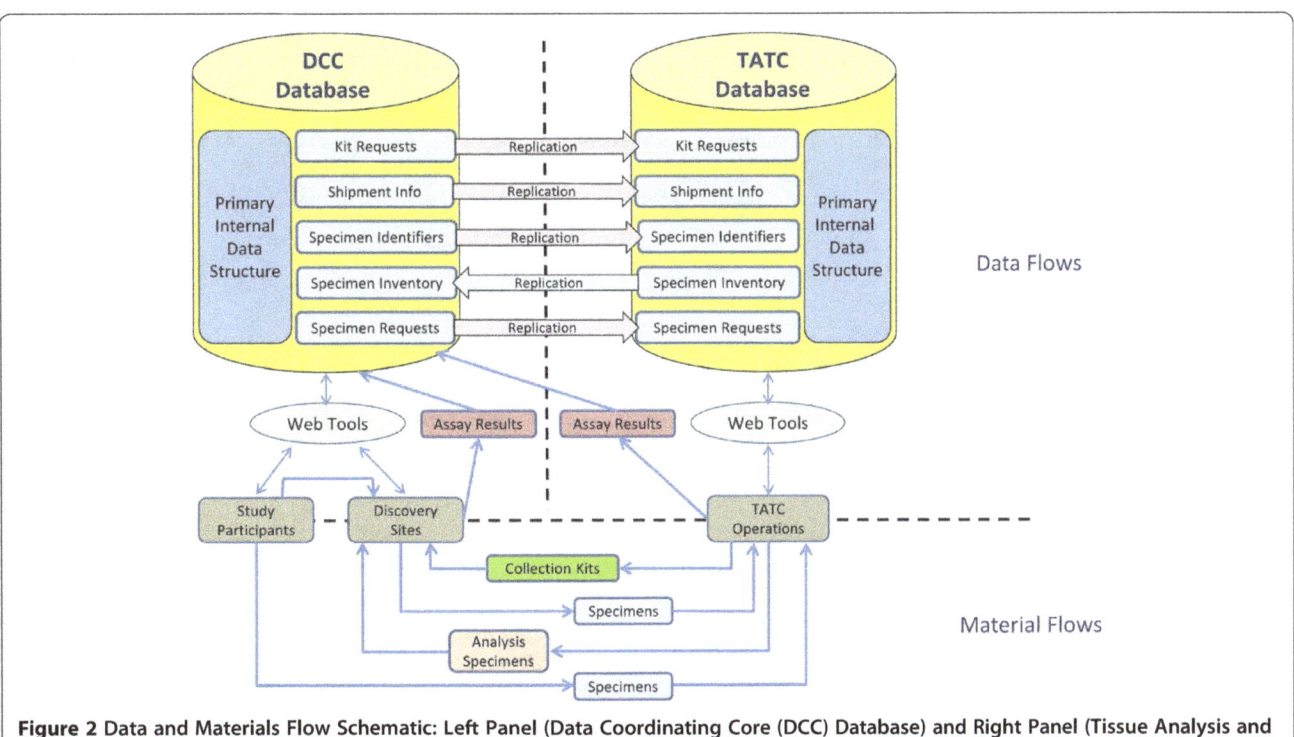

Figure 2 Data and Materials Flow Schematic: Left Panel (Data Coordinating Core (DCC) Database) and Right Panel (Tissue Analysis and Technology Core (TATC) Database).

Quantitative Sensory Testing (QST)

QST is a specialized form of assessment that utilizes Pressure Pain Threshold (PPT) to assess pain sensitivity to standardized evoked stimuli. The PPT was determined by using blunt pressure delivered by a $1\text{-}cm^2$ hard-rubber probe to the thumbnail bed of the participant's non-dominant hand [26-28]. The thumbnail is considered a "neutral site", both because it is distant from the pain that these individuals are experiencing, and this site has been repeatedly shown to be a good measure of overall "central" pain threshold [29]. Evoked pressure pain, rather than heat pain threshold testing was chosen for MAPP studies for several reasons; first, QST studies have found that pressure pain testing differentiates IC from healthy controls better than does heat stimulation [16,30,31], and secondly, pressure testing was more easily deployed in a standardized manner across multiple sites.

Neuroimaging and functional neurobiology

Neuroimaging and functional neurobiology studies support overall participant characterization, as well as specific trans-MAPP brain imaging studies. These studies were designed to identify differences in brain structure and connectivity [32,33] as well as differences in regional intrinsic oscillation frequencies and resting state connectivity of the brain [34] between UCPPS patients and control groups. A standardized protocol was developed to acquire structural (grey matter), diffusion tensor imaging; white matter (integrity and connectivity) and resting state images of the brain, as well as functional neurobiology studies across study sites. The magnetic resonance imaging/functional magnetic resonance imaging (MRI/fMRI) data repository for this study was established at the UCLA Center for Neurobiology of Stress (http://pain.med.ucla.edu/), in close collaboration with UCLA-Laboratory of Neuroimaging (LONI), which has extensive experience in the collection, storage and analysis of large multi-site MRI data sets (loni.usc.edu) [35].

Biomarker and infectious etiology studies

As a component of the Trans-MAPP EP Study protocol, biological samples (urine, plasma, and cheek swab DNA) were collected at Discovery Sites at baseline (UCPPS patients and control cohorts) and the 6- and 12-month in-clinic office visits (UCPPS patients) (see Table 2 for details on samples collected). In addition, a specialized single-use at-home collection kit was developed for use by UCPPS patients at the time of self-reported flare. These samples were archived at the TATC and distributed to MAPP Network investigators, in conjunction with associated clinical data managed at the DCC, to support integrated studies to identify and characterize UCPPS biological markers (biomarkers) and to examine the potential contributions of infectious agents to UCPPS. The biomarker study uses UCPPS and control

Table 2 Number of participants (target, enrolled) by cohort, sex (UCPPS: duration of symptoms), and number of participants with biospecimens by type, MRI scans completed and PPT data collected at baseline visit

Cohorts	No. of participants by cohort		No. of participants with biospecimens						No. of participants with MRI scans	No. of Participants with Pain Pressure Threshold (PPT) measures	
	Target size	Actual enrolled	Cheek swab	Biomarker samples		Infectious etiology urine samples				At baseline	During follow-up
				Plasma	Urine	VB1	VB2	VB3			
UCPPS (Duration of symptoms)											
Male < 2 Yrs	95	90	90	90	90	90	90	39	13	19	20
Male ≥ Yrs	95	101	100	100	101	100	100	42	22	12	20
Female < 2 Yrs	95	89	89	86	89	89	88	0	22	20	19
Female ≥2 Yrs	95	144	144	142	144	142	139	0	41	11	23
Total	380	424	423	418	424	421	417	81	98	62	82
Healthy controls											
Male	190	182	182	177	181	176	174	64	38	40	0
Female	190	233	233	228	232	232	227	0	79	60	0
Total	380	415	415	405	413	408	401	64	117	100	0
Positive controls											
Male	95	44	44	43	43	43	43	10	17	8	0
Female	95	156	156	154	154	154	152	0	47	27	0
Total	190	200	200	197	197	197	195	10	64	35	0
Overall total	950	1,039	1,038	1,020	1,034	1,026	1,013	155	279	197	82

plasma and spot-urine collections (Table 2) to assess the utility of previously identified, candidate markers and to identify new markers in a discovery-based approach using proteomics platforms. The infectious etiology study examines VB1 and VB2 (males and females) and VB3 (males) urine samples (Table 2) through advanced 16S deep sequencing methods to assess UCPPS and control microbial profiles and to address hypotheses regarding an infectious basis for symptom development and fluctuations, including symptom flare. Archived DNA samples will be used for targeted epigenetics and genetic investigations.

Flare assessment in UCPPS

Currently it is unknown what triggers a flare of UCPPS symptomatology. Putative risk factors for flares (e.g., dietary factors, physical activity, stress, sexual activities, recent infections) were assessed for participants reporting a flare (limited to three assessments for subjects reporting >3 flares). The same potential flare risk factors were also collected during randomly selected follow-up contacts for participants when not reporting flares, serving as within-person control data. A home collection kit was designed to allow participants to collect urine samples for biomarker and infectious etiology studies at their first reported "flare". In addition, each participant collected a reference urine sample using the home collection kit at one of the three randomly selected non-flare time points during the first four months. A full set of flare and non-flare biomarker and infectious etiology urine specimens was successfully collected from 188 (44%) of the participants. Another 44 (10%) participants provided only a flare specimen set; whereas 123 (29%) of participants provided only a non-flare specimen set. This reference specimen, together with the urine specimens collected during the in-clinic visits will be analyzed, and compared with the flare specimen, to investigate potential biomarkers and infectious agents that are uniquely present in urine during symptom flares.

Baseline self-report battery characterizing UCPPS and controls

Extensive clinical phenotyping was conducted to characterize UCPPS patients, positive controls and healthy controls at baseline. A description of the self-report battery follows categorized by: General Socio-Demographic and Medical History; Urological Specific Measures; and Non-Urological co-morbidities and diagnostics.

General socio-demographic and medical history

Data on age, sex, race/ethnicity, education, marital status, and income were collected from participant self-report. A directed medical history was gathered on each participant that included co-morbid conditions, early life infection history, concomitant medication use (i.e., name,

dose, frequency and route of administration), previous treatments for UCPPS, and family medical history (i.e., history of chronic pain and psychiatric disorders in parents, grandparents, aunts, uncles, siblings, and children). A physical examination included measurement of height, weight and blood pressure as well as abdominal, pelvic, and rectal examinations. Pelvic floor muscle tenderness (yes/no) and suprapubic tenderness (yes/no) were evaluated in each participant. In women, the presence and degree of pelvic organ prolapse was recorded (above or below the hymenal ring). In men, penile exam (circumcised or not), prostate examination (enlarged, irregular, tender) and scrotal examination (varicocele, hydrocele, mass, hernia) findings were recorded.

Urological specific measures

Urological measures were selected purposefully to provide continuity between MAPP and pre-existing literatures on IC/BPS and IC/CPPS. The urological measures thus sought to assess symptoms that have been historically considered relevant to UCPPS with instruments designed specifically for this population (Table 3).

Symptom and health care utilization Questionnaire (SYM-Q) A 12-item questionnaire was developed specifically for this study. All participants completed this questionnaire at baseline and at bi-weekly intervals throughout the 48-week study period. The SYM-Q inquires about (1) pain, urgency, frequency, (2) the presence of non-urological pain symptoms, (3) mood, (4) health care seeking, (5) last menstrual period, and (6) the occurrence of symptom worsening (flares).

Interstitial Cystitis Symptom Index (ICSI) and problem index (ICPI) (ICINDEX) This instrument consists of two 4-item questionnaires. The ICSI quantifies urinary and pain symptoms in patients with IC/BPS, and the ICPI assesses the degree of bother associated with these symptoms [36].

American Urological Association Symptom Index (AUASI) This validated 8-item questionnaire assesses the severity of voiding symptoms (e.g., frequency, urgency, nocturia, sense of incomplete emptying, intermittency, slow stream, straining to void) and associated bother in either sex [37].

Brief Flare Risk Factor Questionnaire (BFRFQ) Developed specifically for use in the MAPP Research Network as a means of better understanding flares in UCPPS, the BFRFQ contains 33 items documenting potential causes of flares. It includes questions about diet, physical activity, stress, sexual activity, and infection.

Table 3 Baseline phenotyping battery for MAPP: urological self-report questionnaires

Instrument	Subscales
Symptom and Health Care Utilization Questionnaire (SYM-Q)	1. Pain, urgency, frequency
	2. Urologic/Pelvic Pain severity
	3. Non-urologic/Pelvic Pain severity
	4. Mood
	5. Most bothersome symptom
	6. Medical care seeking
	7. Menstrual information
	8. Flare status
Interstitial cystitis symptom and problem index	1. IC Symptom Index (ICSI)
	2. IC Problem Index (ICPI)
American Urological Association Symptom Index Score	1. AUASI total score
Rice case definition questionnaire	1. RICE total score
Brief flare risk factor questionnaire	1. Flare timing, symptoms, and symptom severity
	2. Cause attribution
	3. Foods
	4. Drinks
	5. Physical and sedentary activities
	6. Stress
	7. Sexual activity
	8. Infections
Genitourinary Pain Scale (GUPI)	1. Pain
Male version	2. Urinary symptoms
Female version	3. Quality of life
	4. Total
Female sexual function index	1. FSFI total score
International index of erectile function	1. IIEF total score
University of Washington male sexual function scale	1. Pain with ejaculation
	2. Premature ejaculation
	3. Difficulty reaching ejaculation
Self-esteem and relationship questionnaire	1. SEAR total score
Males	
Females	

Rand Interstitial Cystitis Epidemiology (RICE) case definition The 5-item RICE case definition questionnaire was designed for epidemiological studies to identify the presence of IC/BPS symptoms in men and women [9]. We used it to identify sub-groups with or without bladder pain and urgency due to pain, pressure, or discomfort.

Genitourinary Pain Index (GUPI) This 9-item instrument was developed by modifying the original NIH-Chronic Prostatitis Symptom Index (CPSI) [38]. Several new items about bladder-specific pain were added, and male gender-specific items were replaced with female-gender specific items for women. The GUPI is applicable to men and women to assess pain symptoms, urinary symptoms, and quality of life as separate sub-scales, and overall as a total score [39].

Female Sexual Function Index (FSFI) This 19-item scale provides an overall assessment of female sexual functioning over the past 4 weeks, and includes domain scores in six areas: sexual desire, arousal, lubrication, orgasm, satisfaction, and pain, as well as a total score for sexual dysfunction [40].

International Index of Erectile Function (IIEF) The IIEF is a multidimensional instrument consisting of 15 items and 5 domains of male sexual function: erectile function, orgasmic function, sexual desire, intercourse satisfaction, and overall satisfaction. Total scores indicate greater levels of sexual dysfunction [41].

Washington Male sexual function scale (MSFS) This instrument was used in males to rate the severity of the following symptoms: pain with ejaculation, lack of interest in sexual activity, premature ejaculation, and difficulty reaching ejaculation [42].

Self-Esteem And Relationship questionnaire (SEAR: M & F) The SEAR is a 14-item measure validated to assess psychosocial impact of erectile dysfunction. The measure assesses an overall score, sexual relationship satisfaction, confidence, and self-esteem. The measure was adapted for use in women by omitting the two male-specific items [43].

Non-urologic co-occurring symptoms and diagnostics
Although pain is experienced locally at a site of discomfort, it is often accompanied by other symptoms that influence pain processing, modulation, and ultimately how it is experienced. Understanding these other influential factors can provide insight into the mechanisms associated with the etiology and maintenance of chronic pain. Thus, the following symptoms and traits were assessed in each participant (Table 4).

History of co-occurring somatic symptoms The Complex Multi-Symptom Inventory (CMSI) [44] is a 41-item symptom checklist of past year illnesses specific to functional syndromes (e.g., fibromyalgia (FM), chronic fatigue syndrome (CFS), irritable bowel syndrome (IBS),

Table 4 Baseline phenotyping battery for MAPP: non-urological self-report questionnaires

Instrument	Subscales
Complex Multi-Symptom Inventory (CMSI) (Diagnostics of co-morbid functional disorders and overall symptom burden)	1. Fibromyalgia
	2. Chronic fatigue syndrome
	3. Irritable bowel syndrome
	4. Vulvadynia
	5. Migraine
	6. Temporomandibular disorders
	7. Past year total symptom burden
Brief Pain Inventory (BPI) (General clinical pain)	1. Severity
	2. Interference
	3. Medications
	4. Relief from medications
	5. Body map: overall
	6. Body map: male genital
	7. Body map: female genital
Short Form-12 (Functional status)	1. Physical status
	2. Physical role status
	3. Bodily pain
	4. General health
	5. Energy/vitality
	6. Social functioning
	7. Mental health
	8. Role limitations (emotional)
	9. Composite physical (PCS)
	10. Composite mental health (MCS)
PROMIS: Fatigue	1. Total score (t-score)
PROMIS: Sleep disturbance	1. Total score (t-score)
Multiple Abilities Self-Report Questionnaire (MASQ) (Perceived cognitive problems)	1. Language ability
	2. Visio-spatial ability
	3. Verbal memory
	4. Visual memory
	5. Attention/concentration
Perceived Stress Scale (PSS)	1. Total score
Hospital Anxiety and Depression Scale	1. Depressive symptoms (HADS:D)
	2. Anxiety Symptoms (HADS:A)
PROMIS: Anger	1. Total score (t-score)
Positive and Negative Affect Scale (PANAS)	1. Positive affect
	2. Negative affect
	3. Affect balance

Table 4 Baseline phenotyping battery for MAPP: non-urological self-report questionnaires *(Continued)*

International Personality Item Pool (IPIP)	1. Neuroticism
	2. Extroversion
	3. Agreeableness
	4. Conscientiousness
	5. Openness to experience
Coping Strategies Questionnaire (Catastrophizing scale)	1. Cat score
Beliefs in Pain Control Questionnaire (BPCQ)	1. Internal locus of control
	2. Powerful doctors (external locus)
	3. Chance (external locus)
Childhood Traumatic Events Scale (CTES) Recent Traumatic Events Scale (RTES)	1. Age of each trauma
	2. Intensity of each trauma
	3. Confiding in others for each trauma

vulvodynia (VVD), migraine, and temporomandibular disorders (TMD). The checklist provides a proxy for the presence of these comorbid conditions; whereas the follow–up assessment module uses the standardized diagnostic criteria for each condition [44]. The summed checklist has been interpreted as representing the overall symptom burden from somatic or functional conditions.

Clinical pain The Brief Pain Inventory (BPI) is a 15-item self-report measure that has been validated for use in a wide variety of pain states [45]. The BPI assesses for the presence of pain, pain intensity (i.e., worse, least, average, current), and functional interference from pain. It also catalogues the types of medications being used; the percentage of pain relief obtained from medications, and assesses pain distribution (via a body map). For purposes of the MAPP Research Network, the body map of the BPI was replaced with a more detailed body map used in epidemiological studies to better identify widespread pain by body regions [46]. This more detailed body map was further modified to include larger scale depictions of the pelvic and genital regions. This body map was scored to identify those where pelvic pain was confined to the pelvic region (i.e., pelvic pain only) or was more widespread extending beyond the pelvic region (i.e., pelvic pain and beyond).

Functional status The SF-12 [47], is a 12-item measure of functional status and generic quality of life. The instrument assesses eight domains of health status: physical functioning, role limitations because of physical problems, bodily pain, general health perceptions, energy/vitality, social functioning, role limitations due to emotional problems, and mental health. It also provides both a composite physical functioning score (PCS) and a mental health composite score (MCS). Higher scores on these measures indicate better functioning within the domain.

Fatigue and sleep disturbance The NIH Patient Reported Outcomes Measurement Information System (PROMIS) developed questionnaires for fatigue and sleep disturbance that can be used across disease conditions. Participants completed the following PROMIS short-forms: Fatigue (7-items) and Sleep Disturbance (8-items) [48]. Higher scores on these measures indicate worse symptomatology.

Cognitive difficulties The Multiple Ability Self-Report Questionnaire (MASQ) assessed the self-perception of having cognitive difficulties [49]. This is a 38-item questionnaire comprised of 5 domains of cognitive concerns: language ability, visio-spatial ability, verbal memory, visual memory, and attention/concentration. Validation studies have found the self-reported cognitive difficulties to correspond to performance-based indices of the same constructs [49]. Higher scores on each scale indicate more problematic perceptions.

Stress Perceived stress was measured using the 10-item Perceived Stress Scale (PSS) [50]. The PSS measures the degree to which situations are perceived as being unpredictable, uncontrollable and overwhelming. Higher scores indicate more stress.

Emotional distress Emotional distress was assessed across several affective domains. Depressive and anxiety-related symptoms were assessed using the Hospital Anxiety and Depression Scale (HADS) [51]. The HADS is a 14-item self-report questionnaire developed for use in non-psychiatric settings. This instrument provided both a depressive symptom and anxiety symptom score with validated cut-off scores associated with clinically relevant levels of each affective domain. Anger was assessed with the 8-item anger short form from PROMIS [48]. A potential source of resilience, (i.e., positive affect), was assessed using the Positive and Negative Affect Schedule (PANAS) [52]. This 20-item questionnaire provides both a positive and negative affect score. On each mood measure, higher scores indicate greater problems with mood.

Personality traits Personality was measured using the International Personality Item Pool (IPIP) short form [53]. The IPIP is a public-domain, 120-item instrument that was developed to reflect assessment of five personality domains: extraversion, neuroticism, agreeableness, conscientiousness, and openness to experience. Higher scores indicate greater strength of each personality trait.

Catastrophizing Catastrophizing refers to the perception that pain is overwhelmingly awful and the worst imaginable burden that one can endure. This cognitive perception was assessed using the 6-item Catastrophizing sub-scale from the Coping Strategies Questionnaire (CSQ) [54] a metric for measuring this construct. Higher scores indicate greater catastrophizing.

Locus of control The Beliefs in Pain Control Questionnaire (BPCQ) [55] is a 13-item questionnaire designed to evaluate beliefs regarding whether pain is under personal control or under the control of forces external to the patient. Three scales can be derived: (1) Internal scale – measuring beliefs that pain can be personally controlled (2) Powerful Doctors – an external locus of control scale measuring beliefs that pain control is in the hands of powerful others, and (3) Chance Happenings – a second external locus of control scale measuring beliefs that pain is controlled by chance or misfortune. Higher scores on each scale indicate greater strength of each belief.

Early life trauma history The Childhood Traumatic Events Scale (CTES) [56] is composed of two forms. The first assesses childhood traumatic events that occurred prior to the age of 17. Domains include death of a close family member or friend, parental separation, physical abuse including sexual assault, serious illness, and other. For each question, the age of trauma, perceived intensity of the trauma, and whether or not confiding in others occurred is assessed. The second form is labeled Recent Traumatic Events Scale (RTES). It assesses essentially the same traumatic domains with the exception that the timeframe is within the last 3 years, parental separation is replaced with spouse or significant other separation, and a new category of job change is added. This instrument can be scored to identify the intensity of each type of trauma or intensities can be summed across all traumas. This form is unique in that it also assesses whether the person confided in another individual about the trauma.

The trans-MAPP epidemiology/phenotyping study

The principal study conducted by the MAPP Research Network is a prospective observational study of the treated natural history of UCPPS – the Trans-MAPP Epidemiology/Phenotyping (EP) Study (Figure 3). This study serves as the central clinical phenotyping effort for all MAPP Network participants, and the platform for additional, integrated and complementary phenotyping efforts.

Trans-MAPP EP study participants

As illustrated in Figure 3, the Trans-MAPP EP Study specifically targeted the recruitment of 380 UCPPS

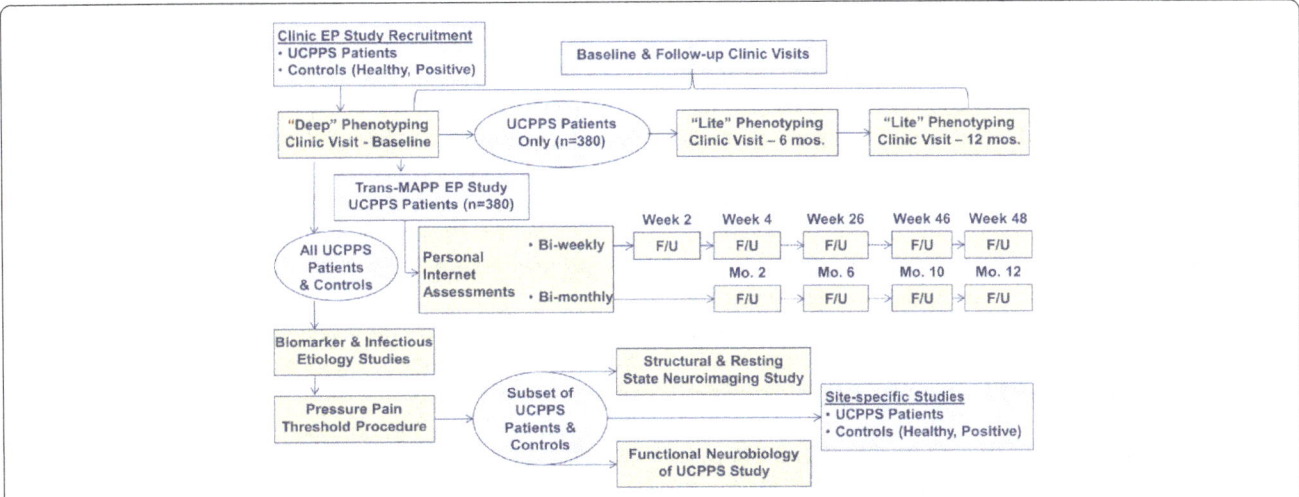

Figure 3 Trans-MAPP Epidemiology and Phenotyping (EP) Study of UCPPS Patients, Control (Healthy, Positive) Groups, Biomarker and Infectious Etiology Studies, Pressure Pain Threshold Study, Structural and Resting State Neuroimaging Study, and Functional Neurobiology of UCPPS Study.

participants for "phenotyping" at baseline and for follow-up. An additional 380 healthy controls matched on sex and age, and 190 "positive" controls, meeting the criteria for one or more of the targeted NUAS were also recruited and phenotyped at baseline. In addition to the self-reported characterization of all study participants at baseline, a standardized protocol for the collection of biological samples (cheek swabs, plasma, urine) was implemented for additional multi-site biomarker and infectious etiology studies, quantitative sensory testing was used to measure pressure pain threshold (PPT), flares were assessed, and structural and resting state neuroimaging and functional neurobiology studies were also conducted to characterize UCPPS patients and controls.

The original recruitment targets were 50% males and 50% females, for both UCPPS and control cohorts. In addition, 50% of both male and female UCPPS participants were targeted to have recent onset of chronic pelvic pain symptoms (operationalized as < two years) and 50% longer symptom duration (operationalized as ≥ two years). Consequently, the recruitment target sample size was 95 for each of these four UCPPS participant subgroups (Table 2). The healthy control group targets were 190 males and 190 females, aiming to balance age and race/ethnicity distributions within the UCPPS subjects. The targets for positive controls were not specified, except for a total of 95 males and 95 females with one or more NUAS.

UCPPS Inclusion criteria

Inclusion criteria for UCPPS participants were: 1) a diagnosis of IC/BPS or CP/CPPS, with urologic symptoms present a majority of the time during any 3 of the past 6 months (CP/CPPS) or the most recent 3 months (IC/BPS); 2) at least 18 years old; 3) reporting a non-zero score for

bladder/prostate and/or pelvic region pain, pressure or discomfort during the past 2 weeks; and 4) consented to provide a blood or cheek swab sample to test DNA for genes related to the main study goals.

UCPPS exclusion criteria

Exclusion criteria for UCPPS consisted of the following: symptomatic urethral stricture, on-going neurological conditions affecting the bladder or bowel, active auto-immune or infectious disorders, history of cystitis caused by tuberculosis or radiation or chemotherapies, history of non-dermatologic cancer, current major psychiatric disorders, or severe cardiac, pulmonary, renal, or hepatic disease. In addition, males diagnosed with unilateral orchalgia without pelvic symptoms, and males with a history of microwave thermotherapy, trans-urethral or needle ablation or other specified prostate procedures were excluded.

Eligibility criteria for controls

To ensure a clearly-defined healthy control subgroup, potential control participants were excluded if they reported any pain in the pelvic or bladder region or chronic pain in more than one non-urologic body region. Like healthy controls, positive controls needed to be free of pain in the pelvic region, but also needed to qualify on the CMSI as having one of the targeted co-morbid conditions.

Screening and baseline procedures

The screening and enrollment process utilized one in-clinic baseline study visit for informed consent and eligibility confirmation. This baseline visit was structured so that essential information, such as brief symptoms analogous to those used in previous UCPPS clinical studies (e.g., pain, pressure, discomfort and sex-specific symptom criteria)

[57,58] and a urine sample dipstick could be acquired prior to the conduct of more intensive, invasive and time-consuming procedures (Figure 4). Persons meeting initial eligibility were then invited to complete the Trans-MAPP EP Study assessments, and were enrolled only after a negative 48-hour urine culture report. Eligible participants then underwent extensive baseline characterization using the standardized battery of urologic and non-urologic assessment instruments described previously. Biosamples, QST, and neuroimaging was also collected concurrently with the self-report information at baseline. Healthy controls, as well as "positive" controls (i.e., individuals with one or more non-urologic associated syndromes of primary interest; Table 2), were also enrolled but only underwent a single phenotyping assessment and biosample collection at baseline identical to that of participants with UCPPS.

Longitudinal phenotyping schedule

After the extensive baseline assessment, participants were administered a small subset of the assessment battery for 48 weeks via internet-based bi-weekly / bi-monthly assessment questionnaires. More extensive assessment was possible at the in-clinic visit occurring at 24 and 48 weeks. Biological samples (e.g., DNA, serum, and urine) were collected in-clinic at baseline and at 24 and 48 weeks, as well as through home collection kits when patients reported symptom worsening ("flares"). The sequence of data and biospecimen collection is illustrated for the Trans-MAPP EP Study in Figure 4.

Recruitment and retention of participants

Participant recruitment was conducted through the urology/urogynecology clinics at each of the clinical sites from 12/14/2009 through 12/14/2012. As summarized in Table 2, the MAPP Research Network enrolled 1,039 men and women, including persons with UCPPS (n = 424); "positive controls" with other NUAS (n = 200 for all conditions); and healthy controls (n = 415), exceeding specified target sizes. Given the success of recruitment and value of this phenotypic data, individuals with

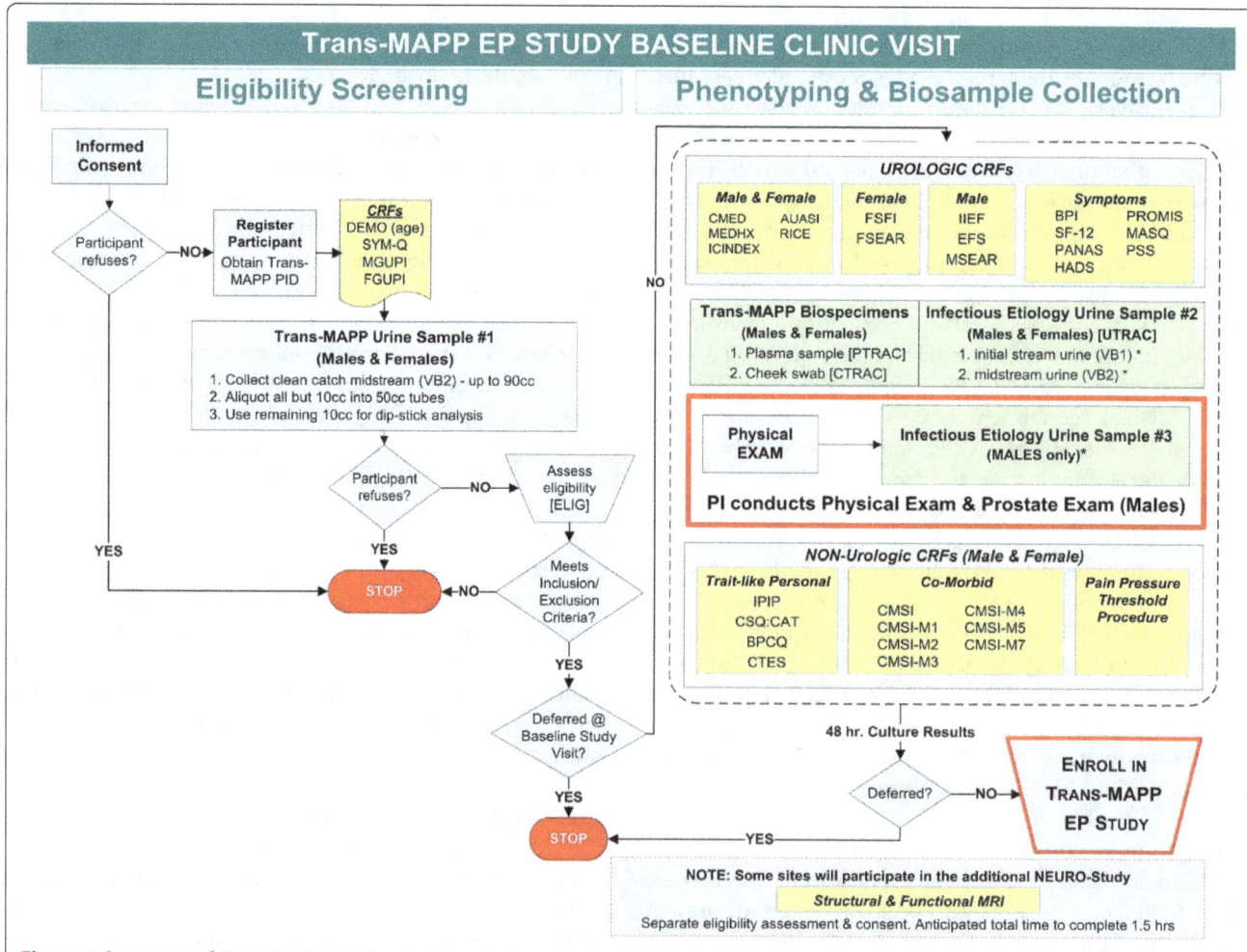

Figure 4 Sequence of Trans-MAPP Epidemiology and Phenotyping (EP) Study Screening, Phenotyping, Biospecimen Collection and Enrollment into the EP Study.

UCPPS will continue to be recruited and characterized in this manner in the subsequent phases of the network.

During the follow-up period, retention was promoted by the research coordinators by sending reminder messages to participants to provide their bi-weekly symptom assessments. Participants who missed these assessments were contacted by phone for further prompting to facilitate ongoing participation. The MAPP Research Network continued follow-up visits through 12/14/2013. The participant retention rate for the final clinic visit at 48 weeks was 83% (349/420), with remarkable adherence (83% missing no more than 3 monthly contacts). Among the 349 UCPPS participants completing the 48-week assessment, 161 (46%) to date have agreed (with re-consent) to participate in an ongoing extended follow-up study with internet-based symptom assessment every 4 months.

Self-report and QST data

Currently, extensive baseline self-report phenotypic data is available on 424 individuals with UCPPS, 200 positive controls, and 415 healthy controls. Longitudinal assessment from all UCPPS participants was initiated with bi-weekly internet-based data capture, with 349 participants completing the 48 week final clinic visit. QST studies were performed on a subset of trans-MAPP EP participants from each site (n = 279) [59].

Biological specimen collection

The biospecimen capture rate at the baseline visit was high, exceeding 98% for the cheek swabs, plasma and urine biomarker samples, and the first-void and infectious etiology mid-stream urine samples (VB1/VB2), as shown in Table 2. Success can be attributed to the tight integration of clinical procedures and biospecimen collection, the design of standardized collection kits, and the data sharing procedures (Figure 2) between the DCC and the TATC. In addition, consistent communication with research coordinators and monthly conference calls developed a strong collaborative environment, promoting timely response to data collection issues. The biosamples are examined in a set of integrated research protocols within the MAPP Network.

Statistical considerations

All data are initially examined using exploratory descriptive methods, investigating potential differences between males and females, and between groups (i.e., UCPPS, healthy and positive controls). Categorical variables, including dichotomous factors, are summarized by proportions and compared among groups using standard chi-square tests of association and generalized Mantel-Haenszel methods, as described in Landis et al. [60].

Extensive baseline phenotype data are being investigated within a multi-stage cluster analysis [61] to construct clinically relevant subgroups, using a distance-dissimilarity matrix and clustering subjects using the average linkage method [62]. For each domain, the variables that are contributing most to the differences among the domain-specific clusters are identified.

Studies aimed at characterizing symptom pattern change over time utilize standard methods for longitudinal data analysis. For measured continuous outcomes, the primary models used are random coefficient growth curve models in which random effects due to subject and/or time are included to account for the correlation among repeated observations on each subject [63,64]. For binary or ordinal outcomes, the methodology of generalized estimating equations are being implemented to evaluate changes over time via logistic models [65,66].

To adjust for regression-to-the-mean effects, data from a pseudo-run-in period from baseline, 2 and 4 weeks of follow-up are being used to construct a baseline measure of variability, and a within-person slope is estimated beginning at 4 weeks through the final visit at 48 weeks. Studies aimed at evaluating factors related to the extent of symptom variability over time are being conducted utilizing subject-specific estimates of mean squared error about the estimated slope of longitudinal symptom outcomes.

Discussion

The MAPP Research Network overall research strategy, and specifically its primary clinical protocol, the Trans-MAPP EP Study, represents a novel investigative direction for the field. Moreover, the integrated approach to systemic phenotyping allows a wealth of clinically important questions to be addressed. Through the use of state-of-the-art research methods developed by network investigators, and adopted from the broader pain field, the MAPP Network seeks to determine if UCPPS patients exhibit similar findings as have been observed for patients with non-urologic chronic pain. The recruitment of a healthy control group (individuals without urologic pain symptoms) and a "positive" control group (those with chronic non-urologic associated functional pain syndromes) allow MAPP Network investigators to search for novel clinical and biological measurements that may be unique to UCPPS, or that define clinically distinct UCPPS subgroups. The bi-weekly longitudinal assessments provide valuable information about UCPPS symptom variability and flares and, indeed, this effort has forged new ground in the highly effective acquisition of extensive, longitudinal clinical data through internet-based platforms developed specifically for this study. These extensive data collection efforts described here were developed to address a series of overarching study hypotheses prioritized by the MAPP Network for their clinical significance and relevance to advancing clinical care for UCPPS patients:

1. Individuals with UCPPS, measured at baseline and followed longitudinally for one year, as well as asymptomatic and disease comparator controls (e.g., CFS, FM, IBS) measured only at baseline, will make it possible to identify biologically-derived UCPPS subsets of individuals with UCPPS who: (a) have differing underlying pathogenesis resulting in their symptoms, and (b) would likely respond to different treatments.

2. There are two subsets of UCPPS patients: those with primarily pelvic symptoms, and those who also display many non-urological symptoms and syndromes. These latter individuals have a more systemic condition, characterized by a different natural history than those with isolated UCPPS symptoms, including a higher likelihood of: (a) symptom progression or continuation, (b) symptom variability, and (c) decreased quality of life and increased healthcare seeking behavior than those with primarily pelvic symptoms.

3. Individuals with UCPPS who have been symptomatic for longer periods of time (operationalized as 2+ years) will have more severe overall symptoms, decreased quality of life, and greater psychological co-morbidities than individuals with more recent (<2 years) onset of symptoms.

4. IC/BPS in females and CP/CPPS in males represent the same underlying condition. Using common phenotyping protocols in males and females, the high rate of non-urological symptoms and syndromes (NUAS) noted previously in women with IC/BPS will also be noted in men with CP/CPPS.

5. A variety of stressors (e.g, dietary, infectious, psychological) will be shown in case-crossover studies to predict worsening of symptoms (flares). Biomarker studies performed during these flares will identify factors in urine that increase with disease activity and decrease during quiescent periods.

6. Groups of individuals with UCPPS exhibit a lower overall pain threshold (i.e., hyperalgesia) compared to asymptomatic controls. This left-shift in stimulus-response function in the entire group of UCPPS patients will be noted, both on quantitative sensory testing, as well as within functional neuroimaging. This finding in the entire group of UCPPS patients will be shown to be driven by the subset of UCPPS patients with the more "systemic" form of the disease noted in Hypothesis 2 above.

7. Specific objective abnormalities (i.e., potential biomarkers, including central pain processing and modulation patterns ("brain signatures") (Hypothesis 6) can be identified that are associated with specific risk factors (Hypothesis 5), reflecting specific pain processing and functional neuroimaging patterns (Hypothesis 6).

8. Disease development in subsets of UCPPS patients' results from an underlying pathogenic process, and symptom exacerbations (flares) may be influenced by changes in pathogen type or quantity.

The phenotyping approach developed in the MAPP Network is the most comprehensive attempt to characterize individuals with UCPPS to date, and one of the most comprehensive phenotyping projects undertaken for any form of chronic pain. Examining not only urological factors, but also non-urological factors consistent with the biopsychosocial model of understanding chronic pain, broadens our ability to explore underlying pathological mechanisms that extend beyond the region of the pelvis. The observed variability across multiple domains within UCPPS suggests the possibility of clinically relevant subgroups that may be used to guide treatment in the future, or be used to understand different causal factors of pain and urinary symptoms. In addition, it is expected that future psychometric analyses will help to translate this extensive phenotyping battery into a set of assessment tools that can be applied in clinical practice so as to guide treatment decisions.

Conclusions

The MAPP Research Network has successfully designed and implemented a 48-week longitudinal, observational study, focused on providing insights into underlying pathophysiology and identifying clinically relevant phenotypes of UCPPS. Healthy control subjects, and positive controls exhibiting NUAS, were also phenotyped to generate comparative data. Both baseline and longitudinal data collection is complete for the Trans-MAPP EP Study, which met or exceeded the original recruitment targets. Protocol adherence proved excellent, especially participant data collection directly through novel internet-based platforms. The biospecimen capture rate reached nearly 100%, and the participant retention rate for the final clinic visit at 48 weeks was 83% (349/420), with remarkable adherence (83% missing no more than 3 monthly contacts). These statistics reveal critical successes in the design and implementation of this complex, multi-site clinical study. A comprehensive, multidimensional battery of self-report measures is at the center of the clinical phenotyping. This was assembled by network investigators and incorporated into the Trans-MAPP Network EP Study to correlate an array of domains, including urologic symptoms, non-urologic pain, psychosocial factors, risk factors, quality of life, among others, in patients with UCPPS. Complementary data from integrated multi-site biomarker studies, neuroimaging, experimental pain testing, and a number of additional efforts were collected and are being used to further inform on pathophysiology and segregate clinically relevant subgroups of individuals with UCPPS, for whom diagnostics, treatments, and further studies of underlying pathological mechanisms can be targeted. These complex data are currently being analyzed to provide a systemic assessment of UCPPS patients and patient groups.

It is expected that information obtained from these studies will significantly aid in our understanding of the pathophysiology and clinical characteristics of UCPPS, inform future clinical efforts, and improve symptom management. Finally, the MAPP Research Network serves as a new model for how large multi-disciplinary efforts may be designed to investigate complex urologic, as well as non-urologic, conditions.

Abbreviations
AUASI: American urological association symptom index; BACH: Boston Area Community Health Survey; BFRFQ: Brief flare risk factor questionnaire; BPCQ: Beliefs in Pain Control Questionnaire; BPI: Brief pain inventory; BPS: Bladder Pain Syndrome; CFS: chronic fatigue syndrome; CNS: Central nervous system; CPC: Chronic Prostatitis Cohort; CP/CPPS: Chronic prostatitis/chronic pelvic pain syndrome; CSQ: Coping Strategies Questionnaire; CTES: Childhood Traumatic Events Scale; DCC: Data coordinating core; DNA: Deoxyribonucleic acid; EEP: External experts panel; FM: Fibromyalgia; FSFI: Female sexual function index; GUPI: Genitourinary pain index; HADS: Hospital Anxiety and Depression Scale; IBS: Irritable bowel syndrome; IC/BPS: Interstitial cystitis/bladder pain syndrome; ICCRN: Interstitial Cystitis Collaborative Research Network; ICCTG: The Interstitial Cystitis Clinical Trials Group; ICDB: Interstitial Cystitis Database study; ICINDEX: Interstitial cystitis symptom index (ICSI) and Problem Index (ICPI); IIEF: International index of erectile function; IPIP: The International Personality Item Pool; LONI: Laboratory of Neuroimaging; MAPP: Multidisciplinary Approach to the Study of Chronic Pelvic Pain; MASQ: Multiple ability self-report questionnaires; MCS: Mental health composite score; MRI/fMRI: Magnetic resonance imaging/functional magnetic resonance imaging; MSFS: Washington male sexual function scale; NIDDK: The National Institute of Diabetes, Digestive, and Kidney Diseases; NUAS: Non-urologic associated syndromes; OPPERA: Orofacial Pain Prospective Evaluation and Risk Assessment (https://www.oppera2.org/OPPERAII/Images/OPPERAIIRecruitmentBrochure.pdf); PANAS: Positive and Negative Affect Schedule; PCS: Physical functioning score; PPT: Pressure pain threshold; PROMIS: The NIH patient reported outcomes measurement information system; PSS: Perceived stress scale; RICE: RAND Interstitial Cystitis Epidemiology Study; RTES: Recent Traumatic Events Scale; SEAR: M & F: Self-esteem and relationship questionnaire; SF-12: The SF-12®: An Even Shorter Health Survey; SYM-Q: Symptom and health care utilization questionnaire; TATC: Tissue analysis and technology core; TMD: Temporomandibular disorders; Trans-MAPP EP: Trans-MAPP epidemiology and phenotyping study; UCLA: University of California at Los Angeles; UCPPS: Urological chronic pelvic pain syndromes; VB1,VB2: Voided bladder 1… 2.

Competing interests
All authors participated in choosing the measures and variables which were collected in the MAPP network studies. All authors participated in the development of the MAPP network protocol. BD Naliboff, JQ Clemens, N Afari, CS Bradley, JW Griffith, P Hanno, BA Hong, JN Krieger, HH Lai, JR Landis, SK Lutgendorf, LV Rodriguez, AJ Schaeffer, S Sutcliffe, CC Yang, JW Kusek, Z Kirkali, EA Mayer, D Buchwald, NA Robinson, A van Bokhoven, and C Mullins declare no competing interests. DA Williams is a Consultant for Health Focus Inc. and has consulted for Pfizer. DJ Clauw has received grants from Pfizer, Cerephex, Lilly, Merck, Nuvo and Furest, and Consulting Fees and Honoraria from Pfizer, Cerephex, Lilly, Merck, Nuvo, Furest, Tonix, Purdue, Therauance, and Johnson & Johnson. DJ Klumpp declares ownership and equity interests in ProbioTx Inc, and Gold Coast Therapeutics Inc. GL Andriole is a Consultant for Augmenix, Bayer, Genomic Health, GlaxoSmithKline, and Myriad Genetics,

and has received research grants from Johnson & Johnson, Medivation, and Wilex. KJ Kreder is a Consultant for Medtronic, Astellas, Symptelligence, and Tengion. MA Pontari is a Consultant for Lilly and Watson and has received Royalties from Up to Date. MS Lucia declares ownership of 3D Biopsy and has consulted for Myriad Genetics and Bayer Healthcare.

Authors' contributions
JRL, DAW and JQC wrote the initial draft manuscript. All authors read and approved the final manuscript.

Acknowledgements
The MAPP Research Network acknowledges support through NIH grants: U01 DK82315, U01 DK82316, U01 DK82325, U01 DK82333, U01 DK82342, U01 DK82344, U01 DK82345, and U01 DK82370. The NIDDK and MAPP Network investigators wish to thank the Interstitial Cystitis Association (ICA) and the Prostatitis Foundation (PF) for their assistance in study participant recruitment and other network efforts.
We thank the participants and staff from the following sites that participated in the study: Northwestern University; University of California, Los Angeles; University of Iowa; Washington University, St. Louis; University of Washington, Seattle; University of Michigan; University of Pennsylvania (Data Coordinating Core); University of Colorado Denver (Tissue Analysis & Technology Core); Stanford University; NIDDK.

MAPP Research Network Study Group
MAPP Network Executive Committee
J. Quentin Clemens, MD, FACS, MSci,
Network Chair, 2013-
Philip Hanno, MD
Ziya Kirkali, MD
John W. Kusek, PhD
J. Richard Landis, PhD
M. Scott Lucia, MD
Chris Mullins, PhD
Michel A. Pontari, MD
Northwestern University
Discovery Site
David J. Klumpp, PhD, Co-Director
Anthony J. Schaeffer, MD, Co-Director
Apkar (Vania) Apkarian, PhD
David Cella, PhD
Melissa A. Farmer, PhD
Colleen Fitzgerald, MD
Richard Gershon, PhD
James W. Griffith, PhD
Charles J. Heckman II, PhD
Mingchen Jiang, PhD
Laurie Keefer, PhD
Darlene S. Marko, RN, BSN, CCRC
Jean Michniewicz
Todd Parrish, PhD
Frank Tu, MD, MPH
University of California, Los Angeles
Discovery Site and PAIN Neuroimaging Core
Emeran A. Mayer, MD, Co-Director
Larissa V. Rodríguez, MD, Co-Director
Jeffry Alger, PhD
Cody P. Ashe-McNalley
Ben Ellingson, PhD
Nuwanthi Heendeniya
Lisa Kilpatrick, PhD
Jason Kutch, PhD
Jennifer S. Labus, PhD
Bruce D. Naliboff, PhD
Fornessa Randal
Suzanne R. Smith, RN, NP
University of Iowa
Discovery Site
Karl J. Kreder, MD, MBA, Director
Catherine S. Bradley, MD, MSCE
Mary Eno, RN, RA II

Kris Greiner, BA
Yi Luo, PhD, MD
Susan K. Lutgendorf, PhD
Michael A. O'Donnell, MD
Barbara Ziegler, BA
University of Michigan
Discovery Site
Daniel J. Clauw, MD, Co-Director; Network Chair, 2008-2013
J. Quentin Clemens, MD, FACS, MSci,
Co-Director; Network Chair, 2013-
Suzie As-Sanie, MD
Sandra Berry, MA
Megan E. Halvorson, BS, CCRP
Richard Harris, PhD
Steve Harte, PhD
Eric Ichesco, BS
Ann Oldendorf, MD
Katherine A. Scott, RN, BSN
David A. Williams, PhD
University of Washington, Seattle
Discovery Site
Dedra Buchwald, MD, Director
Niloofar Afari, PhD, Univ. of California, San Diego
John Krieger, MD
Jane Miller, MD
Stephanie Richey, BS
Susan O. Ross, RN, MN
Roberta Spiro, MS
TJ Sundsvold, MPH
Eric Strachan, PhD
Claire C. Yang, MD
Washington University, St. Louis
Discovery Site
Gerald L. Andriole, MD, Co-Director
H. Henry Lai, MD, Co-Director
Rebecca L. Bristol, BA, BS, Coordinator
Graham Colditz, MD, DrPH
Georg Deutsch, PhD, Univ. of Alabama at Birmingham
Vivien C. Gardner, RN, BSN, Coordinator
Robert W. Gereau IV, PhD
Jeffrey P Henderson, MD, PhD
Barry A. Hong, PhD, FAACP
Thomas M. Hooton, MD, Univ of Miami
Timothy J. Ness, MD, PhD, Univ. of Alabama at Birmingham
Carol S. North, MD, MPE, Univ. Texas Southwestern
Theresa M. Spitznagle, PT, DPT, WCS
Siobhan Sutcliffe, PhD, ScM, MHS
University of Pennsylvania
Data Coordinating Core (DCC)
J. Richard Landis, PhD, Core Director
Ted Barrell, BA
Philip Hanno, MD
Xiaoling Hou, MS
Tamara Howard, MPH
Michel A. Pontari, MD
Nancy Robinson, PhD
Alisa Stephens, PhD
Yanli Wang, MS
University of Colorado Denver
Tissue Analysis & Technology Core (TATC)
M. Scott Lucia, MD, Core Director
Adrie van Bokhoven, PhD
Andrea A. Osypuk, BS
Robert Dayton, Jr
Karen R. Jonscher, PhD
Holly T. Sullivan, BS
R. Storey Wilson, MS
Additional Sites:
Harvard Medical School/Boston Children's Hospital
Marsha A. Moses, PhD, Director
Andrew C. Briscoe

David Briscoe, MD
Adam Curatolo, BA
John Froehlich, PhD
Richard S. Lee, MD
Monisha Sachdev, BS
Keith R. Solomon, PhD
Hanno Steen, PhD
Stanford University
Sean Mackey, MD, PhD, Director
Epifanio Bagarinao, PhD
Lauren C. Foster, BA
Emily Hubbard, BA
Kevin A. Johnson, PhD, RN
Katherine T. Martucci, PhD
Rebecca L. McCue, BA
Rachel R. Moericke, MA
Aneesha Nilakantan, BA
Noorulain Noor, BS
Queens University
J. Curtis Nickel, MD, FRCSC, Director
Drexel University College of Medicine
Garth D.Ehrlich, PhD
National Institutes of Diabetes and Digestive and Kidney Diseases
(NIDDK), National Institutes of Health (NIH)
Chris Mullins, PhD
John W. Kusek, PhD
Ziya Kirkali, MD
Tamara G. Bavendam, MD

This article outlines independent research commissioned by the National Institute for Health (NIH). The views expressed in this article are those of the author(s) and are not necessarily those of the NIH, the NIDDK, or the Department of Health.

Author details

[1]Department of Biostatistics and Epidemiology, Perelman School of Medicine at the University of Pennsylvania, Philadelphia, PA, USA. [2]Departments of Anesthesiology, Medicine and Psychiatry, University of Michigan, Ann Arbor, MI, USA. [3]Department of Pathology, University of Colorado Anschutz Medical Campus, Aurora, CO, USA. [4]Departments of Medicine, Psychiatry, and Gastroenterology, University of California, Los Angeles, CA, USA. [5]Division of Public Health Sciences, Department of Surgery, Washington University, St Louis, MO, USA. [6]Department of Urology, Northwestern University, Chicago, IL, USA. [7]Department of Urology, University of Southern California, Beverly Hills, CA, USA. [8]Division of Digestive Diseases, University of California, Los Angeles, CA, USA. [9]Division of Urologic Surgery, Department of Surgery, Washington University School of Medicine, St. Louis, MO, USA. [10]Department of Urology, University of Washington, Seattle, WA, USA. [11]Department of Urology, University of Iowa, Iowa City, IA, USA. [12]VA Center of Excellence for Stress and Mental Health, University of California San Diego, San Diego, CA, USA. [13]Departments of Obstetrics and Gynecology, Urology and Epidemiology, University of Iowa, Iowa City, IA, USA. [14]Department of Medical Social Sciences, Northwestern University, Chicago, IL, USA. [15]Departments of Psychiatry and Medicine, Washington University School of Medicine, St. Louis, MO, USA. [16]Departments of Epidemiology and Medicine, University of Washington, Seattle, WA, USA. [17]Department of Anesthesiology, Division of Pain Medicine, Stanford University School of Medicine, Palo Alto, CA, USA. [18]Department of Urology, Temple University School of Medicine, Philadelphia, PA, USA. [19]Department of Urology, Perelman School of Medicine at the University of Pennsylvania, Philadelphia, PA, USA. [20]National Institute of Diabetes and Digestive and Kidney Diseases, National Institutes of Health, Bethesda, MD, USA. [21]Department of Urology, Division of Neurourology and Pelvic Reconstructive Surgery, University of Michigan, Ann Arbor, MI, USA.

References

1.   Bogart LM, Berry SH, Clemens JQ: **Symptoms of interstitial cystitis, painful bladder syndrome and similar diseases in women: a systematic review.** *J Urol* 2007, **177**(2):450–456.

2. Clemens JQ, Markossian TW, Meenan RT, O'Keeffe Rosetti MC, Calhoun EA: Overlap of voiding symptoms, storage symptoms and pain in men and women. *J Urol* 2007, **178**(4 Pt 1):1354–1358. discussion 1358.

3. Fall M, Johansson SL, Aldenborg F: Chronic interstitial cystitis: a heterogeneous syndrome. *J Urol* 1987, **137**(1):35–38.

4. Messing E, Pauk D, Schaeffer A, Nieweglowski M, Nyberg LM Jr, Landis JR, Cook YL, Simon LJ: Associations among cystoscopic findings and symptoms and physical examination findings in women enrolled in the Interstitial Cystitis Data Base (ICDB) study. *Urology* 1997, **49**(5A Suppl):81–85.

5. Schaeffer AJ, Knauss JS, Landis JR, Propert KJ, Alexander RB, Litwin MS, Nickel JC, O'Leary MP, Nadler RB, Pontari MA, Shoskes DA, Zeitlin SI, Fowler JE Jr, Mazurick CA, Kusek JW, Nyberg LM, Chronic Prostatitis Collaborative Research Network Study Group: Leukocyte and bacterial counts do not correlate with severity of symptoms in men with chronic prostatitis: the National Institutes of Health Chronic Prostatitis Cohort Study. *J Urol* 2002, **168**(3):1048–1053.

6. Held PJ, Hanno PM, Wein AJ, Pauly MV, Cahn MA: Epidemiology of Interstitial Cystitis. In *Interstitial Cystitis*. Edited by Hanno PM, Stasking DR, Krane RJ, Wein AJ. London: Springer Verlag; 1990:29–48.

7. Berry SH, Elliott MN, Suttorp M, Bogart LM, Stoto MA, Eggers P, Nyberg L, Clemens JQ: Prevalence of symptoms of bladder pain syndrome/ interstitial cystitis among adult females in the United States. *J Urol* 2011, **186**(2):540–544.

8. Link CL, Pulliam SJ, Hanno PM, Hall SA, Eggers PW, Kusek JW, McKinlay JB: Prevalence and psychosocial correlates of symptoms suggestive of painful bladder syndrome: results from the Boston area community health survey. *J Urol* 2008, **180**(2):599–606.

9. Suskind AM, Berry SH, Ewing BA, Elliott MN, Suttorp MJ, Clemens JQ: The prevalence and overlap of interstitial cystitis/bladder pain syndrome and chronic prostatitis/chronic pelvic pain syndrome in men: results of the RAND Interstitial Cystitis Epidemiology male study. *J Urol* 2013, **189**(1):141–145.

10. Daniels NA, Link CL, Barry MJ, McKinlay JB: Association between past urinary tract infections and current symptoms suggestive of chronic prostatitis/ chronic pelvic pain syndrome. *J Natl Med Assoc* 2007, **99**(5):509–516.

11. Shoskes DA, Nickel JC, Dolinga R, Prots D: Clinical phenotyping of patients with chronic prostatitis/chronic pelvic pain syndrome and correlation with symptom severity. *Urology* 2009, **73**(3):538–542. discussion 542-3.

12. Nickel JC, Shoskes D, Irvine-Bird K: Clinical phenotyping of women with interstitial cystitis/painful bladder syndrome: a key to classification and potentially improved management. *J Urol* 2009, **182**(1):155–160.

13. Clemens JQ, Mullins C, Kusek JW, Kirkali Z, Mayer EA, Rodriguez LV, Klumpp DJ, Schaeffer AJ, Kreder KJ, Buchwald D, Andriole GL, Lucia MS, Landis JR, Clauw DJ, The MAPP Research Network Study Group: The MAPP research network: a novel study of urologic chronic pelvic pain syndromes. Accepted to *BMC Urology* on 23 July 2014.

14. Warren JW, Wesselmann U, Morozov V, Langenberg PW: Numbers and types of nonbladder syndromes as risk factors for interstitial cystitis/ painful bladder syndrome. *Urology* 2011, **77**(2):313–319.

15. Warren JW, Howard FM, Cross RK, Good JL, Weissman MM, Wesselmann U, Langenberg P, Greenberg P, Clauw DJ: Antecedent nonbladder syndromes in case-control study of interstitial cystitis/painful bladder syndrome. *Urology* 2009, **73**(1):52–57.

16. Clauw DJ, Schmidt M, Radulovic D, Singer A, Katz P, Bresette J: The relationship between fibromyalgia and interstitial cystitis. *J Psychiatr Res* 1997, **31**(1):125–131.

17. Heitkemper M, Jarrett M: Overlapping conditions in women with irritable bowel syndrome. *Urol Nurs* 2005, **25**(1):25–30. quiz 31.

18. Aaron LA, Herrell R, Ashton S, Belcourt M, Schmaling K, Goldberg J, Buchwald D: Comorbid clinical conditions in chronic fatigue: a co-twin control study. *J Gen Intern Med* 2001, **16**(1):24–31.

19. Clemens JQ, Meenan RT, O'Keeffe Rosetti MC, Kimes TA, Calhoun EA: Case-control study of medical comorbidities in women with interstitial cystitis. *J Urol* 2008, **179**(6):2222–2225.

20. Rodriguez MA, Afari N, Buchwald DS, National Institute of Diabetes and Digestive and Kidney Diseases Working Group on Urological Chronic Pelvic Pain: Evidence for overlap between urological and nonurological unexplained clinical conditions. *J Urol* 2009, **182**(5):2123–2131.

21. van de Merwe JP, Nordling J, Bouchelouche P, Bouchelouche K, Cervigni M, Daha LK, Elneil S, Fall M, Hohlbrugger G, Irwin P, Mortensen S, van Ophoven A, Osborne JL, Peeker R, Richter B, Riedl C, Sairanen J, Tinzl M, Wyndaele JJ: Diagnostic criteria, classification, and nomenclature for painful bladder syndrome/interstitial cystitis: an ESSIC proposal. *Eur Urol* 2008, **53**(1):60–67.

22. Phillips K, Clauw DJ: Central pain mechanisms in chronic pain states–maybe it is all in their head. *Best Pract Res Clin Rheumatol* 2011, **25**(2):141–154.

23. Woolf CJ: Central sensitization: implications for the diagnosis and treatment of pain. *Pain* 2011, **152**(3 Suppl):S2–S15.

24. Tracey I, Bushnell MC: How neuroimaging studies have challenged us to rethink: is chronic pain a disease? *J Pain* 2009, **10**(11):1113–1120.

25. NCI best practices for biospecimen resources. http://biospecimens.cancer.gov/bestpractices/.

26. Petzke F, Clauw DJ, Ambrose K, Khine A, Gracely RH: Increased pain sensitivity in fibromyalgia: effects of stimulus type and mode of presentation. *Pain* 2003, **105**(3):403–413.

27. Giesecke J, Reed BD, Haefner HK, Giesecke T, Clauw DJ, Gracely RH: Quantitative sensory testing in vulvodynia patients and increased peripheral pressure pain sensitivity. *Obstet Gynecol* 2004, **104**(1):126–133.

28. Giesecke T, Gracely RH, Grant MA, Nachemson A, Petzke F, Williams DA, Clauw DJ: Evidence of augmented central pain processing in idiopathic chronic low back pain. *Arthritis Rheum* 2004, **50**(2):613–623.

29. Petzke F, Khine A, Williams D, Groner K, Clauw DJ, Gracely RH: Dolorimetry performed at 3 paired tender points highly predicts overall tenderness. *J Rheumatol* 2001, **28**(11):2568–2569.

30. Ness TJ, Powell-Boone T, Cannon R, Lloyd LK, Fillingim RB: Psychophysical evidence of hypersensitivity in subjects with interstitial cystitis. *J Urol* 2005, **173**(6):1983–1987.

31. Lai HH, Gardner V, Ness TJ, Gereau RW, 4th: Segmental hyperalgesia to mechanical stimulus in interstitial cystitis/bladder pain syndrome: evidence of central sensitization. *J Urol* 2014, **191**(5):1294–1299.

32. Jiang Z, Dinov ID, Labus J, Shi Y, Zamanyan A, Gupta A, Ashe-McNalley C, Hong JY, Tillisch K, Toga AW, Mayer EA: Sex-related differences of cortical thickness in patients with Chronic Abdominal Pain. *PLoS One* 2013, **8**(9):e73932.

33. Labus JS, Gupta A, Coveleskie K, Tillisch K, Kilpatrick L, Jarcho J, Feier N, Bueller J, Stains J, Smith S, Suyenobu B, Naliboff B, Mayer EA: Sex differences in emotion-related cognitive processes in irritable bowel syndrome and healthy control subjects. *Pain* 2013, **154**(10):2088–2099.

34. Hong JY, Kilpatrick LA, Labus J, Gupta A, Jiang Z, Ashe-McNalley C, Stains J, Heendeniya N, Ebrat B, Smith S, Tillisch K, Naliboff B, Mayer EA: Patients with chronic visceral pain show sex-related alterations in intrinsic oscillations of the resting brain. *J Neurosci* 2013, **33**(29):11994–12002.

35. Dinov ID, Petrosyan P, Liu Z, Eggert P, Zamanyan A, Torri F, Macciardi F, Hobel S, Moon SW, Sung YH, Jiang Z, Labus J, Kurth F, Ashe-McNalley C, Mayer E, Vespa PM, Van Horn JD, Toga AW, for the Alzheimer's Disease Neuroimaging Initiative: The perfect neuroimaging-genetics-computation storm: collision of petabytes of data, millions of hardware devices and thousands of software tools. *Brain Imaging Behav* 2014, **8**(2):311–322.

36. O'Leary MP, Sant GR, Fowler FJ Jr, Whitmore KE, Spolarich-Kroll J: The interstitial cystitis symptom index and problem index. *Urology* 1997, **49**(5A Suppl):58–63.

37. Barry MJ, Fowler FJ Jr, O'Leary MP, Bruskewitz RC, Holtgrewe HL, Mebust WK, Cockett AT: The American Urological Association symptom index for benign prostatic hyperplasia. The Measurement Committee of the American Urological Association. *J Urol* 1992, **148**(5):1549–1557. discussion 1564.

38. Litwin MS, McNaughton-Collins M, Fowler FJ Jr, Nickel JC, Calhoun EA, Pontari MA, Alexander RB, Farrar JT, O'Leary MP: The National Institutes of Health chronic prostatitis symptom index: development and validation of a new outcome measure. Chronic Prostatitis Collaborative Research Network. *J Urol* 1999, **162**(2):369–375.

39. Clemens JQ, Calhoun EA, Litwin MS, McNaughton-Collins M, Kusek JW, Crowley EM, Landis JR, Urologic Pelvic Pain Collaborative Research Network: Validation of a modified National Institutes of Health chronic prostatitis symptom index to assess genitourinary pain in both men and women. *Urology* 2009, **74**(5):983–987. quiz 987.e1-3.

40. Rosen R, Brown C, Heiman J, Leiblum S, Meston C, Shabsigh R, Ferguson D, D'Agostino R Jr: The Female Sexual Function Index (FSFI): a multidimensional self-report instrument for the assessment of female sexual function. *J Sex Marital Ther* 2000, **26**(2):191–208.

41. Rosen RC, Riley A, Wagner G, Osterloh IH, Kirkpatrick J, Mishra A: The international index of erectile function (IIEF): a multidimensional scale for assessment of erectile dysfunction. *Urology* 1997, **49**(6):822–830.

42. Lee SW, Liong ML, Yuen KH, Leong WS, Cheah PY, Khan NA, Krieger JN: Adverse impact of sexual dysfunction in chronic prostatitis/chronic pelvic pain syndrome. *Urology* 2008, **71**(1):79–84.

43. Cappelleri JC, Althof SE, Siegel RL, Shpilsky A, Bell SS, Duttagupta S: **Development and validation of the Self-Esteem And Relationship (SEAR) questionnaire in erectile dysfunction.** *Int J Impot Res* 2004, **16**(1):30–38.

44. Williams DA, Schilling S: **Advances in the assessment of fibromyalgia.** *Rheum Dis Clin North Am* 2009, **35**(2):339–357.

45. Cleeland C: *The Brief Pain Inventory: User Guide.* Houston, TX: MD Anderson Cancer Center; 2009.

46. Macfarlane GJ, Croft PR, Schollum J, Silman AJ: **Widespread pain: is an improved classification possible?** *J Rheumatol* 1996, **23**(9):1628–1632.

47. Ware JE Jr, Kosinski M, Keller SD: **A 12-item short-form health survey: construction of scales and preliminary tests of reliability and validity.** *Med Care* 1996, **34**(3):220–233.

48. Cella D, Riley W, Stone A, Rothrock N, Reeve B, Yount S, Amtmann D, Bode R, Buysse D, Choi S, Cook K, Devellis R, DeWalt D, Fries JF, Gershon R, Hahn EA, Lai JS, Pilkonis P, Revicki D, Rose M, Weinfurt K, Hays R, PROMIS Cooperative Group: **The Patient-Reported Outcomes Measurement Information System (PROMIS) developed and tested its first wave of adult self-reported health outcome item banks: 2005-2008.** *J Clin Epidemiol* 2010, **63**(11):1179–1194.

49. Seidenberg M, Haltiner A, Taylor MA, Hermann BB, Wyler A: **Development and validation of a multiple ability self-report questionnaire.** *J Clin Exp Neuropsychol* 1994, **16**(1):93–104.

50. Cohen S, Williamson G: **Perceived Stress in a Probability Sample of the United States.** In *The Social Psychology of Health: Claremont Symposium on Applied Social Psychology.* Edited by Spacapan S, Oskamp S. Newbury Park, CA: Sage; 1988.

51. Snaith RP, Zigmond AS: **The hospital anxiety and depression scale.** *Br Med J (Clin Res Ed)* 1986, **292**(6516):344.

52. Watson D, Clark LA, Tellegen A: **Development and validation of brief measures of positive and negative affect: the PANAS scales.** *J Pers Soc Psychol* 1988, **54**(6):1063–1070.

53. Goldberg LR, Johnson JA, Eber HW, Hogan R, Ashton MC, Cloninger CR, Gough HG: **The international personality item pool and the future of public-domain personality measures.** *J Res Pers* 2006, **40**:84–96.

54. Rosenstiel AK, Keefe FJ: **The use of coping strategies in chronic low back pain patients: relationship to patient characteristics and current adjustment.** *Pain* 1983, **17**(1):33–44.

55. Skevington SM: **A standardised scale to measure beliefs about controlling pain (B.P.C.Q.): A preliminary study.** *Psychol Health* 1990, **4**(3):221–232.

56. Pennebaker JW, Susman JR: **Disclosure of traumas and psychosomatic processes.** *Soc Sci Med* 1988, **26**(3):327–332.

57. Sant GR, Propert KJ, Hanno PM, Burks D, Culkin D, Diokno AC, Hardy C, Landis JR, Mayer R, Madigan R, Messing EM, Peters K, Theoharides TC, Warren J, Wein AJ, Steers W, Kusek JW, Nyberg LM, Interstitial Cystitis Clinical Trials Group: **A pilot clinical trial of oral pentosan polysulfate and oral hydroxyzine in patients with interstitial cystitis.** *J Urol* 2003, **170**(3):810–815.

58. Schaeffer AJ, Landis JR, Knauss JS, Propert KJ, Alexander RB, Litwin MS, Nickel JC, O'Leary MP, Nadler RB, Pontari MA, Shoskes DA, Zeitlin SI, Fowler JE Jr, Mazurick CA, Kishel L, Kusek JW, Nyberg LM, Chronic Prostatitis Collaborative Research Network Group: **Demographic and clinical characteristics of men with chronic prostatitis: the National Institutes of Health chronic prostatitis cohort study.** *J Urol* 2002, **168**(2):593–598.

59. Harte SE, Mitra M, Ichesco EA, Halvorson ME, Clauw DJ, Shih AJ, Kruger GH: **Development and validation of a pressure-type automated quantitative sensory testing system for point-of-care pain assessment.** *Med Biol Eng Comput* 2013, **51**(6):633–644.

60. Landis JR, Sharp TJ, Kuritz SJ, Koch GG: **Mantel-Haenszel Methods.** In *Encyclopedia of Biostatistics.* Edited by Armitage P, Colton T. Chichester; New York: J. Wiley; 1997:2378–2391.

61. Leiby BE, Landis JR, Propert KJ, Tomaszewski JE, Interstitial Cystitis Data Base Study Group: **Discovery of morphological subgroups that correlate with severity of symptoms in interstitial cystitis: a proposed biopsy classification system.** *J Urol* 2007, **177**(1):142–148.

62. SAS Institute: *SAS/STAT User's Guide, Version 8.* Cary, NC: SAS Institute, Inc; 1999.

63. Laird NM, Ware JH: **Random-effects models for longitudinal data.** *Biometrics* 1982, **38**(4):963–974.

64. Lindstrom MJ, Bates DM: **Newton-Raphson and EM Algorithms for linear mixed-effects models for repeated-measures data.** *J Am Stat Assoc* 1988, **83**(404):1014–1022.

65. Liang KY, Zeger SL: **Longitudinal data-analysis using generalized linear-models.** *Biometrika* 1986, **73**(1):13–22.

66. Zeger SL, Liang KY: **Longitudinal data-analysis for discrete and continuous outcomes.** *Biometrics* 1986, **42**(1):121–130.

Primary mucin-producing urothelial-type adenocarcinoma of the prostatic urethra diagnosed on TURP

Elisabeth M Sebesta[1*], Hossein S Mirheydar[2,3], J Kellogg Parsons[2,3], Jessica Wang-Rodriguez[3] and A Karim Kader[2,3]

Abstract

Background: Mucin-producing urothelial-type adenocarcinoma of the prostatic urethra is extremely rare. These lesions must be differentiated from other mucinous tumors including mucin-producing prostatic adenocarcinoma and metastases from either colonic or bladder primaries.

Case presentation: We report here a case of urothelial-type adenocarcinoma arising from the prostatic urethra. The patient is an 81 year-old man with a history of pT1 urothelial cell carcinoma of the bladder status post trans-urethral resection of bladder tumor (TURBT) who initially presented with irritative lower urinary tract symptoms and mucosuria refractory to Flomax and finasteride. A shared decision was made for the patient to undergo trans-urethral resection of prostate (TURP). At the time of surgery, a papillary tumor emanating from the prostatic urethra was found and no urothelial lesions were noted in the bladder. Pathology of the resected prostatic chips revealed an invasive adenocarcinoma with intestinal-type differentiation that stained positive for CK7, CK20, and villin, but negative for PSA, PSAP, uroplakin, and CDX-2. Colonoscopy was normal and CT scan did not show any evidence of colonic lesions nor visceral or lymph node metastases. Thus, the patient was diagnosed with a primary urothelial-type adenocarcinoma of the prostatic urethra.

Conclusion: Herein we review the literature regarding this unusual entity, and discuss the differential diagnosis, immunohistochemistry, and the importance of correctly identifying this rare tumor.

Keywords: Mucin-producing adenocarcinoma, Prostatic urethra, Trans-urethral resection of prostate, Urothelial-type adenocarcinoma, Adenocarcinoma

Background

The most common mucin-producing adenocarcinoma of the prostate gland is a primary prostatic adenocarcinoma with mucin production [1]. The differential diagnosis includes secondary prostatic lesions of primary colonic or bladder origin and urothelial-type adenocarcinoma arising directly from the prostatic urethra or prostatic ducts. The latter diagnosis is exceedingly rare, with only 18 cases identified in the literature to date [1-4]. Urothelial-type adenocarcinoma of the prostatic urethra is histologically identical to nonurachal adenocarcinoma of the bladder, however it arises from urethritis glandularis or glandular metaplasia of the prostatic urethra [1,5]. We describe

a case of primary urothelial-type adenocarcinoma of the prostatic urethra that was initially diagnosed on TURP specimen, with a discussion of its clinical-pathological correlation.

Case presentation

An 81 year-old Caucasian man with past medical history of COPD, on home oxygen, presented with mucosuria, urinary frequency, and nocturia. Digital rectal exam demonstrated a 60 cc benign-feeling gland and the patient's PSA was 0.38. The patient has a history of a 2.5 cm pT1 urothelial cell carcinoma at the bladder dome status post TURBT 19 months prior (Figure 1a, 1b). The patient had two subsequent urine cytology examinations 5 and 2 months prior, both of which were negative for malignant cells. The patient recently noticed mucosuria. His subsequent surveillance cystoscopy demonstrated a normal-appearing

* Correspondence: ems2230@columbia.edu
[1]Columbia University College of Physicians and Surgeons, 630 W. 168th St, New York, NY 10032, USA
Full list of author information is available at the end of the article

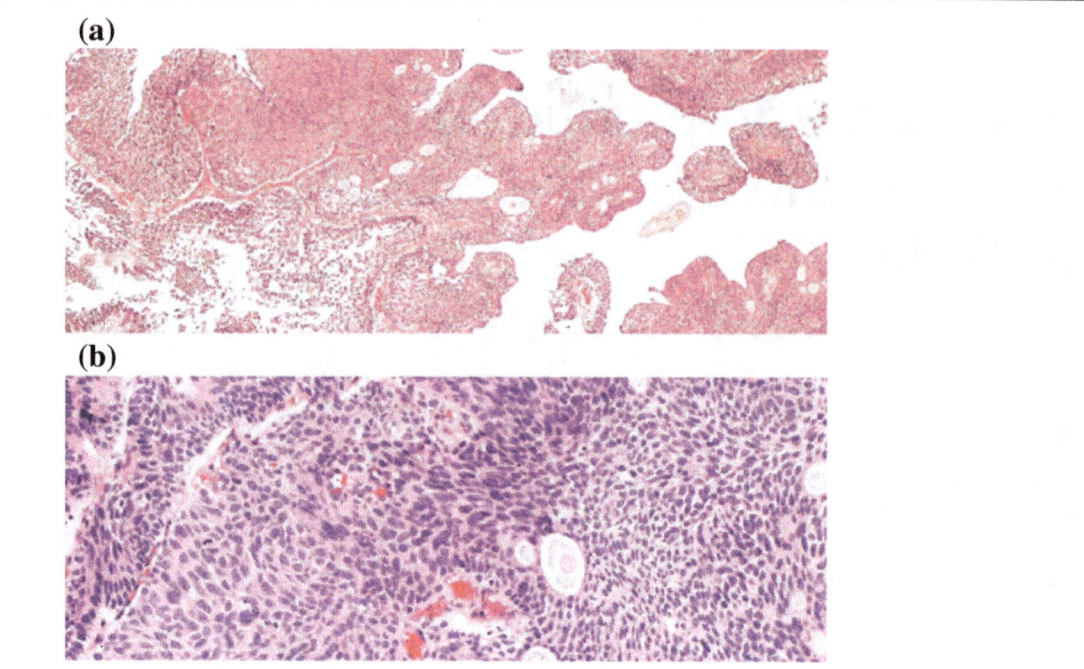

Figure 1 pT1 urothelial cell carcinoma. Patient's original biopsy showing high grade papillary urothelial carcinoma of the bladder. Hematoxylin-eosin stain. **(a)** 40x magnification. **(b)** 100× magnification.

bladder but a fibrinous material emanating from the prostatic urethra and median lobe of the prostate, however no distinct urothelial mass was seen and the bladder urothelium appeared unremarkable. There was evidence of a prostatic adenoma, and the patient was scheduled for TURP via greenlight PVP. During the procedure the prostatic urethra was clearly visualized. The prostatic adenoma seen at the bladder neck was vaporized until the veromontanum was visualized. A white fibrinous material originating from the veromontanum was seen. A prostatic resection was initiated using bipolar TURP. Deep to the fibrinous material, a papillary tumor was visualized. TURP was completed using bipolar without incidence.

Pathological results

Final pathology revealed intestinal type epithelium in a background of necrosis and inflammatory debris together with invasive adenocarcinoma with extensive intestinal differentiation (Figure 2a-d). The specimens were found to stain strongly positive for CK20, CK7, and villin (Figure 3a-c). Beta-catenin showed strong cytoplasmic and membranous staining (Figure 3d). In addition, the tumors were negative for uroplakin, CDX-2, PSA (Figure 4), and PSAP staining. Final urine cytology contained atypical urothelial cells suspicious for malignancy.

Follow-up

Due to the histological appearance of the prostatic tumor, the patient underwent a colonoscopy to rule out a primary colonic malignancy. Multiple diverticula were found in the sigmoid colon and six sessile polyps were biopsied from the ascending and descending colon, all of which were found to be benign. In addition the patient underwent a CT urogram, which was without evidence of a filling defect or bladder primary. The patient was thus given the diagnosis of primary adenocarcinoma of the prostatic urethra. He was evaluated for radical cystectomy and was deemed very high risk for operative management due to his severe chronic pulmonary obstructive disease (COPD). He underwent an oncology evaluation including PET CT scan demonstrating no evidence of metastatic disease. Based on this evaluation, the patient declined to undergo exenterative surgery due to concerns for decreased quality of life. A decision was thus made for him to undergo local aggressive trans-urethral resection with adjuvant multimodal therapy including 42 days of Intensity Modulated Radiotherapy (IMRT) and radiosensitizing oral capecitabine chemotherapy (900 mg po qd × 6 weeks). Capeitabine versus a platinum-based chemotherapy was chosen as the patient had several contraindications to platihum-based chemotherapy including hearing loss, CKD, and peripheral neuropathy. His PSA remains low at 0.074.

Discussion

Mucin-producing urothelial-type adenocarcinoma of the prostate is an exceedingly rare diagnosis, and one that is poorly understood thus far. It is thought to arise from precursor lesions (urethritis glandularis and glandular

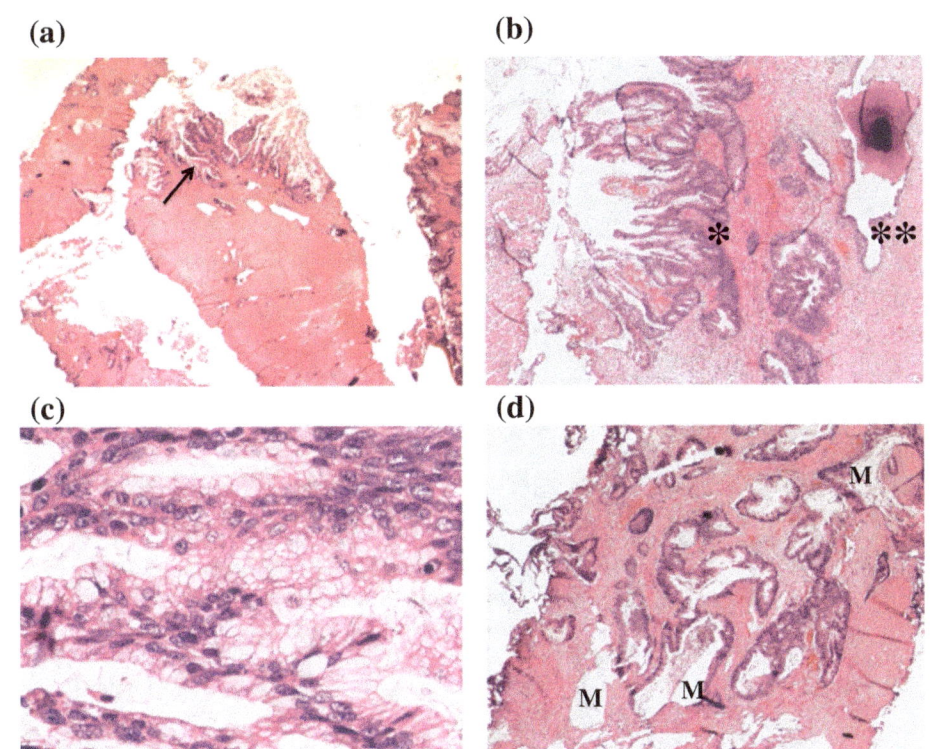

Figure 2 TURP prostate chip specimen. Hematoxylin-eosin stain. **(a)** 10× magnification, arrow demonstrates adenocarcinoma of the prostate with complex glandular arrangement. **(b)** 40× magnification, adenocarcinoma (*) at the edge of the TURP fragments which contrasts with nearby benign prostatic glands (**). **(c)** 400× magnification, demonstrating extensive intestinal differentiation. **(d)** 40× magnification, adenocarcinoma with extensive mucin (M) dissecting into the prostatic stroma.

metaplasia) found in the prostatic urethra or prostatic ducts [1,5]. The published case reports of this disease have helped to determine some of the clinical and pathological features.

In 1996, Tran and Epstein reported the first two cases of mucinous adenocarcinoma arising from the prostatic urethra. In both cases, the patient presented with obstructive urinary symptoms. The gross pathology of the tumors revealed mucin lakes lined by tall columnar epithelium, one specimen of which contained mucin-positive signet ring cells. Both patients had a negative colonoscopy and cystoscopy to rule out bladder and colon primaries, and both had low PSA values. The patients remained without evidence of disease with short-term follow-up following radical retropubic prostatectomy in the first patient and external beam radiotherapy in the second [2].

Curtis, et al. in 2005 described an additional two cases. One man presented with urinary retention, bilateral flank pain, microhematuria, and renal insufficiency and the other with a nodule on digital rectal exam. Again the patients had a low PSA and a negative cystoscopy and colonoscopy work-up. The first patient underwent TURP for bladder outlet obstruction, and shortly after was found have liver metastases and died from disseminated intravascular coagulation. The second patient was treated with

radical prostatectomy with bilateral lymph node dissections, and remained with no evidence of disease for 16 months of follow-up [3].

Osunkoya, et al. in 2007 published 15 cases identified between 1990 and 2006, the largest collection to date. All patients presented with an element of urinary obstructive symptoms, however other symptoms included mucosuria (20%), hematuria (13.3%), and urinary tract caliculi (20%). The PSA remained <1.5 in 9/10 patients throughout follow-up. Treatment included TURP in 7/15 and radical pelvic resection in 8/15, including 5 radical prostatectomies (3 of which underwent adjuvant therapy), 2 cystoprostatecomies, and 1 pelvic exenteration. Among these men, 53% died of their disease at an average of 49.2 months from presentation, and all 8 men undergoing radical resection had evidence of extraprostatic extension, 4 of whom developed metastatic disease to the lungs, liver, pelvic side wall, and/or testes. The two men initially described by Tran and Epstein as having no evidence of disease at short-term follow-up both eventually died of their disease at 13 and 63 months [4].

This large collection of cases encompassed only 0.02% of their consult service for prostate cancer. In addition, this description of cases was the first to truly highlight the aggressiveness of the disease with a clinical course

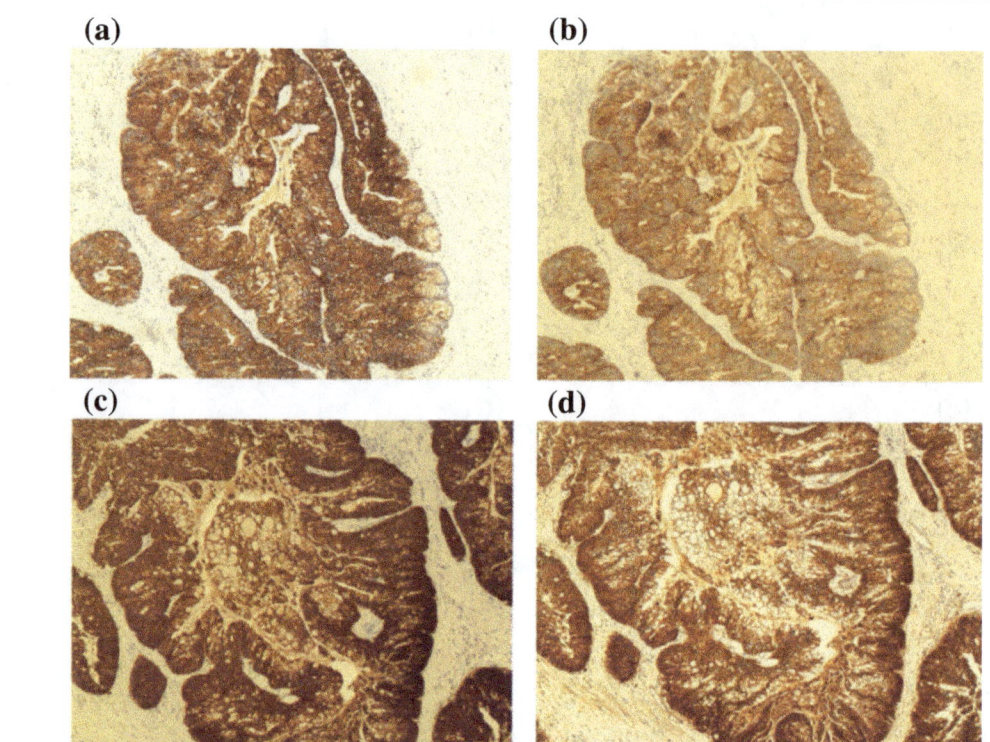

Figure 3 Surgical specimen and positive pathological staining. (a) Diffusely positive staining for CK20. **(b)** Diffusely positive staining for CK7. **(c)** Diffusely positive staining for villin. **(d)** Mostly cytoplasmic positive staining for beta-catenin.

that differs drastically from the common adenocarcinoma of the prostate. In these cases, bone metastases were not present at time of progression, and progression of disease to death was more common and rapid [4].

All case reports thus far have helped to identify the histologic features and the immunohistochemical staining that can help differentiate this disease on pathology. Precursor lesions identified in men include glandular metaplasia of the prostatic urethra (53%) and villous features

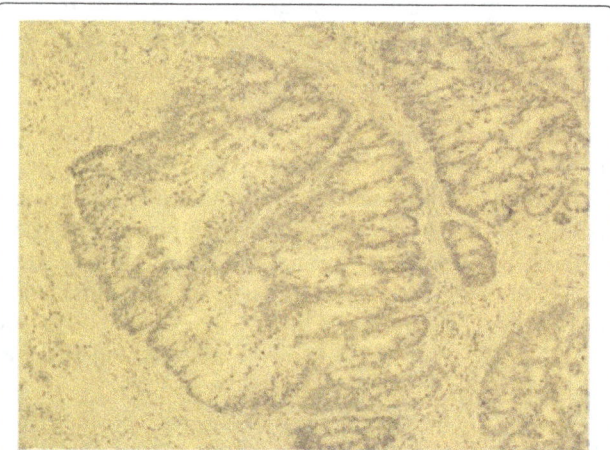

Figure 4 Surgical specimen and negative pathological staining. Diffusely negative staining for PSA.

(47%). All specimens contained mucin pools lined by pseudostratified columnar mucinous epithelium with varying degrees of cytologic atypia. Other less commonly demonstrated patterns include necrosis, signet ring cells, and perineural invasion [1-4].

Curtis, et al. identified that in comparison to prostatic adenocarcinoma with mucin production, both urothelial-type adenocarcinoma arising in the prostatic urethra and secondary adenocarcinoma of colonic origin involving the prostate were PSA and PSAP negative and CK20 positive. In addition they proposed that a colonic primary would stain negative for CK7 and 34βE12 (high molecular weight cytokeratin) while a prostatic primary would stain positive [3]. Osunkoya, et al. corroborated these findings, in addition to identifying that 10/15 specimens in their study also stained negative for beta-catenin and CDX-2 [4]. Tamboli, et al. demonstrated that villin staining was useful in differentiating the primary tumor, as it was positive in colonic adenocarcinoma but negative in urothelial carcinoma with glandular differentiation [6]. However villin is also positive in primary enteric-type adenocarcinoma of the urinary tract, and therefore not helpful in distinguishing this diagnosis from colonic metastases.

Conclusion

Using the work of our predecessors, we were able to diagnose the case reported here with primary mucin-producing urothelial-type adenocarcinoma of the prostatic urethra. We obtained an immunohistochemical profile including PSA, PSAP, CK7, CK20, CDX-2, and villin. This in addition to a negative colonoscopy and CT urogram helped to differentiate between prostatic adenocarcinoma with mucin production from secondary lesions from colon or bladder to suggest a diagnosis of primary urothelial-type adenocarcinoma of the prostatic urethra. As evidenced by previous case reports, making the correct diagnosis in this disease early is crucial. First, it may save the patient multiple invasive procedures and work-up to exclude other primaries. In addition, the distinction from prostatic adenocarcinoma with mucin production is critical, as the disease described here is more aggressive and deadly. It cannot be treated with hormonal therapy and assigning a Gleason score is rendered useless. Continuing to gather data and case reports will be crucial to help determine the clinical behavior and to identify the optimal treatment for this rare and aggressive disease.

Consent

Written informed consent was obtained from the patient for publication of this case report and any accompanying images. A copy of the written consent is available for review by the Series Editor of this journal.

Abbreviations

TURP: Trans-urethral resection of prostate; TURBT: Trans-urethral resection of bladder tumor; PSA: Prostate-specific antigen; PSAP: Prostatic-specific acid phosphatase; CK7: Cytokeratin 7; CK20: Cytokeratin 20; CDX-2: Caudal type homeobox 2.

Competing interests

The authors declare that they have no competing interests.

Authors' contributions

EMS wrote the manuscript and made the revisions. JWR performed the pathological evaluation and provided the slides for pathology. HAM, JKP, and AKK treated the patient. HAM obtained written informed consent from the patient for submission of this case report. All authors read and approved the final manuscript.

Author details

[1]Columbia University College of Physicians and Surgeons, 630 W. 168th St, New York, NY 10032, USA. [2]UC San Diego Health System, 200 W. Arbor Drive #8897, San Diego, CA 92103-8897, USA. [3]VA San Diego Healthcare System, 3350 La Jolla Village Dr. (113), San Diego, CA 92161, USA.

References

1. Bohman KD, Osunkoya AO: **Mucin-producing tumors and tumor-like lesions involving the prostate: a comprehensive review.** *Adv Anat Pathol* 2012, **19**:374–387.
2. Tran KP, Epstein JI: **Mucinous adenocarcinoma of urinary bladder type arising from the prostatic urethra. Distinction from mucinous adenocarcinoma of the prostate.** *Am J Surg Pathol* 1996, **20**:1346–1350.
3. Curtis MW, Evans AJ, Srigley JR: **Mucin-producing urothelial-type adenocarcinoma of the prostate: report of two cases of a rare and diagnostically challenging entity.** *Mod Pathol* 2005, **18**:585–590.
4. Osunkoya AO, Epstein JI: **Primary mucin-producing urothelial-type adenocarcinoma of prostate: report of 15 cases.** *Am J Surg Pathol* 2007, **31**:1323–1329.
5. Uchijima Y, Ito H, Takahashi M, Yamashina M: **Prostate mucinous adenocarcinoma with signet ring cell.** *Urology* 1990, **36**:267–268.
6. Tamboli P, Mohsin SK, Hailemariam S, Amin MB: **Colonic adenocarcinoma metastatic to the urinary tract versus primary tumors of the urinary tract with glandular differentiation: a report of 7 cases and investigation using a limited immunohistochemical panel.** *Arch Pathol Lab Med* 2002, **126**:1057–1063.

15

Testicular prostheses in patients with testicular cancer - acceptance rate and patient satisfaction

Klaus-Peter Dieckmann[1*†], Petra Anheuser[1†], Stefan Schmidt[2], Benjamin Soyka-Hundt[1], Uwe Pichlmeier[3], Philipp Schriefer[4], Cord Matthies[2], Michael Hartmann[4] and Christian G Ruf[2]

Abstract

Background: The loss of a testicle to cancer involves much emotional impact to young males. Little is known about the number of patients with testicular germ cell tumour (GCT) who would accept a testicular prosthesis. Also, knowledge about the satisfaction of implant recipients with the device is limited.

Methods: A retrospective chart analysis was performed on 475 consecutive GCT patients. Prior to orchiectomy, all patients were offered prosthesis insertion. Acceptance of implant was noted along with age, clinical stage, histology and year of surgery. 171 implant recipients were interviewed using an 18 item questionnaire to analyze satisfaction with the prosthesis. Statistical analysis involved calculating proportions and 95% confidence intervals. Multivariate analysis was performed to look for interrelations between the various items of satisfaction with the implant.

Results: 26.9% of the patients accepted a prosthesis. The acceptance rate was significantly higher in younger men. Over-all satisfaction with the implant was "very high" and "high" in 31.1% and 52.4%, respectively. 86% would decide again to have a prosthesis. Particular items of dis-satisfaction were: implant too firm (52.4%), shape inconvenient (15.4%), implant too small (23.8%), position too high (30.3%). Living with a permanent partner had no influence on patient ratings. Multivariate analysis disclosed numerous inter-relations between the particular items of satisfaction.

Conclusions: More than one quarter of GCT patients wish to have a testicular prosthesis. Over-all satisfaction with implants is high in more than 80% of patients. Thus, all patients undergoing surgery for GCT should be offered a testicular prosthesis. However, surgeons should be aware of specific items of dis-satisfaction, particularly shape, size and consistency of the implant and inconvenient high position of the implant within the scrotum. Appropriate preoperative counselling is paramount.

Keywords: Testicular cancer, Testicular prosthesis, Orchiectomy, Masculinity, Quality of life, Body appearance

Background

The loss of a testicle due to cancer has considerable impact on the sexual life and over-all quality of life in survivors of patients with testicular germ cell tumour (GCT) because this is felt to be a threat to masculinity by many patients [1]. That loss is associated with feelings of uneasiness or shame about impaired body appearance in one quarter of the patients and roughly one third of GCT patients do actually miss or have previously missed their lost testicle [2]. Not surprisingly, younger men perceive the loss of a testicle more often a humiliating situation than older men do [3]. From a practical point of view, replacement of a testicle by a testicular prosthesis is technically simple, and only few surgical complications are to be expected [4,5]. Generally, questions surrounding the quality of life have increasingly gained attention among physicians caring for GCT patients [6]. However surprisingly, despite the ever increasing total number of reports relating to GCT, the issue of testicular implants has been addressed only sporadically. The first testicular prosthesis was implanted in 1941 [7]. Technical refinements regarding the material of the device were reported subsequently [8] until the silicone-made testicular prosthesis was introduced in 1973 [9]. That type of implant is still in use with only few modifications made [10,11]. There are some reports on the technical feasibility of testicular

* Correspondence: DieckmannKP@t-online.de
†Equal contributors
[1]Department of Urology, Albertinen-Krankenhaus Hamburg, Hamburg, Germany
Full list of author information is available at the end of the article

prosthesis insertion and on surgical problems relating to this procedure [12-15], but very few studies have systematically explored the patient view on testicular implants. In particular, little information exists as to how many patients would accept an implant in the case of orchiectomy for GCT and how those having received such a device are satisfied with it. Remarkably, none of the current international guidelines on treatment of GCT address the option of prosthesis implantation subsequent to orchiectomy [16-19]. We retrospectively looked to our sample of testis cancer patients to find out how many of them accepted an implant and if there were any associations with age and oncological characteristics. Further, we asked recipients of testicular prostheses about their satisfaction with the implant using a questionnaire.

Methods

Since 1997, it was the policy of our department to offer the implantation of a testicular prosthesis to patients undergoing surgery for GCT and who were not older than 60 years. From January 1997 to June 2014 a total of 507 patients underwent inguinal orchiectomy for testicular cancer. We retrospectively analyzed the patient files and noted whether or not the patient had been offered and if so whether they had accepted a testicular prosthesis. To look for any association of prosthesis acceptance with clinical characteristics, the following parameters were registered additionally: patient's age, histology of GCT, and clinical stage. To look for any temporal association of implant acceptance, the year of orchiectomy was noted. 475 patients (293 pure seminoma, 183 nonseminoma) qualified for further analysis.

The patient perception of living with a testicular implant was studied by interviewing the recipients with a structured questionnaire after obtaining written informed consent from the patients. Only adult patients were asked to participate in the study. To obtain a sufficient number of patients for a meaningful statistical analysis, the questionnaire was sent to implant recipients of three Hamburg based testicular cancer units (Albertinen-Krankenhaus, Bundeswehr-Krankenhaus, Universitätsklinikum Eppendorf). Candidates for interview were defined by the diagnosis of unilateral testicular germ cell tumour and by having the implant for at least half a year and no longer than 10 years. The response rate was 41% and a total of 171 questionnaires were available for analysis. The questionnaire involved 18 questions (see Additional file 1) with multiple choice answers and one question with free-text answering. The study had been approved by the institutional ethical committee of the Theologisches Seminar Elstal (Wustermark).

Statistical analysis

The data of both parts of the study were filed in a commercially available system (Microsoft Excel) prior to

further analysis. The final statistical analysis was accomplished by using descriptive statistical methods performed with the SAS software package (version 9.3, SAS Institute, Inc., Cary, NmC, USA) on Windows platform. To derive exact confidence intervals for multinominal parameters, StatXact (Version 9.0, Cytel Software Corporation) was applied. Pre-defined hypotheses were subjected to statistical analysis. For nominal variables, Chi-square tests were applied. Exact Cochran-Armitage trend tests were employed for testing ordered binominal populations and the exact Jonckhere Terpstra tests for doubly ordered contingency tables, respectively. Ordinal variables between two groups were tested using Mann-Whitney tests. For multivariable assessment of the probability of acceptance logistic regression models were derived [20].

Results

A total of 128 patients of the unselected GCT cohort accepted a testicular prosthesis (26.9%). Tables 1 and 2 show the acceptance rates in subgroups and the associations with clinical parameters. The acceptance rate did not change over time. The only significant association was with age (Cochran Armitage Trend Test p = 0.0058). The acceptance rate was 30.5% in patients younger than

Table 1 Acceptance rate of testicular prostheses in unselected cohort of GCT patients

	Total	With prosthesis	
	n (%)	n (%)	95% CI
Total sample	475 (100)	128 (26.9)	23.0%; 31.2%
Histology*			
Seminoma	293 (100)	81 (27.6)	22.6%; 33.1%
Nonseminoma	182 (100)	47 (25.8)	19.6%; 32.8%
Clinical stage* *			
CS1	313 (100)	91 (29.1)	24.1%; 24.4%
CS 2	138 (100)	32 (23.2)	16.4%; 31.1%
CS 3	24 (100)	5 (20.8)	7.1%; 42.2%
Age at diagnosis§			
≤20 years	16 (100)	4 (25.0)	7.3%; 52.2%
>20 - ≤ 30 years	103 (100)	34 (33.0)	24.1%; 43.0%
>30 - ≤ 40 years	206 (100)	61 (29.6)	23.5%; 36.4%
>40 - ≤ 50 years	113 (100)	25 (22.1)	14.9%; 30.9%
>50 - ≤ 60 years	37 (100)	4 (10.8)	3.0%; 25.4%
Treatment#			
1997 - 2003	143 (100)	35 (24.5)	17.7%; 32.4%
2004 – 2009	167 (100)	55 (32.9)	25.9%; 40.6%
2010 – 2014	165 (100)	38 (23.0)	16.8%; 30.2%

*histology: chi-square test p = 0.66.
**clinical stage: Cochran-Armitage Trend Test p = 0.07.
§age at diagnosis: Cochran-Armitage Trend Test p = 0.006, significant.
#episode of treatment: Cochran-Armitage Trend Test p = 0.38.
CI 95% confidence intervals.

Table 2 Acceptance of prosthesis – logistic regression model

Parameter	Odds ratio	95% Wald CI		p-value*
Age (years)				0.05
≤20 vs. > 30 - ≤ 40	1.06	0.31	3.62	
>20 - ≤ 30 vs. > 30 - ≤ 40	1.28	0.75	2.17	
>40 - ≤ 50 vs. > 30 - ≤ 40	0.64	0.37	1.11	
>50 - ≤ 60 vs. > 30 - ≤ 40	0.28	0.09	0.82	
Histology				0.50
Seminoma yes vs. no	0.84	0.52	1.38	
Clinical stage				0.33
CS2 vs. CS1	0.71	0.43	1.15	
CS3 vs. CS1	0.70	0.23	1.93	
Year of treatment				0.09
2004 - 09 vs. 1997 – 2003	1.65	0.99	2.74	
2010-14 vs. 1997 – 2003	1.06	0.61	1.82	

*Wald chi square; CS clinical stage; CI confidence intervals.

40 years while it was 19.3% in the older age group. The parameter "age" remained almost significant (p = 0.0503) upon multivariate analysis.

The statistical analysis of the questionnaire was somewhat hampered by the fact that some of the 171 patients did not answer to every question. So, sample size varies with each question (Table 3). The majority of implant recipients (77.4%) were living with a permanent partner and the majority had the device for more than 2 years (74.3%). 4.8% required additional surgery. To "look normal with regard to the genital region" was rated "extremely important" or "important" in 53% and 32% of patients, respectively. Accordingly, 98% of the responders regarded the preoperative offer of an implant important. However, preoperative counseling with respect to testicular prosthesis insertion was valued "too short" by 31% and even "insufficient" by 8.5%. With respect to the physical appearance of the implant, 52.4% valued the consistency "too firm" and 15.4% rated the shape of the implant "not convenient" with most of the dissatisfied men saying it was "too round". 9.8% sensed the implant as a foreign body. Size of the implant was regarded "too small" by 23.8% while 30.3% criticized a "too high" position of the implant within the scrotum.

Despite dissatisfaction with several particular items, the over-all satisfaction with the implant was very high and high in 31.1% and 52.4%, respectively. Accordingly, 86.1% would opt again for receiving an implant in the case of orchiectomy.

Living with or without a permanent partner had no influence on any of the patient ratings. However, multivariate analysis disclosed several significant associations between the physical attributes of the implant (Table 4). Inappropriate size of the implant was associated with perceived excess weight of the device and with inconvenient shape, respectively. Inappropriate position within the scrotum correlated with insufficient weight of prosthesis. The appraisal "too firm" was associated with inconvenient shape and with inappropriate position. Over-all satisfaction was significantly higher in patients having the prosthesis for more than two years (p = 0.015; exact Jonckhere-Terpstra Test). Over- all satisfaction was 54.5% in patients who required additional treatment, while it was 85.6% among those without such procedures (p = <0.001, exact Mann-Whitney Test). Likewise, 87.3% of the patients opting again for a prosthesis were (very well and well) satisfied while only 60.8% deciding against redoing the implant were so. Over-all satisfaction was significantly associated with appropriate size of the implant, as well as with shape and consistency (Table 5).

Discussion

Surprisingly few studies have so far explored patient attitudes to receiving a prosthesis to replace a testicle that has been lost to cancer. It is thus valuable to note that more than one quarter of GCT patients (26.9%) in the present series decided to have such a device. Expectedly, testicular implants are more frequently requested by younger patients. This observation has already been made previously [15,21,22] and it is also in close accordance with the experience that body appearance is of greater importance to younger men [3].

Adshead et al. noted lower acceptance rates in married men and in those living in steady relationship [23]. We could not directly confirm this observation because we did not look to the marital status of the patients in our retrospective analysis. The inverse association of steady relationship and prosthesis acceptance appears probable as older men are more frequently married or live in steady relationship than younger men.

The likelihood of accepting a prosthesis decreases with age and likewise with the probability of living in steady relationship. Clinical stage and histology of the GCT did not influence the decision to have an implant in the present study.

The acceptance rate of 26% in our series is somewhat lower than the rates of 55% [15], 46% [24], and 43% [25] reported earlier. Our report is in line with the 24% rate found in a large and unselected GCT population from Swedish hospitals [3] and it is not significantly different from the rate of 30% reported in a British series [23]. The reasons for the large differences regarding the acceptance rates among the reported series remain elusive. Selection in favour of young patients [24] could represent one possible bias, and chance due to small sample size [25] another. A patient's wish to have a prosthesis is a complex decision [26]. As documented in a Swedish survey on survivors of GCT, 32% of patients reported

Table 3 Results of questionnaire regarding patients' satisfaction with testicular implant

Question	Eligible (n)	Answer	(%)	95% CI
Married	167	yes	50.3	41.4%; 59.2%
Living with permanent partner	164	yes	77.4	69.5%; 84.0%
Time living with implant	168	<1 year- 2 years > 2 years	14.9	9.3%; 22.3%
			10.7	5.8%; 17.4%
			74.4	65.7%; 81.8%
Additional surgery after implant insertion	170	yes	4.7	2.1%; 9.6%
Normal appearance with two testicles: important?	168	very important	53.6%	44.1%; 62.6%
		important	31.3	23.2%; 40.6%
Being offered a prosthesis, preoperatively	169	important	98.2	94.2%; 99.6%
Size of the implant	164	too large	9.8	5.0%; 16.3%
		too small	23.8	16.3%; 32.3%
Weight of the implant	166	too heavy	6.6	2.9%; 12.5%
		Just right	91	84.4%; 95.2%
Shape of implant	169	not right	15.4	9.7%; 22.5%
Consistence of implant	164	too firm	52.4	43.4%; 61.1%
Position of implant within scrotum	165	too high	30.3	22.0%; 39.6%
Any particular feeling with the implant	164	convenient	16.5	10.0%; 24.6%
		inconvenient	4.3	1.5%; 9.7%
		strange	9.1	4.6%; 16.0%
Problems with implant during physical exercise	164	no	92.1	85.8%; 96.1%
Concerns about future problems with the implant	164	no	89.0	82.7%; 93.6%
Counseling before implant placement	164	too short	31.1	22.7%; 40.5%
		Insufficient	8.5	4.2%: 14.9%
After all, would you have an implant again?	165	yes	86.1	79.1%; 91.4%
Over-all satisfied with implant	164	very well	31.1	22.2%; 41.0%
		satisfied	52.4	42.1%; 62.4%
		just so	12.2	6.5%; 20.0%
		no	4.3	7.4%; 1.2%

feelings of loss and uneasiness or even shame secondary to the excision of a testicle. Acceptance rates of testicular prostheses are in close accordance with the prevalence of feelings of reduced masculinity secondary to orchiectomy.

As revealed in the second part of the present study, preoperative counselling is highly valued by the patients. Thus, the way and extent of professional advice prior to orchiectomy for TC will probably represent one cornerstone in patient decision-making regarding testicular implants [27].

In contrast to other reports, we did not find a trend to higher acceptance rates in recent years [3,24].

With regard to surgical complications, 4.7% of our patients required additional surgery. This result is well in line with the previously reported incidence of surgical complications of 2.6% to 8% following testicular prosthesis insertion [4,14,15,28-30] and noteworthy, it is not higher than the 8% complication rate encountered after inguinal orchiectomy [31]. We did not experience ruptures of prosthesis or spontaneous extrusion but we did replace three devices because of shrinkage (Figure 1).

The over-all aesthetic results of testicular implants are far from ideal and this is probably the most important result of the present study. Dissatisfaction mostly relates to consistency (too firm), inappropriate size (too small), shape (too round), and to the position within the scrotum (too high). As revealed by multivariate analysis, there are numerous cross-associations between these items of satisfaction. Noteworthy, most of the previous studies reported very similar results (Table 6) [21,23,24,28,32,33]. Only one study from France revealed a somewhat higher degree of satisfaction with the particular aesthetic results [34]. The reasons for unfavourable aesthetic outcome are probably

Table 4 Significant associations between various items of satisfaction with prosthesis

	Size of prosthesis			
	Too much	Just right	Too small	
Weight of prosthesis				p = 0.032*
Too heavy	18.8%	4.6%	7.9%	
Right	81.3%	95.4%	81.6%	
Too light	-	-	10.5%	
Shape of prosthesis				p = 0.002#
Inconvenient	31.3%	8.3%	28.2%	
Just right	68.8%	91.7%	71.8%	
	weight of prosthesis			
Position within scrotum				p = 0.023§
Right	81.8%	69.6%	-	
Not right	18.2%	30.4%	100%	
	shape of prosthesis			
Consistency of prosthesis				p = 0.017#
Too firm	75%	48.6%		
Convenient	25%	51.4%		
	consistency of prosthesis			
Position of prosthesis				p = 0.035*
Right	61.6%	76.9%		
Too high	38.4%	23.1%		

*Exact Jonckhere Terpstra test.
#chi square test.
§Exact Cochran Armitage Trend Test.

three-fold: iatrogenic (i.e. physician-made), manufacturer-made, and nature-related. Consistency (too firm) and shape (too round) are probably related to technical and economic aspects of the manufacturing process but (hopefully), improvement should be possible as soon as

manufacturing companies acknowledge the problem. Inappropriate size of implants appears to be an avoidable problem because it is the surgeon's duty to insert the best-fitting prosthesis intra-operatively. A 33% dissatisfaction rate regarding the size (too small and too large) of the implants as noted in our series is rather surprising because, it is quite simple to select the appropriate size of the device from three or four available sizes. Yet, four previous studies also reported a very similar degree of dissatisfaction with size indicating that this kind of criticism is not uncommon. Dissatisfaction with size is much influenced by the patient's emotional appraisal of the implant. It is likely that dissatisfaction with prosthetic size is based on both, surgeon-related and patient-related misconceptions. To minimize such discontent, patients should be invited to actively participate in preoperative decision-making upon implant-size.

The inconvenient position of many of the implants (mostly too high within the scrotum) is probably related to two reasons. First, it could be a surgical failure to create a scrotal pouch not large enough to host the implant. The proper surgical procedures have been extensively reviewed [24,35]. However, inescapable biological processes i.e. tissue reactions to the synthetic material introduced into the scrotal cavity do possibly account for shrinkage of the scrotal wall and thus cause upward migration of the prosthesis. Analogous scarring reactions are known from breast implants [36]. It is thus paramount for the surgeon to both, employ the appropriate surgical technique to ensure the right position of the implant and to advise the patient preoperatively about biological processes that may cause inadvertent high position. Noteworthy, inappropriate high scrotal position of implants has been observed in 27-39% by two previous studies [21,23]. Positioning of the prosthesis appears to be a major problem and every surgeon performing such operations should be aware of the issue [37].

Table 5 Significant associations of over-all satisfaction with particular items of patients' satisfaction

	Over-all satisfaction with testicular implant					
	Very well	Well	Just so	Not much	Not at all	
Size						p < 0.001*
Too large	7.8%	13.3%	-	-	33%	
Right	82.4%	65.1%	31.6%	100%	-	
Too small	9.8%	21.7%	68.4%	-	66.6%	
Shape						p = 0.001**
Inconvenient	5.9%	14.0%	35.0%	-	66.7%	
Convenient	94.1%	86.0%	65.0%	100%	33.3%	
Consistence						p < 0.001**
Too firm	20.0%	62.8%	75.0%	100%	100%	
Convenient	80.0%	37.2%	25.0%	-	-	

All numbers represent percentages, *Jonckhere-Terpstra Test, **Cochran-Armitage Trend Test.

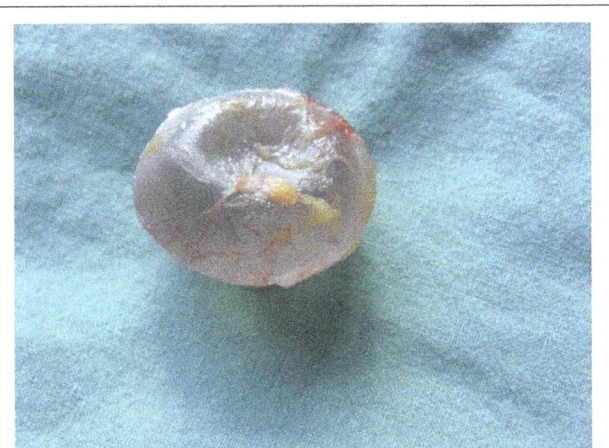

Figure 1 Silicone testicular prosthesis removed from scrotum because of shrinkage: note prune-like appearance of the device.

The answers to the more general questions of the questionnaire indicated a high rate of over-all contentment with the implant. No more than 10% of patients are concerned about potential health problems originating from the implant. Only few patients complained of inconvenient feelings with the implant (3.7%). Some bother with the device upon physical activity was reported by 8.6% which is less than the 15% rate reported previously [21]. Accordingly, the over-all satisfaction rate is 83% (very high and high satisfaction). But noteworthy, over-all satisfaction is significantly influenced by contentment with the particular items of size, shape and consistency of the implant.

86% of patients would decide again to have a prosthesis. This rate is identical to the result reported by Yossepowitch et al. [21] and it is similar to other studies reporting rates of slightly more than 90% [23,24,28,32-34] (Table 6).

Limitations of our study include the lack of a control group of patients who declined the offer of a prosthesis. Exploring the particular reasons for deciding against a prosthesis could aid in obtaining a clearer image of young men's emotions when they are confronted with the necessity of losing a testicle to cancer. Another drawback could be the lack of information regarding the manufacturer of the prostheses. Thus, relating specific items of dissatisfaction to the products of particular companies is not possible. On the other hand, strengths of our investigation include, first, the multicentric method of obtaining data on patients' perception of testicular implants and second, the investigation of the largest patient sample studied for this purpose to date. The latter two issues probably aid to keep selection bias low. The employment of multivariate statistical methods to reveal cross-associations of various items of satisfaction with implants is perhaps another strength of the present study.

Conclusions

More than one quarter of all testis cancer patients wish to receive a prosthesis to replace the excised testicle. Over-all satisfaction with the testicular implant is very high. All patients undergoing surgery for testis cancer should be advised about the availability of a testicular implant. However, it must be noted that there is considerable dissatisfaction with several particular attributes of the implants, e.g. shape, consistency, size, and high intrascrotal position. Urologic surgeons performing prosthesis insertion should be aware of these issues. Appropriate preoperative counselling with participation of the patient upon selection of implant size is paramount.

Table 6 Survey of the literature – patients' satisfaction with testicular implants

Author	Year	Country	(n)	Method	Over-all satisfaction	Have it again	Shape	Position	Size	Consistency	Other
Petersen [24]	1992	Ger	119	I	93%	93%	-	high 11%	19% too large / 14% too small	10% too firm	-
Lynch [32]	1992	UK	19	Q	79%	95%	-	-	-	-	—
Incrocci [33]	2001	NL	22	Q	95%	95%	-	-	-	29% inconvenient	–
Adshead [22]	2001	UK	71	Q	73%	90%	32% not right	27% not right	37% inconvenient	-	30% weight inconvenient
Boy [28]	2002	Ger	39	Q	97%	-	-	3% too high	36% not right	3% too firm	partners' rating: 55% satisfied
Xylinas [34]	2008	F	63	Q	96%	96%	12% not right	3% not right	5% too small	12% too firm	2% too cold
Yossepowitch [21]	2011	Isr	86	I	88%	86%	-	39% too high	27% not right	73% too firm	after 2005 better results

I interview; Q questionnaire.

Competing interests
The authors declare that they have no competing interests.

Authors' contributions
KPD conceived the study, designed the study, made substantial contributions to analyzing and interpreting the data, main contributor to drafting of manuscript. PA contributed to patient enrolment, made substantial contributions to analyzing and interpreting the data, coordinated multicentric data collection. SS contributed substantially to patient enrolment, contributed to drafting of manuscript, BSH contributed substantially to patient enrolment, made substantial contributions to analyzing and interpreting the data. UP contributed to designing of the study, carried out the statistical analysis, contributed to drafting and revising the manuscript. PS contributed substantially to patient enrolment, contributed in analyzing data. CM contributed to conceiving and designing of the study, contributed to patient enrolment, contributed to coordination of multicentric data collection. MH contributed to patient enrolment, contributed to drafting and critically revising the manuscript. CGR participated in designing of the study and contributed substantially to establishing of the questionnaire, contributed to analyzing data, contributed to drafting of manuscript. All authors read and approved the final manuscript.

Acknowledgements
Dr. Olaf Netzband and Raphael Ikogho substantially contributed to recruitment of patients.

Author details
[1]Department of Urology, Albertinen-Krankenhaus Hamburg, Hamburg, Germany. [2]Department of Urology, Bundeswehrkrankenhaus Hamburg, Hamburg, Germany. [3]Institute of Medical Biometry and Epidemiology, Universitätsklinikum Eppendorf, Hamburg, Germany. [4]Department of Urology, Universitätsklinikum Eppendorf, Hamburg, Germany.

References
1. Rossen P, Pedersen AF, Zachariae R, von der Maase H. Sexuality and body image in long-term survivors of testicular cancer. Eur J Cancer. 2011;48(4):571–8.
2. van Basten JP, Jonker-Pool G, van Driel MF, Sleijfer DT, van de Wiel HB, Mensink HJ, et al. Fantasies and facts of the testes. Br J Urol. 1996;78(5):756–62.
3. Skoogh J, Steineck G, Cavallin-Ståhl E, Wilderäng U, Håkansson UK, Johansson B, et al. Feelings of loss and uneasiness or shame after removal of a testicle by orchidectomy: a population-based long-term follow-up of testicular cancer survivors. Int J Androl. 2011;34(2):183–92.
4. Marshall S. Potential problems with testicular prostheses. Urology. 1986;28(5):388–90.
5. Beer M, Kay R. Testicular prostheses. Urol Clin North Am. 1989;16(1):13313–8.
6. Kim C, McGlynn KA, McCorkle R, Erickson RL, Niebuhr DW, Ma S, et al. Quality of life among testicular cancer survivors: a case-control study in the United States. Qual Life Res. 2011;20(10):1629–37.
7. Girdansky J, Newman HF. Use of a vitallium testicular implant. Am J Surg. 1941;53:514.
8. Prentiss RJ, Boatwright DC, Pennington RD, Hohn WF, Schwarzt MH. Testicular prosthesis: materials, methods and results. J Urol. 1963;90(2):208–10.
9. Lattimer JK, Vakili BF, Smith AM, Morishima A. A natural-feeling testicular prosthesis. J Urol. 1973;110(1):81–3.
10. Rosen JS, Benson RCJ. Testicular prostheses. Semin Urol. 1984;2(3):176–9.
11. Böhm WD, Biedermann M, Hackel W, Baumann I, Knoch HG. Hodenprothesen-Chirurgie. Ergebnisse einer ambulanten klinischen Prüfstudie. Z Urol Nephrol. 1989;82:253–8.
12. Bodiwala D, Summerton DJ, Terry TR. Testicular prostheses: development and modern usage. Ann R Coll Surg Engl. 2007;89(4):349–53.
13. Weissbach L, Janssen PL, Bach D. Die Implantation von Hodenprothesen unter Berücksichtigung psychischer Aspekte. Urologe A. 1979;18(3):151–6.
14. Herrinton LJ, Brox T, Greenland S, Finkle WD, Cattolica E, Shoor S. Regarding: a cohort study of systemic and local complications following implantation of testicular prostheses. Ann Epidemiol. 2003;13(1):73–7.
15. Robinson R, Tait C, Clarke N, Ramani V. Is it safe to insert a testicular prosthesis at the time of radical orchidectomy for testis cancer - an Audit of 904 Men Undergoing Radical Orchidectomy. BJU Int 2014, Aug 28. doi:10.1111/bju.12920. [Epub ahead of print].
16. Albers P, Albrecht W, Algaba F, Bokemeyer C, Cohn-Cedermark G, Fizazi K, et al. EAU guidelines on testicular cancer: 2011 update. Eur Urol. 2011;60(2):304–19.
17. Oldenburg J, Fosså SD, Nuver J, Heidenreich A, Schmoll HJ, Bokemeyer C, et al. Testicular seminoma and non-seminoma: ESMO Clinical Practice Guidelines for diagnosis, treatment and follow-up. Ann Oncol. 2013;24 Suppl 6:vi125–32.
18. Beyer J, Albers P, Altena R, Aparicio J, Bokemeyer C, Busch J, et al. Maintaining success, reducing treatment burden, focusing on survivorship: highlights from the third European consensus conference on diagnosis and treatment of germ-cell cancer. Ann Oncol. 2013;24(4):878–88.
19. Motzer R, Agarwal N, Beard C, Bhayani S, Bolger GB, Buyyounouski MK, et al. Testicular cancer. J Natl Compr Canc Netw. 2012;10(4):502–35.
20. Armitage P, Berry G, Matthews JNS. Statistical methods in medical research. 4th ed. Oxford: Blackwell Scientific; 2002.
21. Yossepowitch O, Aviv D, Wainchwaig L, Baniel J. Testicular prostheses for testis cancer survivors: patient perspectives and predictors of long-term satisfaction. J Urol. 2011;186(6):2249–52.
22. Schmidt S, Wagner W, Ruf CG. Evaluation der persönlichen Entscheidungskriterien für oder gegen die Implantation einer Hodenprothese. J Reproduktionsmed Endokrinol. 2013;10(5):309. Abstract.
23. Adshead J, Khoubehi B, Wood J, Rustin G. Testicular implants and patient satisfaction: a questionnaire-based study of men after orchidectomy for testicular cancer. BJU Int. 2001;88:559–62.
24. Petersen W, Hartmann M. Erfahrungen mit Hodenprothesen. Sexualmedizin. 1992;21:168–72.
25. Gritz ER, Wellisch DK, Wang HJ, Siau J, Landsverk JA, Cosgrove MD. Long-term effects of testicular cancer on sexual functioning in married couples. Cancer. 1989;64(7):1560–07.
26. Chapple A, McPherson A. The decision to have a prosthesis: a qualitative study of men with testicular cancer. Psychooncology. 2004;13:654–64.
27. Rieker PP. How should a man with testicular cancer be counselled and what information is available to him? Semin Urol Oncol. 1996;14:17–23.
28. Boy D, Carl P. Akzeptanz von Silikonhodenprothesen im Langzeitverlauf. Urologe A. 2002;41:462–9.
29. Turek PJ, Master VA, Group TPS. Safety and effectiveness of a new saline filled testicular prosthesis. J Urol. 2004;172(4 Pt 1):1427–30.
30. Auberget JL, Bourlaud G, Timbal Y. Testicular prosthesis. Study of complications, apropos of 63 cases].[Article in French]. J Urol (Paris). 1989;95(8):505–6.
31. Anheuser P, Kranz J, Will J, Dieckmann KP. Complications associated with inguinal orchiectomy and scrotal orchiectomy].[Article in German]. Urologe A. 2014;53(5):676–82.
32. Lynch MJ, Pryor JP. Testicular prostheses: the patient's perception. Br J Urol. 1992;70:420–2.
33. Incrocci L, Bosch JL, Slob AK. Testicular prostheses: body image and sexual functioning. BJU Int. 1999;84:1043–5.
34. Xylinas E, Martinache G, Azancot V, Amsellem Ouazana D, Saighi D, Flam T, et al. Testicular implants, patient's and partner's satisfaction: a questionnaire-based study of men after orchidectomy].[Article in French]. Prog Urol. 2008;18(13):1082–6.
35. Lawrentschuk N, Webb DR. Inserting testicular prostheses: a new surgical technique for difficult cases. BJU Int. 2005;95:1111–4.
36. Zahavi A, Sklair ML, Ad-El DD. Capsular contracture of the breast: working towards a better classification using clinical and radiologic assessment. Ann Plast Surg. 2006;57(3):248–51.
37. Foster RS. Role of urologist in testis cancer management. Editorial Comment. J Urol. 2013;186:1251.

16

Procalcitonin and C-reactive protein in urinary tract infection diagnosis

Rui-Ying Xu[*], Hua-Wei Liu, Ji-Ling Liu and Jun-Hua Dong

Abstract

Background: Urinary infections are a common type of pediatric disease, and their treatment and prognosis are closely correlated with infection location. Common clinical manifestations and laboratory tests are insufficient to differentiate between acute pyelonephritis and lower urinary tract infection. This study was conducted to explore a diagnostic method for upper and lower urinary tract infection differentiation.

Methods: The diagnostic values of procalcitonin (PCT) and C-reactive protein (CRP) were analyzed using the receiver operating characteristic curve method for upper and lower urinary tract infection differentiation. PCT was determined using chemiluminescent immunoassay.

Results: The PCT and CRP values in children with acute pyelonephritis were significantly higher than those in children with lower urinary tract infection (3.90 ± 3.51 ng/ml and 68.17 ± 39.42 mg/l vs. 0.48 ± 0.39 ng/ml and 21.39 ± 14.92 mg/l). The PCT values were correlated with the degree of renal involvement, whereas the CRP values failed to show such a significant correlation. PCT had a sensitivity of 90.47% and a specificity of 88% in predicting nephropathia, whereas CRP had sensitivity of 85.71% and a specificity of 48%.

Conclusions: Both PCT and CRP can be used for upper and lower urinary tract infection differentiation, but PCT has higher sensitivity and specificity in predicting pyelonephritis than CRP. PCT showed better results than CRP. PCT values were also correlated with the degree of renal involvement.

Keywords: Urinary tract infections, Acute pyelonephritis, Receiver operating characteristic curve, Procalcitonin

Background

Urinary infections are a common pediatric disease and their treatment and prognosis are closely correlated with infection location. Common clinical manifestations and laboratory indices are insufficient for acute pyelonephritis and lower urinary tract infection (UTI) differentiation. Differentiating between these diseases is particularly difficult for infants and children, but is necessary because pyelonephritis poses a risk of renal parenchyma involvement, which can lead to renal scar formation, as well as high blood pressure and end stage renal failure in adults [1-4]. Smellie et al. conducted a retrospective analysis of 52 patients with neo-development or progressive renal scars and revealed that 50 of these patients had a medical history of urinary infection diagnosis or treatment delay [5]. Therefore, finding a technically easy and practical method for differentiating between upper and lower UTIs is urgently required.

As of this writing, ^{99m}Tc-dimercaptosuccinic acid (DMSA) scintigraphy is a commonly adopted method for diagnosing severity degrees of renal involvement and pyelonephritis. However, this method is costly and is radioactive to sick children [6,7]. Procalcitonin (PCT) is a type of hormonal activity-free calcitonin precursor protein that can serve as an early diagnosis index of serious bacterial infections and septicemia; PCT is also correlated with the severity of bacterial infections [8-10]. PCT is a satisfactory predictor of renal parenchymal involvement in acute and late renal scars [11-13].

We retrospectively analyzed the diagnostic value of PCT in differentiating upper and lower UTIs, and the serum PCT level was determined and compared with C-reactive protein (CRP) and peripheral blood leukocyte count; the results were subsequently analyzed using the receiver operating characteristic (ROC) method [14,15].

* Correspondence: zjqqcn@126.com
Department of Pediatrics, Qilu Hospital of Shan Dong University, Jinan 250012, China

Methods

Clinical data

A total of 46 patients with suspected acute pyelonephritis (APN) were enrolled in the study from December 1999 to April 2002. Twenty-eight females and 18 males were included, and their ages ranged from 2 months old to 14 years old. Inclusion criteria were as follows: fever (≥38.5°C, axillary), pyuria (≥10 white blood cells per high-power field on a spun urine), and positive urine culture (≥100,000 colonies/ml of a single organism, clean catch). Exclusion criteria included the presence of renal calculi, obstructive uropathy, and a neurogenic bladder.

We performed a retrospective analysis of 46 admitted patients, who underwent a DMSA renal scan for suspected APN within 5 d of admission.

APN was confirmed using radioactive nuclide ^{99m}Tc-DMSA scanning. Diagnostic criteria were based on literature [16]. APN is indicated when radioactive renal parenchyma distributional sparse or loss areas are present and accompanied with swelling or a normal kidney profile. Renal scar formation is diagnosed when the kidney volume decreases (manifested by cortex attenuation, renal morphologic abnormality, or profile shrinkage) with wedge-shaped defects. Renal involvement was graded as follows: renal injury <25% was considered mild; renal injury between 25% and 50% was considered moderate; and renal injury >50% was considered serious. Lower UTI was diagnosed by normal DMSA scanning. If the first DMSA findings were abnormal, another analysis was performed six months later. All patients underwent renal ultrasonography within 48 h of admission, and eight recurrent patients underwent voiding cystourethrography within 7 d of admission.

Experimental methods

The patients were divided into APN and lower UTI groups and treated as follows: two weeks of antibiotic treatment for APN patients, 7 d of antibiotic treatment for Lower UTI. PCT was determined using chemiluminescent immunoassay, and CRP was scored using nephrometry scoring. PCT, CRP, and white blood cell (WBC) count were determined within 24 h of admission and 24 h of therapy.

Statistical analysis

All data were normally distributed and were presented as mean ± standard error ($\bar{x} \pm s$). *T*-tests were performed to compare the means between groups. Cut points were selected and then graded according to normal, basically normal, susceptible, basically abnormal, and abnormal classifications. Se and Sp of each point were calculated. Taking Se as the ordinate, which represented true positive rate, and (1-Sp) as the abscissa, which represented false positive rate. ROC curves were drawn by the SPSS 10.0 software to calculate the area under curve and standard errors. The cut-off value was selected

Table 1 Comparisons of the laboratory outcomes between groups ($\bar{x} \pm s$)

Group	PCT (ρ/ng · ml^{-1})	CRP (ρ/mg · l^{-1})	WBC number (/mm^3)
Lower urine tract infection	0.48 ± 0.39	21.39 ± 14.92	14068 ± 6870
Acute pyelonephritis	3.90 ± 3.51	68.17 ± 39.42	15882 ± 7350
p value	< 0.01	< 0.01	> 0.05

depending on $(Sp + Se)_{max}$. Values of different indices were also compared.

This study was conducted in accordance with the declaration of Helsinki and with approval from the Ethics Committee of Qilu Hospital of Shan Dong University. Written informed consent was obtained from all parent or guardian of participants.

Results

Clinical data

A total of 46 children with urinary infection who received treatment between December 1999 and April 2002 were enrolled. Among the patients, 18 were males and 28 were females. Their ages ranged from 2 months old to 14 years old: six males and two females were <1 year old, seven males and 11 females were between 1 year old and 3 years old, and five males and 15 females were ≥3 years old. A total of 38 patients had primary urinary infection, and eight had recurrent infection. Their courses of disease ranged from 3 d to 1 yr. These patients did not receive antibiotic treatment within half a month before hospitalization. A total of 40 patients had body temperatures between 38.5°C and 40.0°C. Twenty-eight patients presented UTI symptoms, such as frequent micturition, urgent micturition, odynuria, and crying while urinating. Twelve patients had lumbago and percussion pain

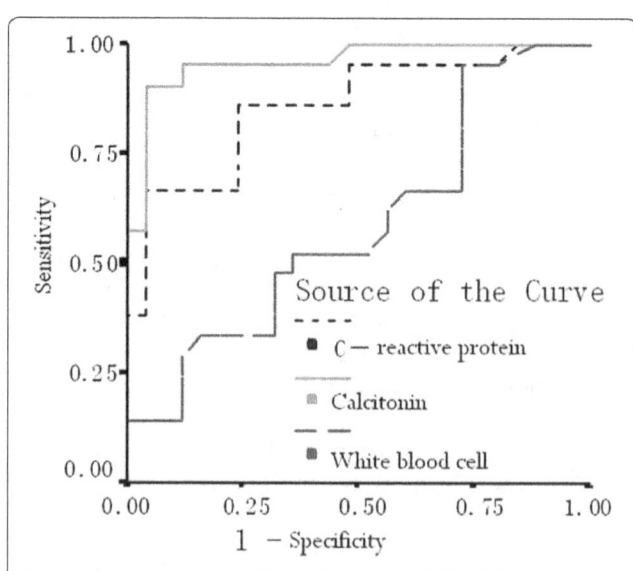

Figure 1 Comparison of the ROC curves of PCT, CRP and WBC.

Table 2 Comparisons of the diagnostic values of PCR, CRP, and WBC for acute pyelonephritis (%)

Index	Diagnostic reference value	Sensitivity	Specificity	Accuracy	Positive predictive value	Negative predictive value
PCT	1 ng/ml	90.47	88	89	87	95
CRP	20 mg/l	85.71	48	86.9	58	80
WBC	15000/mm^3	57	44	71	46	55

on kidney region. Four patients had macroscopic hematuria. Eight patients, six of whom were less than 2 years old, presented non-specific signs and symptoms, such as emesis, diarrhea, abdominal pain, poor disposition and appetite, icterus, and irritability. All patients had WBC count >10/HP, 12 had red blood cell count of >5/HP, and 11 had urine protein between + and ++, according to routine urine examination. Urine culture outcomes of all patients were positive.

Radioactive nuclide scanning

Twenty-one out of the 46 patients were diagnosed with APN. Among these patients, two had non-obstructive hydronephrosis, one presented renal scar formation, and two presented vesico-ureteral reflux.

PCT and CRP

The serum PCT and CRP levels of the APN group were significantly higher than those of the lower UTI group $(3.90 \pm 3.51$ ng/ml and 68.17 ± 39.42 mg/l vs. 0.48 ± 0.39 ng/ml and 21.39 ± 14.92 mg/l, $P < 0.01$, Table 1). Correlation analysis demonstrated that PCT and CRP were in a significantly positive correlation with a correlation coefficient of 0.729 $(P < 0.01)$.

Curve analysis

As shown in Figure 1, the areas under the PCT, CRP, and WBC curves were 0.958, 0.858, and 0.588, respectively. Group comparison analysis showed no significant difference between the areas under the PCT and CRP curves $(P > 0.05)$, whereas the areas under these curves were significantly larger than that under the WBC curve $(P < 0.01)$. PCT and CRP are highly accurate in diagnosing APN.

Diagnostic values

The diagnostic values of PCT, CRP, and WBC were 1.0 ng/ml, 20 mg/l, and 15,000/mm^3, respectively. The sensitivity and specificity of PCT in predicting nephropathia were 90.47% and 88%, whereas those of CRP were 85.71% and 48%, respectively. PCT had the highest sensitivity and specificity in diagnosing APN among the three methods. The results are summarized in Table 2.

Renal involvement degrees

The PCT level in children with serious renal involvement $(8.60 \pm 2.80$ ng/ml) was noticeably higher than that in children with mild and moderate renal involvement $(2.02 \pm 1.24$ ng/ml; $P < 0.01)$, whereas the WBC counts and serum

CRP levels among children with different renal involvement degrees did not show significant differences $(P > 0.05)$. High PCT value indicates a serious degree of renal involvement. The results are summarized in Table 3.

PCT and CRP outcome analysis

The pre- and post-treatment PCT levels were 3.90 ± 3.51 and 1.78 ± 2.07 ng/ml, respectively, and the pre- and post-treatment CRP levels were 68.17 ± 39.42 and 26.13 ± 15.14 mg/l. Great differences in the PCT and CRP were observed before and after treatment $(P < 0.05)$. Follow-up DMSA scanning at six months after treatment showed that 15 children completely recovered, three showed great improvement, two showed little improvement, and one failed to show noticeable improvement. The child who failed to show noticeable improvement had renal scars with vesico-ureteral reflux before the hospitalization, whereas all other patients had no new scars. The serum PCT levels (>10 ng/ml) in three patients before treatment were still higher than 5 ng/ml after treatment.

Discussion and conclusion

Urinary infections are a common type of pediatric disease, and their treatment and prognosis are closely associated with infection position. Differentiating APN from lower UTI is difficult based on common clinical manifestations and laboratory indices, and thus, an easier and more practical method is necessary. ^{99m}Tc-DMSA scintigraphy is currently a commonly adopted method for the diagnosis of renal involvement degree and pyelonephritis; this method is costly and radioactive to children [6,7].

PCT is a hormonal activity-free calcitonin precursor protein [17]. Studies have proven that PCT serves as an early diagnosis index for bacterial infections and septicemia, and that PCT is also correlated with the severity of bacterial infections; thus, PCT can predict prognosis [18-20]. Normally, PCT does not increase when local

Table 3 Comparisons between laboratory outcomes and renal involvement degrees

Index	Mild and moderate degrees (n = 15; DMSA scanning)	Serious degree (n = 6; DMSA scanning)	p values
PCT (ρ/ng·ml^{-1})	2.02 ± 1.24	8.60 ± 2.80	< 0.01
CRP (ρ/mg·l^{-1})	62.0 ± 42.83	82.02 ± 28.56	> 0.05
WBC (cells/mm^3)	14990 ± 2611	15980 ± 3220	> 0.05

bacterial infection occurs unless the infection is accompanied by systemic inflammatory reactions [20-22]. Most authors conclude that PCT has satisfactory diagnostic accuracy and an interesting clinical value for APN, with a sensitivity and a specificity ranging from 70% to 100% and 70% to 97%, respectively, across studies and thresholds [23-28]. However, a Belgium team found lower sensitivity and specificity (68% and 23%, respectively) with no obvious difference regarding the cut-off of the characteristics of the population [29]. The average PCT and CRP levels of children with APN were greatly higher than those of children with lower UTI ($P < 0.01$). In contrast, peripheral blood WBC counts were not significant in predicting renal involvement.

The areas under the PCT, CRP, and WBC curves were 0.958, 0.858, and 0.588, respectively, and the group analysis shows that the areas under both PCT and CRP curves displayed significant differences compared with those under the WBC curve. Both PCT and CRP can serve as laboratory indices for APN diagnosis, but PCT has a higher diagnostic value than CRP. The ROC curves in this study illustrate the same findings.

This study shows that PCR and CRP have a significant correlation with a Pearson's correlation coefficient of 0.729 ($P < 0.01$). CRP also has a diagnostic value for APN diagnosis, but its sensitivity, specificity, and accuracy are low. The sensitivity and specificity of CRP, PCT, and WBC are related to a real positive patient's threshold determination. Based on the results in this study, 1 ng/ml PCT can be considered the reference value because PCT has sensitivity of 90.47%, specificity of 88%, accuracy of 89%, a positive predictive value of 87%, and a negative predictive value of 95% in predicting APN.

The PCT and CRP levels after treatment significantly decreased compared with those before treatment ($P < 0.05$). Both PCT and CRP can be used for observing pathogenesis and curative effect. The serum PCT value in children with serious renal involvement was significantly higher than in those with mild and moderate renal involvement. A high PCT value indicates serious renal involvement. Therefore, PCT can be applied in predicting renal involvement. The CRP values in children with serious renal involvement were higher than those in children with mild and moderate renal involvement, but no significant difference was observed.

Serum PCT determination is an easy and cheap method for diagnosing APN, and only a small amount of blood is required. Furthermore, PCT is highly stable in serum, and the entire PCT determination process can be completed in 2 h. PCT determination can also be used for the observing curative effect and follow-up pathogenic condition sequelae, prognostic judgment, and renal involvement degree prediction. Serum PCT determination can be used in clinical settings.

The following are the limitations of this study. First, the sample size used was small. Second, PCT was initially measured with a quantitative immunoluminometric assay, but this assay was progressively replaced by PCT-sensitive KRYPTOR. Third, validation studies, threshold analyses, and studies on various effects are required before PCT is deemed safe for daily use.

Competing interests
I declare that we have no financial competing interests.

Authors' contributions
R-YX participated in the design of the study, statistical analysis and drafting the manuscript. H-WL helped to carry out the immunoassays and data analysis. J-LL helped collecting blood samples. J-HD has given medical instruction. All authors read and approved the final manuscript.

Acknowledgements
We thank Xiang-Dong Jian who provided medical writing services and technical help.

References

1. Jacobson SH, Eklöf O, Eriksson CG, Lins LE, Tidgren B, Winberg J: Development of hypertension and uraemia after pyelonephritis in childhood: 27 year follow up. *BMJ* 1989, **299**:703–706.
2. Martinell J, Jodal U, Lidin-Janson G: Pregnancies in women with and without renal scarring after urinary infection in childhood. *BMJ* 1990, **300**:840–844.
3. Ransley PG, Risdon RA: Reflux nephropathy: effects of antimicrobial therapy on the evolution of the early pyelonephritic scar. *Kidney Int* 1981, **20**:733–742.
4. Sacks SH, Verrier Jones K, Roberts R, Asscher AW, Ledingham JG: Effect of symptomless bacteriuria in childhood on subsequent pregnancy. *Lancet* 1987, **2**:991–994.
5. Smellie JM, Poulton A, Prescod NP: Retrospective study of children with renal scarring associated with reflux and urinary infect. *BMJ* 1994, **308**:1193–1196.
6. Jakobsson B, Nolstedt L, Svensson L, Söderlundh S, Berg U: 99 m Technetium-dimercaptosuccinic acid scan in the diagnosis of acute pyelonephritis in children: relation to clinical and radiological findings. *Pediatr Nephrol* 1992, **6**:328–334.
7. Ilyas M, Mastin ST, Richard GA: Age-related radiological imaging in children with acute pyelonephritis. *Pediatr Nephrol* 2002, **17**:30–34.
8. Hatherill M, Tibby SM, Sykes K, Turner C, Murdoch IA: Diagnostic markers of infection: comparison of procalcitonin with C reactive protein and leucocyte count. *Arch Dis Child* 1999, **81**:417–421.
9. Tang BM, Eslick GD, Craig JC, Mclean AS: Accuracy of procalcitonin for sepsis diagnosis in critically ill patients: systematic review and meta-analysis. *Lancet Infect Dis* 2007, **7**(3):210–7.
10. Moulin F, Raymond J, Lorrot M, Marc E, Coste J, Iniguez JL, Kalifa G, Bohuon C, Gendrel D: Procalcitonin in children admitted to hospital with community acquired pneumonia. *Arch Dis Child* 2001, **84**:332–336.
11. Mori F, Lakhanpanul M, Verrier-Jones K: Diagnosis and management of urinary tract infection in children: summery of NICE guidance. *Br Med J* 2007, **335**(7616):395–397.
12. Bressans S, Andreola B, Zucchetta P, Montini G, Burei M, Perilongo G, Da Dalt L: Procalcitonin as a predictor of renal scarring in infants and young children. *Pediatr Nephrol* 2009, **24**(6):1199–1204.
13. Nikfar R, Khotaee G, Ataee N, Shams S: Usefulness of procalcitonin rapid test for the diagnosis of acute pyelonephritis in children in the emergency department. *Pediatr Int* 2010, **52**(2):196–198.
14. John AS: Measuring the accuracy of diagnostic systems. *Science* 1988, **240**:1285–1293.
15. Zweig MH, Campbell G: Receiver operating character (ROC) curve plots: a fundamental evaluation toll in clinical medicine. *Clin Chem* 1993, **39**:561–577.

16. Majdm M, Rushton H: **Renal cortical scintigraphy in the diagnosis of acute pyelonephritis.** *Semin Nucl Med* 1992, **22**:98–111.

17. Meisner M, Tschaikowsky K, Schnabel S, Schmidt J, Katalinic A, Schüttler J: **Procalcitonin-influence of temperature, storage, anticoagulation and arterial or venous asservation of blood samples on procalcitonin concentrations.** *Eur J Clin Chem Clin Biochem* 1997, **35**:597–601.

18. Harbarth S, Holeckova K, Froidevaux C, Pittet D, Ricou B, Grau GE, Vadas L, Pugin J: **Geneva Sepsis Network: diagnostic value of Precalcitonin, Interleukin-6, and Interlerkin-8 in critically ill patients admitted with suspected sepsis.** *Am J Respir Crit Care Med* 2001, **164**:396–402.

19. Monneret G, Pachot A, Laroche B, Picollet J, Bienvenu J: **Procalcitonin and calcitonin gene-related peptide decrease LPS-induced TNF production by human circulating blood cells.** *Cytokine* 2000, **12**:762–764.

20. Whang KT, Steinwald PM, White JC, Nylen ES, Snider RH, Simon GL, Goldberg RL, Becker KL: **Serum calcitonin precursors in sepsis and systemic inflammation.** *J Clin Endocrinol Metab* 1998, **83**:3296–3301.

21. Assicot M, Gendrel D, Carsin H, Raymond J, Guilbaud J, Bohuon C: **High serum procalcitonin concentrations in patients with sepsis and infection.** *Lancet* 1993, **341**:515–518.

22. Oberhoffer M, Stonans I, Russwurm S, Stonane E, Vogelsang H, Junker U, Jäger L, Reinhart K: **Procalcitonin expression in human peripheral blood mononuclear cells and its modulation by lipopolysaccharides and sepsis related cytokines in vitro.** *J Lab Clin Med* 1999, **134**:49–55.

23. Karavanaki K, Haliotis FA, Sourani M, Kariyiannis C, Hantzi E, Zachariadou L, Avlonitis S, Papassotiriou I: **DMSA scintigraphy in febrile urinary tract infections could be omitted in children with low procalcitonin levels.** *Infect Dis Clin Pract* 2007, **15**(6):377–381.

24. Kotoula A, Gardikis S, Tsalkidis A, Mantadakis E, Zissimopoulos A, Kambouri K, Deftereos S, Tripsianis G, Manolas K, Chatzimichael A, Vaos G: **Procalcitonin for the early prediction of renal parenchymal involvement in children with UTI: preliminary results.** *Int Urol Nephrol* 2009, **41**(2):393–399.

25. Mantadakis E, Please E, Vouloumanou EK, Karageorgopoulos DE, Chatzimichael A, Falagas ME: **Serum procalcitonin for prediction of renal parenchymal involvement in children with urinary tract infections: a meta-analysis of prospective clinical studies.** *J Pediatr* 2009, **55**(6):875–881.

26. Van Nieuwkoop C, Bonten TN, Van't Wout JW, Kuijper EJ, Groeneveld GH, Becker MJ, Koster T, Wattel-Louis GH, Delfos NM, Ablij HC, Leyten EM, van Dissel JT: **Procalcitonin reflects bacteremia and bacterial load in urosepsis syndrome : a prospective observational study.** *Crit Care* 2010, **14**(6):R206.

27. Shen JN, Chang HM, Chen SM, Hung TW, Lue KH: **The role of procalcitonin for acute pyelonephritis and subsequent renal scarring in infants and young children.** *J Urol* 2011, **186**(5):2002–8.

28. Leroy S, Fernandez-Lopez A, Nikfar R, Romanello C, Bouissou F, Gervaix A, Gurgoze MK, Bressan S, Smolkin V, Tuerlinckx D, Stefanidis CJ, Vsos G, Leblond P, Gungor F, Gendrel D, Chalumeau M: **Association of procalcitonin with acute pyelonephritis and renal scars in pediatric UTI.** *Pediatrics* 2013, **131**(5):870–9.

29. Tuerlinckx D, Vander Borght T, Glupczynski Y, Galanti L, Roelants V, Krug B, de Bilderling G, Bodart E: **Is procalcitonin a good marker of renal lesion in febrile urinary tract infection?** *Eur J Pediatr* 2005, **164**(10):651–652.

Expression of brain derived-neurotrophic factor and granulocyte-colony stimulating factor in the urothelium: relation with voiding function

Seung Mo Yuk[1], Ju Hyun Shin[2], Ki Hak Song[2], Yong Gil Na[2], Jae Sung Lim[2] and Chong Koo Sul[2*]

Abstract

Background: We designed this experiment to elucidate the relationship between the expression of brain derived-neurotrophic factor (BDNF), the expression of granulocyte-colony stimulating factor (G-CSF), and the development of overactive bladder (OAB). In our previous study, the urothelium was observed to be more than a simple mechanosensory receptor and was found to be a potential therapeutic target for OAB. Moreover, neuregulin-1 and BDNF were found to be potential new biomarkers of OAB. Here, we investigated the relationship between changes in the voiding pattern and the expression of BDNF and G-CSF in the urothelium and evaluated the effects of 5-hydroxymethyl tolterodine (5-HMT) on rats with bladder outlet obstruction (BOO).

Methods: A total of 100 Sprague–Dawley rats were divided into the following groups: 20 control rats; 40 BOO rats; and 40 BOO rats administered 5-HMT (0.1 mg/kg). After BOO was induced for 4 weeks, the rats were assessed by cystometrography. The changes in BDNF and G-CSF expression were examined in both separated urothelial tissues and in cultured urothelial cells by reverse transcription polymerase chain reaction (RT-PCR).

Results: BOO rats showed increased non-voiding activity [NVA; (number/10 voidings)] and bladder weight and decreased micturition volume (MV), micturition interval (MI), and micturition time (MT) relative to the controls. Moreover, the 5-HMT administration rats showed decreased NVA and bladder weight and increased MV and MI in comparison to the BOO rats. BDNF and G-CSF expression was increased in BOO rats and decreased following 5-HMT administration. In this model, voiding dysfunction developed as a result of BOO. As a therapeutic agent for OAB, the administration of 5-HMT improved the voiding dysfunction.

Conclusions: BDNF and G-CSF might modulate voiding patterns through micturition pathways and might be involved only in the urothelium. Moreover, the expression of both genes in the urothelium might be related to voiding dysfunction in OAB patients. Thus, the urothelium has an important role in the manifestation of voiding symptoms.

Keywords: Bladder, Brain derived-neurotrophic factor, Granulocyte-colony stimulating factor, Overactivity

Background

Overactive bladder (OAB) is a clinical syndrome that is characterized by the presence of urinary urgency, with or without urgency incontinence, and is usually accompanied by daytime frequency and nocturia in the absence of proven infection or other obvious pathologies [1]. Bladder outlet obstruction (BOO) results in changes in bladder structure and function that include detrusor hypertrophy, elevated detrusor contractile pressure, and detrusor instability, which can result in OAB [2]. Prolonged BOO can also influence the occurrence and severity of OAB by increasing the production of nerve growth factors (NGF) and thereby inducing neuronal enlargement [3].

The urothelium has specialized sensory and signaling properties through which it responds to the chemical and physical environment and engages in reciprocal chemical communication with neighboring nerves in the

* Correspondence: doctor6@daum.net
[2]Department of Urology, Korea Chungnam National University Hospital, College of Medicine, Chungnam National University, Daejeon, South Korea
Full list of author information is available at the end of the article

bladder wall. The detrusor muscle has traditionally been known for having a significant influence on voiding function. However, the urothelium also plays an important role in this process, as evidenced by the effect of changes in urothelial characteristics on the regulation of voiding function. To elucidate the role of the urothelium in voiding function, we have focused solely on this tissue in the absence of the detrusor muscle. In our previous report, we suggested that urothelium-expressed neuregulin-1 and BDNF are potential new biomarkers of OAB [4]. Based on these findings, we believe that the urothelium is more than a simple mechanosensory receptor and may be a potential therapeutic target for OAB treatment. The present study builds upon the work from our previous study by evaluating the relation between voiding dysfunction and the expression of growth factors.

Previous studies has discovered a significant link between BDNF and OAB [4, 5]; however, little is known about whether a significant relationship exists between G-CSF and OAB. Fesoterodine (Pfizer Central Research, Sandwich, UK) is an antimuscarinic drug approved for the treatment of OAB, and is hydrolyzed by a nonspecific esterase to 5-hydroxymethyl tolterodine (5-HMT) [6]. 5-HMT is the active metabolite and is responsible for the antimuscarinic activity of this drug [6]. Antimuscarinics have been found to act in response to muscarinic receptors on detrusor smooth muscle cells to reduce spontaneous myocyte activity during the storage phase [7], thus eventually decreasing the frequency and intensity of detrusor contractions. Hence, the use of 5-HMT as a therapeutic agent of OAB can be used to confirm the presence of OAB, examine the role of BDNF and G-CSF in OAB, and evaluate changes in the urothelium. Here, we evaluated BDNF and G-CSF expression in a BOO rat model and the effect of 5-HMT on their expression both in the urothelium and in cultured urothelial cells (UCs) to understand the relationship between the expression of BDNF and G-CSF and voiding dysfunction. We aimed to test whether 1) OAB occurrence and treatment are related to the BDNF and G-CSF expression, 2) 5-HMT would affect the expression of growth factors on the urothelium, and 3) the urothelium functions as more than a simple mechanosensory receptor in regulating bladder functions.

Methods
Animals
Female Sprague–Dawley rats (250–300 g; Daehan Biolink Co. Ltd, Daejeon, Korea) were used in this study. The experimental protocol was approved by the Animal Ethics Committee of the University of Chungnam, South Korea. The rats were handled according to the NIH guidelines. The sample size needed for evaluating the expression of the different growth factors, as affected by BOO, was

determined. To achieve a power of 0.8, alpha value of 0.05, and sample size rate of 2 for detecting statistical differences, 11 animals would be required as controls.

Group I (20 rats) was the control group, group II (40) comprised BOO rats, and group III (40) comprised BOO rats injected with 5-HMT (0.1 mg/kg) in the rat tail vein (2 times/weeks) for 3 weeks. These doses of 5-HMT generally correspond to the doses used clinically in humans [8]; the 5-HMT was generously provided by Pfizer. The BOO rats were injected with 5-HMT as described by Melman et al. [9]. For inducing BOO, a lower midline incision was made to approach the bladder of each anesthetized rat and to expose the proximal urethra. A 3–0 polypropylene suture was used to tie the proximal urethra with a 24-G angioneedle sheath. After suturing, the angioneedle sheath was removed, leaving the urethra partially obstructed.

Cystometry investigations
The BOO rats were anesthetized 4 weeks after they were injected with 5-HMT. Polyethylene catheters were implanted through the bladder dome and exteriorized at the scapular level. A cystometry procedure was performed in conscious rats 4 days after catheter implantation. A tube was connected to a pressure transducer (Powerlab, ADInstrument, Sydney, NSW, Australia) and an infusion pump (Promed-Tech., Bellingham, Massachusetts, USA) via a 3-way stopcock to record intravesical pressure (IVP) and to infuse saline into the bladder, respectively. Micturition volumes (MV) were recorded with a fluid collector connected to a force displacement transducer (Grass Inst. Co., Quincy, MA, USA). Room-temperature saline was infused into the bladder continuously at a rate of 0.2 ml/min. After the voiding pattern stabilized, the micturition cycles were recorded. The IVP and MV were recorded continuously with a data acquisition system (Chart software v5.5.6, ADInstrument) at a sampling rate of 2000 Hz.

In addition to MV, the following parameters were analyzed based on the cytometry results: micturition pressure (MP, maximum bladder pressure during micturition), basal pressure (BP, minimum bladder pressure between two micturitions), micturition interval (MI), micturition time (MT), and bladder weight (Fig. 1). Pressure values were compared by calculating the difference between BP values.

Tissue preparation
After cystometry, the bladder of each rat was excised at the level of the ureteric orifices and proximal urethral and subsequently weighed. The urothelium and detrusor muscles were separated under microscopic vision with microscissors and microforces. The separated layers from half of the bladder were stored in liquid nitrogen

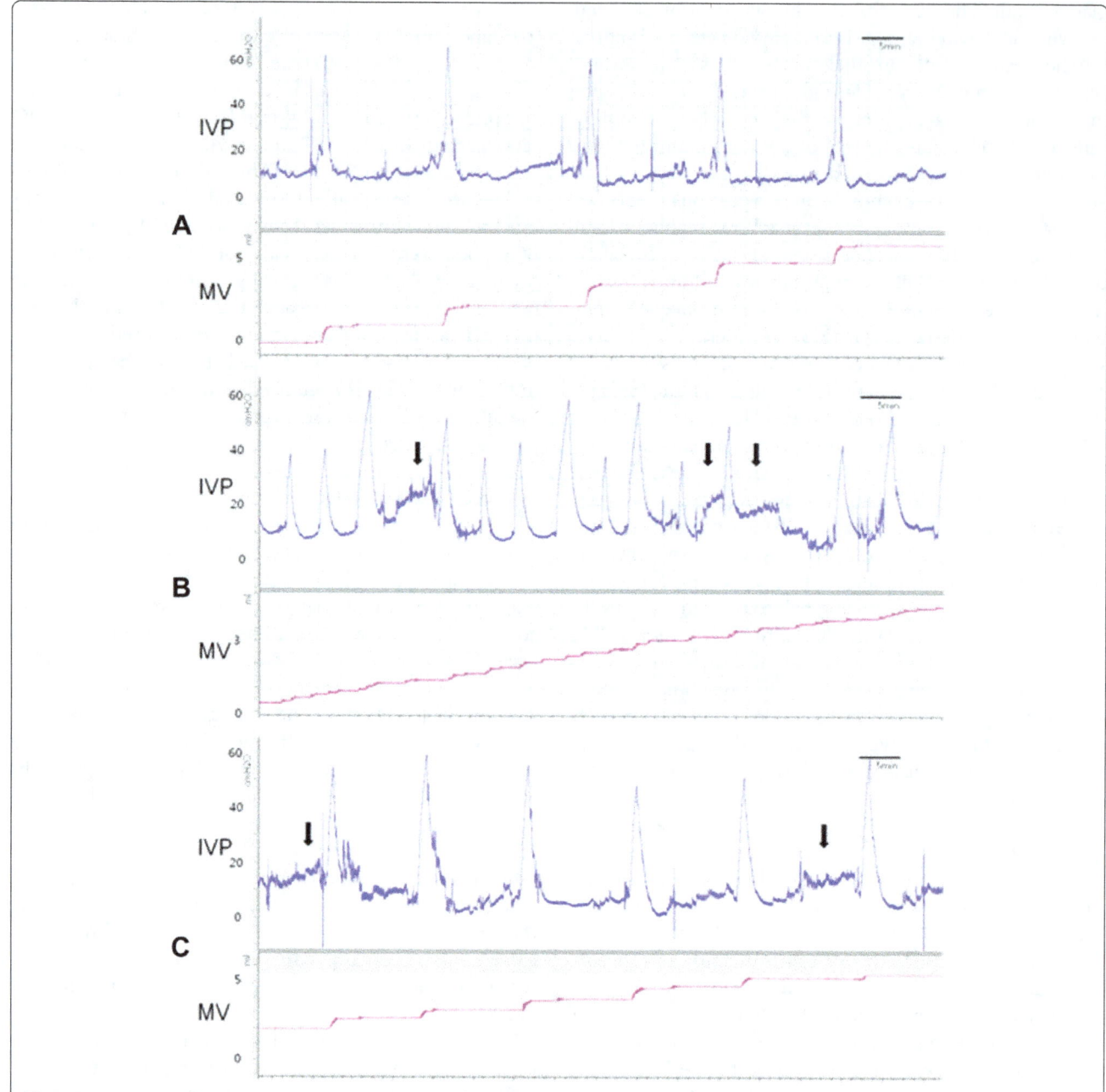

Fig. 1 Representative cystometry results for the different study groups. Representative tracing of the cystometry parameters for intravesical pressure (IVP; cmH2O) and micturition volume (MV; ml). Black arrows represent non-voiding activity (NVA). **A**. Group I (controls). **B**. Group II (BOO rats). **C**. Group III (BOO rats administered 5-HMT)

for reverse transcription polymerase chain reaction (RT-PCR) until needed. The other half of the bladder was used as soon as possible for primary cell cultures.

RT-PCR of urothelium-expressed RNA

Total RNA was extracted from the frozen urothelium using Trizol (Invitrogen, Carlsbad, CA, USA). One milliliter of Trizol was added to the urothelium and homogenized in a 5-ml glass tube. The homogenate was transferred to a 1.0-ml tube and was mixed with 0.2 ml

of 99 % chloroform (Sigma-Aldrich, St. Louis, MO, USA). After incubation for 5 minutes at room temperature, the homogenate was centrifuged at $13,200 \times g$ for 10 minutes at room temperature. The supernatant was transferred to a clean tube, and 1 ml of isopropyl alcohol (Sigma-Aldrich) was added, followed by further centrifugation. After the supernatant was discarded, the pellet was mixed with 0.5 ml of diethylpyrocarbonate (DEPC; Sigma-Aldrich) and centrifuged at $13,200 \times g$ for 10 minutes at room temperature. After discarding the supernatant, the pellet was dried at room temperature, dissolved with DEPC-treated water, and stored at −75 °C. cDNA was then prepared from 1 μg of random priming by using a First-Strand cDNA synthesis kit (Enzynomics, Korea), in accordance with the manufacturer's protocol. It was incubated at 50 °C for 50 minutes, 70 °C for 10 minutes, and finally stored at −20 °C. The primer pair sequences are listed in Table 1. GAPDH was used as the reference gene. After an initial denaturation step at 95 °C for 5 min, an annealing procedure of 35 cycles (58 °C for 30 s), and an extension step (72 °C for 30 s and 72 °C for 5 min), were performed. The PCR products were separated on 1.2 % ethidium-containing agarose gels and photographed under an ultraviolet transilluminator. The band intensities were quantified by densitometry and qualified by Bio-ID (Vilber Lourmat, France).

Urothelial cell culture

UCs were harvested from the bladders of each group using a previously described trypsin-based method (GIbco, Invitrogen, Carlsbad, CA, USA) [10]. The bladder was removed and placed in cold minimal essential medium (MEM; Invitrogen, Carlsbad, CA) supplemented with HEPES (2.5 g/l; Sigma, St. Louis, MO) and containing 1 % penicillin/streptomycin/fungi zone (PSF; Sigma). The bladder was turned inside out and incubated in dispase (2.5 mg/ml; Worthington Biochemical, Lakewood, NJ) overnight at 4 °C. UCs were gently scraped from the underlying tissue, placed in trypsin (0.25 % wt/vol; Sigma) for 10–15 min at 37 °C, and dissociated by trituration. Cells were suspended in MEM containing 10 % FBS (Invitrogen) and centrifuged at 416 × g for 10 min. After the supernatant was removed, the cells were suspended in keratinocyte media (bovine pituitary extract: 60 g/ml, hydrocortisone: 0.5 g/ml, insulin: 5 g/ml, epidermal growth factor: 0.1 ng/ml, gentamicin: 30 g/ml, amphotericin [Bio Whittaker, Walkersville, Maryland]: 15 ng/ml, and human recombinant cholera toxin [Calbiochem, San Diego, California]: 8.3 ng/ml, 2 % FBS [Invitrogen]) with 1 % PSF, centrifuged again, and resuspended in fresh media. Cells were plated on collagen-coated glass coverslips at densities of 50–70 × 10^4 cells/ml. Media was added after 4 hours of

incubation at 37 °C following cell isolation and changed every other day. Cultured UCs were analyzed 48 hours after dissociation.

RT-PCR of primary cultured UCs

RNA was prepared using the Cells-to-cDNA II kit (Ambion Europe Ltd, Huntingdon, UK). The lysates of the cell layer were processed according to the instructions until just before the RT step (i.e., 75 °C for 10 minutes, DNase I digestion at 37 °C for 15 minutes, and 75 °C for 5 minutes). The RNA preparations were stored at −20 °C for a short period. RT was also performed using the kit, according to the instructions using the random decamers provided as well as 5 μl of cell lysate (RNA). The resultant cDNA was diluted 5 times with water and stored at −20 °C. PCR was conducted using primer sets in accordance with the above-described method (Table 1).

Data analysis

All statistical analysis was performed using SPSS, version 20.0 for windows (SPSS Inc., Chicago, IL, USA). A nonparametric Kruskal-Wallis test followed by a post-hoc test (Scheffe's multiple comparison test) were performed for comparisons between the 3 groups. Differences were considered statistically significant when $P < 0.05$. The results are expressed as the mean ± sd.

Results
Animals

One hundred rats were used in the study: group I (20 rats), group II (40 rats), and group III (40 rats). Two rats each died in groups II and III after the BOO procedure. All control groups had a sham operation, and the cystometric investigations were performed after 4 weeks. Two rats in group II and 3 rats in group III were excluded because of failed BOO (i.e., no change in bladder weight and no difference in the voiding pattern compared to the control group). In the final analysis, groups I, II, and III had 20, 36, and 35 rats, respectively.

Cystometry

Group II rats showed increased non-voiding activity [NVA; (number/10 voidings)] and bladder weight and decreased MV, MI, and MT relative to the control group (Table 2). Group III rats showed reduced NVA and bladder weight and increased MV and MI in comparison to group II rats.

RT-PCR results for the urothelium

Group II showed the highest expression of BDNF in the urothelium in comparison to groups I and III. G-CSF expression was significantly higher in group II relative to groups I and III, but did not significantly differ between

Table 1 List of primer sequences used for RT-PCR

Gene	Primer sequence	Product
GAPDH	Forward: CAC GGC AAG TTC AAC GGC AC	189 bp
	Reverse: AGC GGA AGG GGC GGA GAT GA	
BDNF	Forward: CAT TCT TTC CCT CCC TCC TC	360 bp
	Reverse: CAG CTC CAC TTA GCC TCC AC	
G-CSF	Forward: TTG GCC ACT CTC TGG GTA TC	348 bp
	Reverse: GGT GAG CTG TCT CCA GGA AG	

Table 2 Comparison of cystometric parameters and bladder weight between the experimental groups. The results of various cystometric parameters and bladder weight for group I (control), group II (BOO rats), and group III (BOO rats after 5-HMT administration) are shown

Group (n)	TP-BP	MP-BP	MV	MI	MT	NVA	Bladder weight
I (20)	14.0 (a) ±0.97	55.4 (a) ±4.64	0.61 (a) ±0.06	64.7 (a) ±4.36	11.6 (a) ±1.33	0.15 (a) ±0.37	116.5 (a) ±8.26
II (26)	9.5 (b) ±6.95	55.2 (a) ±8.31	0.19 (b) ±0.05	27.4 (b) ±4.26	10.6 (b) ±0.85	2.36 (b) ±0.49	212.1 (b) ±12.00
III (25)	4.9 (c) ±3.51	49.24 (b) ±4.65	0.27 (c) ±0.64	39.3 (c) ±5.91	10.7 (b) ±1.45	1.31 (c) ±0.47	197.4 (c) ±10.66
p-value[1]	0.000	0.001	0.000	0.000	0.017	0.000	0.000

TP, BP, MP: cmH_2O; MV: mL; MT: seconds; bladder weight: mg; NVA (number/10 voidings)
The same letters indicate non-significant differences between groups based on Scheffe's multiple comparison tests
1) Statistical significance among the different groups was tested by a nonparametric Kruskal-Wallis test

groups I and III (Fig. 2). The injection of 5-HMT injection suppressed and partially suppressed the up-regulated mRNA expression of BDNF and G-CSF in BOO rats, respectively. Therefore, the changes in the voiding patterns were related to the expression of BDNF and G-CSF in the urothelium.

Culturing and RT-PCR of UCs
In culture, the UCs proliferated and formed small islands (5–30 cells/island) (Fig. 3). No significant differences were observed in the number of living UCs between groups, indicating that no problems had resulted from the cell harvesting and culturing methods. The results for the cultured UCs were similar to those of the urothelium. The expression of BDNF and G-CSF was upregulated in the UCs of group II compared to that in the control, but was downregulated in group III (Fig. 4). The changes in both growth factors were related to the changes in the voiding patterns.

Discussion
The changes in urothelial BDNF and G-CSF have not been previously observed in other OAB models. This might be due to the fact that neurogenic or myogenic BOO was assessed in these previous studies. This is an experimental model where, in particular, the BOO is "quickly" made instead of clinical OAB-BOO. Detrusor overactivity (DO) is the urodynamic hallmark of OAB,

and the BOO rat can be useful for assessing potential pharmacotherapeutic concepts of DO in humans [11].

Moreover, various voiding patterns following BOO have been reported in this model. DO was identified and recorded as non-micturition-related increases in IVP [12], and a significant increase in MP was observed with this condition [2]. The common result of DO is a markedly shortened MI. The NVA in the present cystometry data consisted of small phasic contractions in the filling bladder. NVA is believed to represent the motor component of a motor/sensory system [13-15] and is accentuated in BOO. Moreover, NVA shows characteristics similar to DO in patients with OAB. Furthermore, tolterodine has been shown to significantly decrease the number and amplitude of NVA [16, 17]. In line with the cystometry results, the voiding pattern of groups II and III had characteristics similar to those for OAB and the treated condition. Hence, the present model is suitable as an experimental model.

In the storage phase, mechanical stretch stimulates the bladder afferents. This mechanosensory information is constantly sent to the central nervous system [18]. Alterations in afferent activity may lead to lower urinary tract dysfunction and is one of the possible mechanisms for OAB [18]. As the urothelium is a mechanosensory receptor, bladder function is influenced according to the changing state of the urothelium. Growth factors also may play a role in bladder function. Moreover, growth

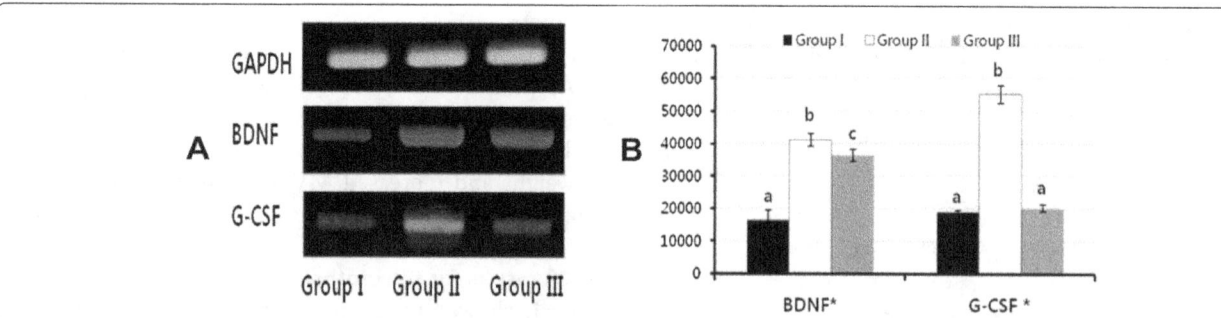

Fig. 2 RT-PCR expression of BDNF and G-CSF in the urothelium. **A.** RT-PCR results. **B.** Densitometry measurements. *indicates statistical significance between groups (p < 0.001) as tested by a nonparametric Kruskal-Wallis test. The same letters indicate non-significant differences between groups based on Scheffe's multiple comparison tests

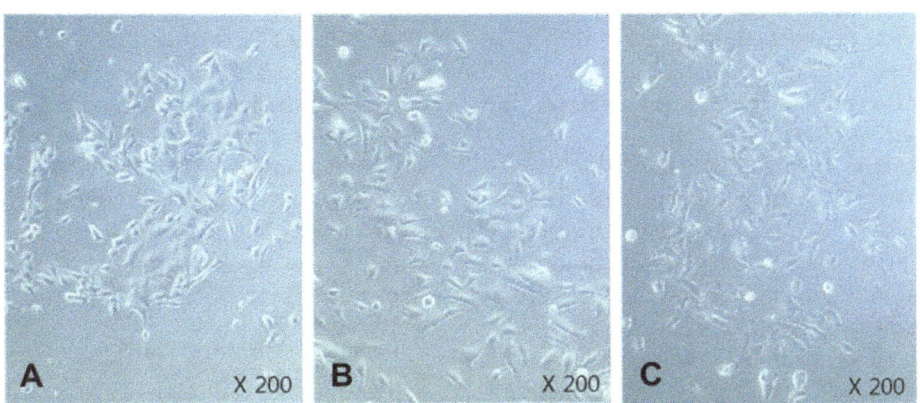

Fig. 3 Cultured urothelial cells from each study group. **A**. Group I (controls). **B**. Group II (BOO rats). **C**. Group III (BOO rats administered 5-HMT)

factors have been found to play a crucial role in various cellular processes such as proliferation, differentiation, migration, apoptosis, and neurodegeneration [19]. Previous research has examined the correlation between OAB and NGF. It was observed that increased NGF expression in the bladder may contribute to storage symptoms (e.g., urgency and frequency) in patients with OAB [20, 21]. In addition, NGF expression in the bladder was found to be associated with the clinical symptoms of OAB [22]. It has become clear that NGF modulates neuronal function along micturition pathways, is involved in multiple bladder pathologies, and serves as a urinary marker of OAB [21]. BDNF, a member of the NGF family, is primarily present in the sensory neuronal cell body in the dorsal root ganglion and is involved in sensory neuronal activation in a variety of animal models [23]. Of note, BDNF synthesis has been shown to be stronger in the bladder after chronic bladder inflammation [5]. Moreover, in patients with bladder pain syndrome/interstitial cystitis, the urinary concentration of BDNF was high at baseline but was significantly reduced after botulinum toxin administration to the bladder trigone [24]. Consistent with this previous finding, BDNF sequestration improved voiding function in rats with

chronic cystitis [5]. Accordingly, BDNF has been found to be a sensitive indicator of the resolution of lower urinary tract disorders by therapeutic management [4].

On the other hand, the G-CSF receptor is markedly upregulated in neurons during cerebral ischemia and has direct effects on neurons, including the reduction of neuronal apoptosis and the stimulation of endogenous neural progenitors [25]. A further mechanism of action for G-CSF in stroke is the mobilization of bone marrow-derived stem cells to participate in neurogenesis and angiogenesis [26]. G-CSF has also been shown to have neuroprotective effects after peripheral axotomy [27]. Previous studies have also investigated G-CSF in terms of the diagnosis and treatment of bladder cancer. However, no prior research has confirmed the relevance of G-CSF to voiding function. In the present study, the functions of G-CSF and BDNF in the urothelium were evaluated at the tissue and cellular level by specifically using only the urothelium and UCs. A similar upregulation of G-CSF and BDNF expression and subsequent downregulation following 5-HMT treatment was observed in BOO rats for both the urothelium and UCs. BOO has been found to induce inflammation, multiple nerve injury, and changes in nerve density [28]. One

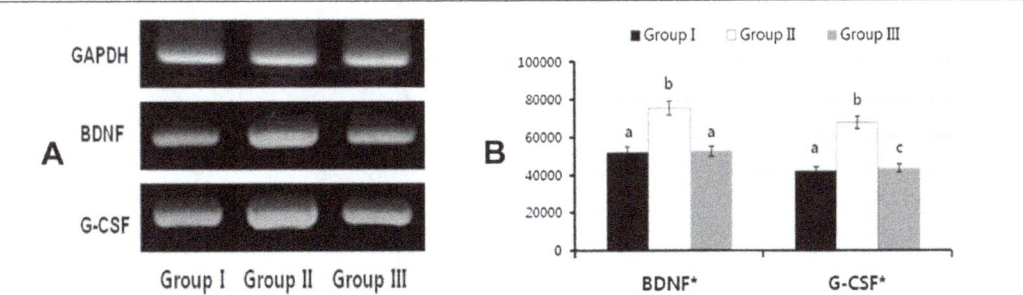

Fig. 4 RT-PCR expression of BDNF and G-CSF in UCs. **A**. RT-PCR results. **B**. Densitometry measurements. *indicates statistical significance between groups (p < 0.001) as tested by a nonparametric Kruskal-Wallis test. The same letters indicate non-significant differences between groups based on Scheffe's multiple comparison tests

effect stemming from neural damage inflicted by BOO might be an increase in the neuroprotective activity of G-CSF. Nonetheless, a clear mechanism, in terms of changes in the expression of these growth factors and their attendant roles, remains unknown.

DO might be attributable to an increase in afferent activation. The proximity of the afferent nerves to the urothelium suggests that chemicals released by the urothelium might alter afferent excitability. Hence, the urothelium could be important in the manifestation of voiding symptoms, and changes in the expression of various urothelial receptors might play a key pathophysiological role in OAB occurrence. At therapeutic doses, muscarinic antagonists do not seem to inhibit bladder contractility [29]. Hence, OAB appears to be affected by factors other than those involved in bladder muscle contractile dysfunction, thus also suggesting that the urothelium potentially plays an important role in voiding function. Based on these findings and additional previous ones, the investigation of urothelium-expressed G-CSF and BDNF in voiding function seemed suitable for further exploring urothelial function. In particular, previous studies have indicated that NGF, BDNF, prostaglandins, cytokines, and C-reactive protein may be suitable biomarkers of OAB [4, 30-32]. Furthermore, the evaluation of urine samples from OAB patients revealed that G-CSF is upregulated by several different molecules [33]. Within the present experimental context, the use of the urothelium and cultured UCs from the bladder allowed a more robust examination of the changes in these growth factors. In both rats and humans, the M1 to M5 muscarinic receptors are distributed throughout the urothelium [34], and Kullmann et al. detected the expression of all 5 muscarinic receptors subtypes in UCs [35]. We chose 5-HMT as a non-selective agent that could serve as a competitive blocking agent for all muscarinic receptors [6, 36]. Following 5-HMT administration, both growth factors were altered in the control as voiding dysfunction improved. Because the changes in the growth factors were observed in the urothelium and UCs, they will also presumably affect bladder function. Hence, based on the present findings, the urothelium may not only function simply as a mechanosensory receptor, but also play an important role in bladder function. Our study also provides new evidence that 5-HMT has a significant effect on the expression of growth factors in addition to its antimuscarinic tendencies.

A limitation of the present study is that quantitative tests could not be performed because of the small number of UCs. However, the use of RT-PCR with the cell culture allowed an examination of the changes in the characteristics of the UCs. The results showed that BDNF and G-CSF expression was altered in each group and that these alterations had a significant relationship with voiding function.

Conclusions

BDNF and G-CSF expressions were increased in BOO rats and decreased following 5-HMT administration in both the urothelium and UCs. The expression of BDNF and G-CSF in the urothelium might be related to voiding dysfunction in OAB patients. As a therapeutic agent for OAB, 5-HMT improves voiding dysfunction. Based on the present findings, the urothelium plays an important role in the manifestation of voiding symptoms.

Abbreviations
5-HMT: 5-Hydroxymethyl tolterodine; BP: Basal pressure; BOO: Bladder outlet obstruction; BDNF: Brain derived-neurotrophic factor; UCs: Cultured urothelial cells; G-CSF: Granulocyte-colony stimulating factor; IVP: Intravesical pressure; MEM: Minimal essential medium; MI: Micturition interval; MP: Micturition pressure; MT: Micturition time; MV: Micturition volume; NGF: Nerve growth factor; NVA: Non-voiding activity; OAB: Overactive bladder; RT-PCR: Reverse transcription polymerase chain reaction.

Competing interests
The authors declare that they have no competing interests.

Authors' contributions
SMY conceived of the study, participated in its design and coordination, carried out the cystometry, performed the statistical analysis, and helped draft and critically revise the manuscript. JHS conducted the immunoassays and participated in the design of the study. KHS, YGN, and JSL participated in the design of the study, performed the statistical analysis, and helped draft and critically revise the manuscript. CKS conceived of the study, participated in its design and coordination, and helped draft and revise the manuscript. All authors read and approved the final manuscript.

Acknowledgements
The funding source had no role in the design, in the collection, analysis, and interpretation of data; in the writing of the manuscript; and in the decision to submit the manuscript for publication.

Author details
[1]Department of Urology, Korea St. Mary's Hospital, College of Medicine, The Catholic University of Korea, Seoul, South Korea. [2]Department of Urology, Korea Chungnam National University Hospital, College of Medicine, Chungnam National University, Daejeon, South Korea.

References
1. Abrams P, Cardozo L, Fall M, Griffiths D, Rosier P, Ulmsten U, et al. The standardisation of terminology of lower urinary tract function: report from the Standardisation Sub-committee of the International Continence Society. Neurourol Urodyn. 2002;21(2):167–78.
2. Kim JC, Yoo JS, Park EY, Hong SH, Il Seo S, Hwang TK. Muscarinic and purinergic receptor expression in the urothelium of rats with detrusor overactivity induced by bladder outlet obstruction. BJU Int. 2008;101(3):371–5.
3. Steers WD, De Groat WC. Effect of bladder outlet obstruction on micturition reflex pathways in the rat. J Urol. 1988;140(4):864–71.
4. Fry CH, Sahai A, Vahabi B, Kanai AJ, Birder LA. What is the role for biomarkers for lower urinary tract disorders? ICI-RS 2013. Neurourol Urodyn. 2014;33(5):602–5.
5. Pinto R, Frias B, Allen S, Dawbarn D, McMahon SB, Cruz F, et al. Sequestration of brain derived nerve factor by intravenous delivery of TrkB-Ig2 reduces bladder overactivity and noxious input in animals with chronic cystitis. Neuroscience. 2010;166(3):907–16.
6. Michel MC. Fesoterodine: a novel muscarinic receptor antagonist for the treatment of overactive bladder syndrome. Expert Opin Pharmacother. 2008;9(10):1787–96.
7. Andersson KE. Storage and voiding symptoms: pathophysiologic aspects. Urology. 2003;62(5 Suppl 2):3–10.

8. Fullhase C, Soler R, Gratzke C, Brodsky M, Christ GJ, Andersson KE. Urodynamic evaluation of fesoterodine metabolite, doxazosin and their combination in a rat model of partial urethral obstruction. BJU Int. 2010;106(2):287–93.

9. Melman A, Tar M, Boczko J, Christ G, Leung AC, Zhao W, et al. Evaluation of two techniques of partial urethral obstruction in the male rat model of bladder outlet obstruction. Urology. 2005;66(5):1127–33.

10. Kurzrock EA, Lieu DK, de Graffenried LA, Isseroff RR. Rat urothelium: improved techniques for serial cultivation, expansion, freezing and reconstitution onto acellular matrix. J Urol. 2005;173(1):281–5.

11. Lluel P, Duquenne C, Martin D. Experimental bladder instability following bladder outlet obstruction in the female rat. J Urol. 1998;160(6 Pt 1):2253–7.

12. Lee T, Andersson KE, Streng T, Hedlund P. Simultaneous registration of intraabdominal and intravesical pressures during cystometry in conscious rats–effects of bladder outlet obstruction and intravesical PGE2. NeurourolUrodyn. 2008;27(1):88–95.

13. Streng T, Hedlund P, Talo A, Andersson KE, Gillespie JI. Phasic non-micturition contractions in the bladder of the anaesthetized and awake rat. BJU Int. 2006;97(5):1094–101.

14. Gillespie JI. The autonomous bladder: a view of the origin of bladder overactivity and sensory urge. BJU Int. 2004;93(4):478–83.

15. Gillespie JI, van Koeveringe GA, de Wachter SG, de Vente J. On the origins of the sensory output from the bladder: the concept of afferent noise. BJU Int. 2009;103(10):1324–33.

16. Gillespie JI, Palea S, Guilloteau V, Guerard M, Lluel P, Korstanje C. Modulation of non-voiding activity by the muscarinergic antagonist tolterodine and the beta(3)-adrenoceptor agonist mirabegron in conscious rats with partial outflow obstruction. BJU Int. 2012;110(2 Pt 2):E132–42.

17. Kaiho Y, Nishiguchi J, Kwon DD, Chancellor MB, Arai Y, Snyder PB, et al. The effects of a type 4 phosphodiesterase inhibitor and the muscarinic cholinergic antagonist tolterodine tartrate on detrusor overactivity in female rats with bladder outlet obstruction. BJU Int. 2008;101(5):615–20.

18. Yoshimura N. Bladder afferent pathway and spinal cord injury: possible mechanisms inducing hyperreflexia of the urinary bladder. Prog Neurobiol. 1999;57(6):583–606.

19. McCubrey JA, Steelman LS, Chappell WH, Abrams SL, Wong EW, Chang F, et al. Roles of the Raf/MEK/ERK pathway in cell growth, malignant transformation and drug resistance. Biochim Biophys Acta. 2007;1773(8):1263–84.

20. Lowe EM, Anand P, Terenghi G, Williams-Chestnut RE, Sinicropi DV, Osborne JL. Increased nerve growth factor levels in the urinary bladder of women with idiopathic sensory urgency and interstitial cystitis. Br J Urol. 1997;79(4):572–7.

21. Steers WD, Tuttle JB. Mechanisms of Disease: the role of nerve growth factor in the pathophysiology of bladder disorders. Nat Clin Pract Urol. 2006;3(2):101–10.

22. Kim JC, Park EY, Seo SI, Park YH, Hwang TK. Nerve growth factor and prostaglandins in the urine of female patients with overactive bladder. J Urol. 2006;175(5):1773–6. discussion 1776.

23. Tao X, Finkbeiner S, Arnold DB, Shaywitz AJ, Greenberg ME. Ca2+ influx regulates BDNF transcription by a CREB family transcription factor-dependent mechanism. Neuron. 1998;20(4):709–26.

24. Pinto R, Lopes T, Frias B, Silva A, Silva JA, Silva CM, et al. Trigonal injection of botulinum toxin A in patients with refractory bladder pain syndrome/interstitial cystitis. Eur Urol. 2010;58(3):360–5.

25. Schneider A, Kruger C, Steigleder T, Weber D, Pitzer C, Laage R, et al. The hematopoietic factor G-CSF is a neuronal ligand that counteracts programmed cell death and drives neurogenesis. J Clin Invest. 2005;115(8):2083–98.

26. McCubrey JA, Steelman LS, Chappell WH, Abrams SL, Montalto G, Cervello M, et al. Mutations and Deregulation of Ras/Raf/MEK/ERK and PI3K/PTEN/Akt/mTOR Cascades. Oncotarget. 2012;3(9):954–87.

27. Kawada H, Takizawa S, Takanashi T, Morita Y, Fujita J, Fukuda K, et al. Administration of hematopoietic cytokines in the subacute phase after cerebral infarction is effective for functional recovery facilitating proliferation of intrinsic neural stem/progenitor cells and transition of bone marrow-derived neuronal cells. Circulation. 2006;113(5):701–10.

28. Liu F, Yao L, Yuan J, Liu H, Yang X, Qin W, et al. Protective effects of inosine on urinary bladder function in rats with partial bladder outlet obstruction. Urology. 2009;73(6):1417–22.

29. Finney SM, Andersson KE, Gillespie JI, Stewart LH. Antimuscarinic drugs in detrusor overactivity and the overactive bladder syndrome: motor or sensory actions? BJU Int. 2006;98(3):503–7.

30. Bhide AA, Cartwright R, Khullar V, Digesu GA. Biomarkers in overactive bladder. Int Urogynecol J. 2013;24(7):1065–72.

31. Antunes-Lopes T, Carvalho-Barros S, Cruz CD, Cruz F, Martins-Silva C. Biomarkers in overactive bladder: a new objective and noninvasive tool? Adv Urol. 2011;2011:382431.

32. Wang LW, Han XM, Chen CH, Ma Y, Hai B. Urinary brain-derived neurotrophic factor: a potential biomarker for objective diagnosis of overactive bladder. Int Urol Nephrol 2014.46(2):341–7.

33. Ghoniem G, Faruqui N, Elmissiry M, Mahdy A, Abdelwahab H, Oommen M, et al. Differential profile analysis of urinary cytokines in patients with overactive bladder. Int Urogynecol J. 2011;22(8):953–61.

34. Zarghooni S, Wunsch J, Bodenbenner M, Bruggmann D, Grando SA, Schwantes U, et al. Expression of muscarinic and nicotinic acetylcholine receptors in the mouse urothelium. Life Sci. 2007;80(24–25):2308–13.

35. Kullmann FA, Artim D, Beckel J, Barrick S, de Groat WC, Birder LA. Heterogeneity of muscarinic receptor-mediated Ca2+ responses in cultured urothelial cells from rat. Am J Physiol Renal Physiol. 2008;294(4):F971–81.

36. Ney P, Pandita RK, Newgreen DT, Breidenbach A, Stohr T, Andersson KE. Pharmacological characterization of a novel investigational antimuscarinic drug, fesoterodine, in vitro and in vivo. BJU Int. 2008;101(8):1036–42.

18

The resonance® metallic ureteric stent in the treatment of chronic ureteric obstruction

C. Patel[1*] 🆔, D. Loughran[1], R. Jones[1], M. Abdulmajed[1] and I. Shergill[1,2]

Abstract

Background: We evaluate the efficacy and safety of metallic ureteric stenting using the Cook Resonance® stent in the treatment of chronic ureteric obstruction of benign and malignant aetiology. Published experience of using this stent in this context is limited. We add to the body of literature on this topic.

Methods: All patients who had a Resonance® metallic stent inserted between April 2009 and November 2014 in our institution were identified from a prospectively maintained stent-database. Primary outcome was relief of ureteric obstruction, defined by successful clinical and radiological treatment of hydronephrosis/hydroureter. Secondary outcome measures included operative time, radiological exposure, total stent dwell time (defined as the cumulative time in months for which a Resonance® metallic stent was in situ), and early and late complications.

Results: Twenty-one patients underwent 52 stent insertion episodes (SIE). Median age was 58 years (range 39–90). Stent insertion resulted in successful treatment of hydronephrosis/hydroureter in 96% (2 SIE resulted in failure to relieve ureteric obstruction). Median operative time was 21 min (range 12–90) Median radiation exposure was 815. 3 cGy/cm2 (range 192.9–5366.3). Median stent dwell time was 19.5 months (range 6–52) in non-malignant and 12 months (range 2–48) in malignant ureteric obstruction. One stent migrated proximally during insertion and had to be retrieved using an antegrade approach. 5 patients re-admitted with haematuria: all resolved without intervention or blood transfusion. 3 episodes of post-operative urinary infection were recorded; all were successfully treated with oral antibiotics.

Conclusion: Metallic ureteric stenting using the Resonance® stent is safe and effective for treating ureteric obstruction from both malignant and benign causes. The success rate in our series is 96%.

Background

Ensuring adequate long term renal drainage in the context of chronic ureteric obstruction can be a challenge for the urologist. Traditionally, the two main options available for treatment are indwelling polymeric ureteral stents (polyurethane, silicone or hydrogel) and percutaneous nephrostomies. Percutaneous nephrostomy is more invasive and often susceptible to tube blockage and dislodgement and a reduced quality of life. Indwelling-stent failure rates in extrinsic compression are reported at 36–58% [1–5]. They are also commonly associated with device encrustation (thereby requiring bi-annual exchange), biofilm development and subsequent urinary tract infection, and reduced intra-luminal flow in the context of extrinsic compression [6].

The all-metal Cook Resonance® stent has been shown to have much better intraluminal flow compared to polymeric stents (5.15 vs. 0.64 mls/min) [6] and reduced stent encrustation (requiring annual exchange only and more cost effective than standard polymer stenting [7]). The improved intraluminal flow is explained by the Resonance® stent's spiral coil design resulting in bending of the coils as opposed to buckling, which requires much higher external force to cause compression (it maintains

* Correspondence: chigsypatel@doctors.org.uk
[1]Department of Urology, Wrexham Maelor Hospital, Croesnewydd Rd, Wrexham LL13 7TD, Wales
Full list of author information is available at the end of the article

50% of its internal diameter with 31 pounds of compressive force placed at its' proximal, middle and distal segments [8]). The occluded end design means urine drains into the lumen of the stent through small gaps between the spirally wound coils. Stent encrustation led to polymer stent manufacturers advising bi-annual stent changes. Due to reduced stent encrustation, the Resonance® stent requires annual exchange only.

Published experience with the Cook Resonance® stent to date is limited and includes case series' with small numbers of patients [9–19]. The aim of our study was to evaluate the efficacy and safety of the Resonance® stent in our experience in the treatment of chronic ureteric obstruction from both benign and malignant causes, and add to the body of literature on this topic.

Methods

From our prospectively maintained electronic stent database, we identified all patients in whom a Cook Resonance® metallic stent was inserted between April 2009 and Nov 2014. In total 21 patients underwent 52 stent insertion episodes (SIE) during this study. Follow up data was obtained from detailed review of patient casenotes and electronic records.

The primary outcome measure was relief of ureteric obstruction as defined by successful clinical and radiological treatment of hydronephrosis +/- hydroureter. Treatment failure was also defined as removal of the stent before the recommended removal date. Secondary outcome measures included surgical operative time, radiological exposure during fluoroscopy, total *stent dwell time* (defined as the cumulative time period in months for which a Cook Resonance® metallic stent was in situ) as well as early and late post-procedural complications, defined using the modified Clavien-Dindo classification [20].

All patients had previously had their ureteric obstruction managed by either Double J® polymer stenting or nephrostomy. The decision to change to a Cook Resonance® metallic stent was consultant led and based on the patient's individual experience with previous stent/nephrostomy, clinical indication, life expectancy and patient preference.

Cook Resonance® metallic stent was performed as previously described [21]. Briefly, under general anaesthesia, a guidewire was inserted using a combination of cystoscopic and fluoroscopic guidance, followed by a coaxial introduction of the Resonance® sheath and catheter, which contains a radio-opaque tip. The guidewire and catheter were then exchanged for the closed ended Cook Resonance® stent through the sheath, with the aid of the catheter as a pusher. The Resonance® sheath is then finally removed to leave the stent in position. The length of the stent used was based on published literature [22].

Follow up included urine microscopy and imaging (ultrasound or CT depending on clinical indication), and all hospital visits in the post-operative period were recorded. Routine stent exchanges due at 12 months were triggered by the electronic stent register.

Results

Of the patients 7 were male and 14 female. Median age was 58 years (range 39 to 90). Of all the SIE, 35 (67%) had a benign cause (see Table 1). All patients had 6Fr stents of varying lengths (Table 2). Median stent duration was 12 months (range 0.5–14). Median clinical follow up was 12 months (range 2–52) (Table 3).

Primary outcome results

The stent failure rate in our experience was 4%–; 2 SIE resulted in failure to successfully relieve hydronephrosis +/- hydroureter. Success rate of initial retrograde insertion was 98%, with no intraoperative complications. 1 stent had to be inserted in an antegrade fashion after percutaneous renal access.

Secondary outcome results

Median surgical time was 21 min (range 12–90) (this included 15 bilateral stent insertions at the same procedure). Median radiation exposure (measured as kerma-air-product, P_{ka}) was 815.3 cGy/cm^2 (range 192.9–5366.3).

Success rate of initial retrograde insertion was 98%, with no intraoperative complications. 1 stent had to be inserted in an antegrade fashion after percutaneous renal access.

Median stent duration was 12 months (range 2–52). However, when sub-categorised into benign versus malignant aetiology, median stent dwell time (cumulative time period in months for which a Resonance® stent was in-situ) was 19.5 months (range 6–52) for the former and 12 months (range 2–48) for the latter (in all non-deceased patients). 10 (47%) patients died during the follow up period with a metallic stent in-situ. The median stent dwell time in these patients was 7.5 months (range 0.5–14).

Urine microscopy was performed within the first 14 days post-operatively in thirty-eight (73%) of fifty-two stent episodes. Thirty-five (92%) showed no infection, two cultured *E. coli* (both on the same patient with poorly-controlled diabetes) and one grew *Pseudomonas aeruginosa* (patient with an indwelling catheter). These required oral antibiotic treatment only (grade I complication according to the modified Clavien classification system). Haematuria requiring hospital admission occurred in five (24%) patients. All were managed conservatively without the need for intervention or transfusion (grade I). One stent had to be retrieved through an antegrade approach due to incorrect placement of the distal end into the ureter at the time of retrograde insertion

Table 1 Stent Insertion Episode (SIE) by underlying cause

Underlying cause of extrinsic ureteric compression	Associated Number of SIE
Retroperitoneal fibrosis	24
Neuropathic bladder	4
PUJ stricture	3
Duplex kidney	2
Obstructed transplant kidney	2
Malignancy (direct or nodal compression on ureter)	17

Table 3 Number of stent exchanges analysed by patient

Total number of Stent Exchanges	Number of patients
0 (i.e., removed/deceased ≤ 12 months)	13 (9 deceased, 4 removed)
1	5
2	1
3	2

(grade III-a). Removal of stents (bilateral in situ) was performed in one patient due to significant pain (grade III-b). All the remaining stent episodes (96%) successfully relieved hydronephrosis +/− hydroureter on subsequent imaging (ultrasound or CT). 9 patients died within 12 months of stent insertion. Malignancy accounted for 5 (56%) of these and underlying medical co-morbidities for the remainder.

Duration of surgery and radiation exposure to the patient were both seen to reduce as more experience was gained of performing the procedure (Figs. 1 and 2).

Discussion

Since its' introduction in 2006, the Cook Resonance® metallic ureteric stent has gained increasing popularity as an option for relieving ureteric obstruction from malignant and benign pathologies. It is the design that lends itself to this purpose. This case series contributes significantly to the limited literature published on the safety, efficacy and tolerability of this stent in clinical practice.

Retrograde insertion was achieved for the closed-ended Resonance® stent (using a coaxial technique of sheath and introduction catheter) in 51 of 52 episodes. Antegrade insertion was performed in 1 episode due to failed retrograde insertion from inability to pass a guidewire past the distal ureter. Liatsikos et al. [9] have previously chosen the antegrade approach in patients with long strictures or lower ureteric strictures. They safely used balloon-dilatation over an antegradely inserted standard 0.0035 in. guidewire to allow passage of the 8.3Fr outer introducer sheath. Patient selection to

Table 2 Stent length distribution for SIE

Resonance Stent length (cm)	Number of SIE
26	14
24	23
22	11
18	2
14	1
12	1

identify potentially difficult retrograde insertion would avoid a general anaesthetic in a high risk patient. 'Stent failure' as defined by failure of decompression of hydronephrosis/hydroureter occurred in only 2 (4%) of stent episodes. This was despite uncomplicated retrograde insertion and as a result of the individuals' underlying malignant disease. Published figures for stent failure from case series' of greater than fifteen patients vary from 16–35% [7, 9, 10, 18]. This wide variation can be explained by the different study sample sizes, which on the whole remains relatively low. The largest series to date only had 50 patients and reported a 16% stent failure rate, interestingly all with a non-cancerous cause of renal or ureteric obstruction [9]. We believe our low stent failure rate was due to case selection in our series, rather than all comers.

Cook advise stent exchange at 12 months. This is therefore our departmental policy. Overall median stent duration was noted as being 12 months (range 0.5–14). Due to our long follow-up period (upto 52 months), some patients had multiple stent exchanges. When this was factored in to the analysis of sub-categorisation by aetiology, median *stent dwell time* (cumulative time period in months for which a Resonance® stent was in-situ) was longer in benign compared to malignant cases. This difference can be explained by the higher mortality rate amongst the group with an underlying malignancy as a cause of ureteric obstruction. To our knowledge, this series has the longest follow-up duration to date. Stent patency at 14 months has previously been reported [9] and therefore raises the potential for a longer time duration between exchanges.

Radiation exposure associated with this procedure was low at a median of 815 cGy/cm2. A significant dose (requiring patient follow-up) for interventional radiology procedures is defined as a kerma-air-product of greater than 50,000 cGy/cm2 [23]. Furthermore, both radiation exposure to the patient and procedure duration reduced in a linear fashion from 2009 to 2014.

The overall majority of complications were grade I according to the modified Clavien classification system. Urinary tract infection (UTI) within the first 2 weeks post-stenting occurred in 3 (8%) cases, twice in the same patient but after different stent insertion episodes. Underlying co-morbidities are likely to have increased this risk (poorly controlled diabetes and an indwelling

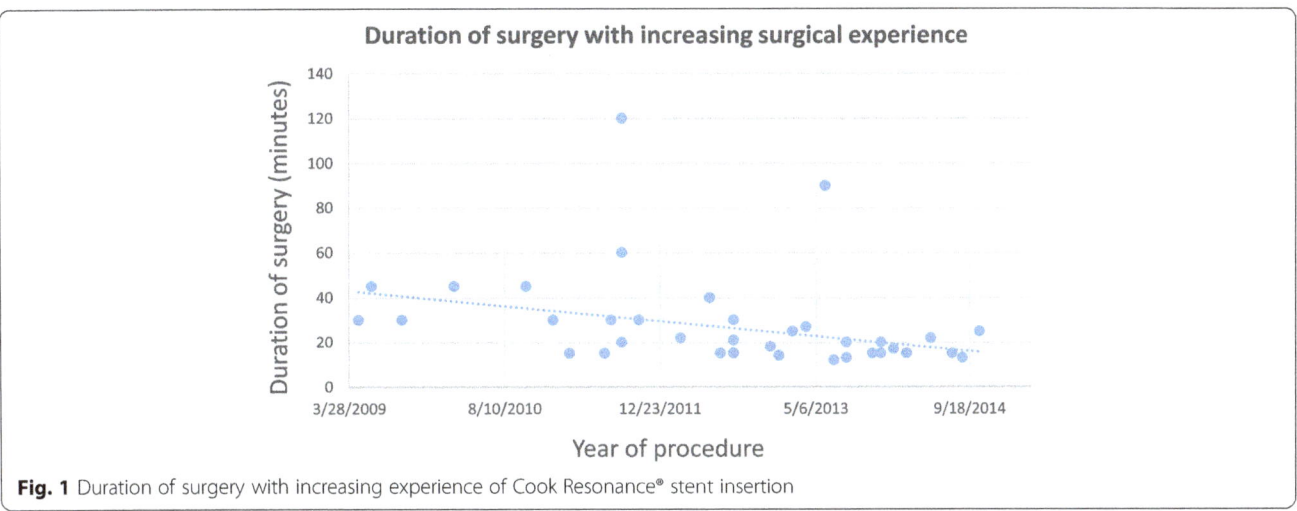

Fig. 1 Duration of surgery with increasing experience of Cook Resonance® stent insertion

catheter). The British Association of Urological Surgeons quote a UTI rate of 2–10% post cystoscopy and ureteric stenting. Our figures for the Resonance® metallic stent are comparable but on a very limited study size and in patients with risk factors for infection. Haematuria requiring hospital admission was seen in 5 (25%) patients. They were all managed conservatively. It can be argued that counselling for primary care to better inform them on post-stenting care could reduce unnecessary, and costly, hospital admission. Similarly it is possible that some patients may have experienced transient haematuria but not reported it. Previous studies with greater than 15 patients have reported haematuria in 6–21% of patients [9, 14].

Pain has not been identified as a major issue, with only one patient requiring stent removal (bilateral stents) as a result.

Nine patients died within 12 months of stent insertion. Malignancy accounted for greater than half of these and all deaths were secondary to the underlying disease process. As can be expected the median *stent dwell time* was higher in benign compared to malignant cases.

Sample size can be viewed as a limitation of our study. Whereas our database continues to expand, this is at a relatively slow rate given that metallic stenting is still on the whole reserved for a select group of patients. We hope that changing clinicians' thinking through this critical analysis of the safety, efficacy and tolerability of this stent will lead to a larger number of patients being made eligible.

A further limitation is that we did not perform a cost analysis to compare the Resonance® stent with the standard polymeric stent. The convenience to the patient is an annual as opposed to bi-annual stent exchange. Only one study to date has performed a cost analysis [7]. In it Lopez-Huertas et al. reported a significant (43%) cost saving with the Resonance® metallic stent compared to the Percuflex™ stent in a thirteen patient cohort.

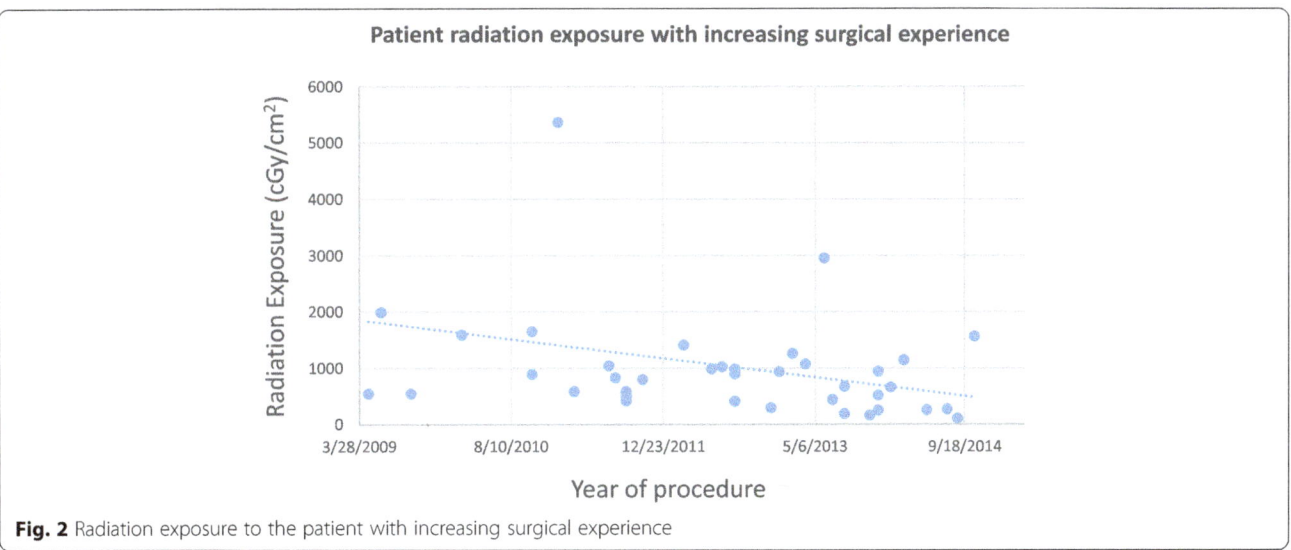

Fig. 2 Radiation exposure to the patient with increasing surgical experience

Conclusion

We conclude that the Resonance® metallic stent is safe and effective for treating ureteric obstruction from both malignant and benign causes. Increased awareness of this potential will allow more patients to benefit from an annual (as opposed to bi-annual) stenting procedure.

Abbreviations

CGY: Centi-gray; CT: Computed tomography; Fr: French; Pka: Kerma-air-product; PUJ: Pelvi-ureteric junction; SIE: Stent insertion episodes

Acknowledgements

Not applicable.

Funding

No funding.

Availability of data and materials

The datasets generated during and/or analysed during the current study are available from the corresponding author on reasonable request.

Author's contributions

CP and IS acquired, analysed and interpreted the data. CP drafted the manuscript. CP and IS revised the manuscript critically for important intellectual content. DL, RJ and MA assisted in acquisition of data and manuscript revision. All authors gave final approval of the version to be published.

Competing interests

The authors declare that they have no competing interests.

Author details

[1]Department of Urology, Wrexham Maelor Hospital, Croesnewydd Rd, Wrexham LL13 7TD, Wales. [2]North Wales and North West Urological Research Centre, Croesnewydd Rd, Wrexham LL13 7TD, Wales.

References

1. Ganatra AM, Loughlin KR. The management of malignant ureteral obstruction treated with ureteral stents. J Urol. 2005;174(6):2125–8.
2. Chung SY, Stein RJ, Landsittel D, et al. 15-year experience with the management of extrinsic ureteral obstruction with indwelling ureteral stents. J Urol. 2004;172(2):592–5.
3. Docimo SG, Dewolf WC. High failure rate of indwelling ureteral stents in patients with extrinsic obstruction: experience at 2 institutions. J Urol. 1989; 142:277.
4. Yossepowitch O, Lifshitz DA, Dekel Y, et al. Predicting the success of retrograde stenting for managing ureteral obstruction. J Urol. 2001;166:1746.
5. Feng MI, Bellman GC, Shapiro CE. Management of ureteral obstruction secondary to pelvic malignancies. J Endourol. 1999;13:521.
6. Blaschko SD, Deane LA, Krebs A, et al. In-vivo evaluation of flow characteristics of a novel metal ureteral stent. J Endourol. 2007;21:780–3.
7. Lopez-Huertas H, Polcari AJ, Acosta-Miranda A, et al. Metallic ureteral stents: A cost-effective method of managing benign ureteral obstruction. J Endourol. 2010;24:483–5.
8. Christman MS, L'Esperance JO, Choe CH, et al. Analysis of ureteral stent compression force and its role in malignant obstruction. J Urol. 2009;181: 392–6.
9. Liatsikos E, Kallidonis P, Kyriazis I, et al. Ureteral obstruction: is the full metallic double-pigtail stent the way to go? Eur Urol. 2010;57(3):480–7.
10. Kadlec AO, Ellimoottil CS, Greco KA, et al. Five-year experience with metallic stents for chronic ureteral obstruction. J Urol. 2013;190(3):937–41.
11. Li CC, Li JR, Huang LH, et al. Metallic stent in the treatment of ureteral obstruction: experience of single institute. J Chin Med Ass. 2011;74(10):460–3.
12. Wah TM, Irving HC, Cartledge J. Initial experience with the Resonance metallic stent for antegrade ureteric stenting. Cardiovasc Intervent Radiol. 2007;30:705–10.
13. Nagele U, Kuczyk MA, Horstmann M, et al. Initial clinical experience with full-length metal ureteral stents for obstructive ureteral stenosis. World J Urol. 2008;26:257–62.
14. Wang HJ, Lee TY, Luo HL, et al. Application of resonance metallic stents for ureteral obstruction. BJU Int. 2010;108:428–32.
15. Modi AP, Ritch CR, Arend D, et al. Multicenter experience with metallic ureteral stents for malignant and chronic benign ureteral obstruction. J Endourol. 2010;24:1189–93.
16. Garg T, Guralnick ML, Langenstroer P, et al. Resonance metallic ureteral stents do not successfully treat ureteroenteric strictures. J Endourol. 2009;23: 1199–202.
17. Benson AD, Taylor ER, Schwartz BF. Metal ureteral stent for benign and malignant ureteral obstruction. J Urol. 2011;185:2217–22.
18. Goldsmith ZG, Wang AJ, Bañez LL, et al. Outcomes of metallic stents for malignant ureteral obstruction. J Urol. 2012;188:851–5.
19. Gayed BA, Mally AD, Riley J, et al. Resonance metallic stents do not effectively relieve extrinsic ureteral compression in pediatric patients. J Endourol. 2012;27:154–7.
20. Dindo D, Demartines N and Clavien PA. Classification of surgical complications: A new proposal with evaluation in a cohort of 6336 patients and results of a survey. Ann Surg. 2004;240(2):205–213.
21. Shergill ISS, Abdulmajed M, Jones R et al. Cook Resonance metallic ureteric stent insertion technique and North Wales clinical experience. J Endourol Part B Videourol. 2013; doi:10.1089/vid.2012.0020.
22. Pilcher JM, Patel U. Choosing the correct length of ureteric stent: a formula based on the patient's height compared with direct ureteric measurement. Clin Radiol. 2002;57(1):59–62.
23. Stecker MS, Balter S, Towbin RB, et al. Guidelines for patient radiation dose management. J Vasc Interven Radiol. 2009;20:s263–73.

19

Successful bilateral pudendal neuromodulation to treat male detrusor areflexia following severe pubic symphysis fracture

Serge P. Marinkovic*, Brandi Miller, Scott Hughes, Christina Marinkovic and Lisa Gillen

Abstract

Background: A Drum Dock Manager in an auto manufacturing company suffers a pelvic fracture, severing the bulbar urethra and completely fracturing the right side of his pelvis.
He is unable to void without catheterization but has a complete sensation to void. Can neuromodulation help him achieve spontaneous voiding?

Case presentation: We reviewed the electronic medical record of Mr. M.E. from Detroit Medical Center following his 2012 forklift accident and subsequent orthopedic surgeries. He successfully underwent bilateral sacral neuromodulation, with a resulting max flow of 16.8 mls/sec and post-void residual urine of 50–100 mls. Unfortunately, he later presented with bilateral pocket and sacral lead infection, and both systems had to be removed. Six weeks later, M.E. had bilateral pudendal neurostimulation placement to avoid the previously infected areas. Max flow improved to 14.5 mls/sec and 0–50 mls residual urine. However, urodynamics proved that his P_{det} at max flow was in excess of 120 cm of H20 pressure while he had been on finesteride and tamsulosin for the preceding five years for the management of his documented benign prostate hyperplasia symptoms. He underwent Green light laser transurethral resection of the prostate and had max flow improvement to 22.5 mls/second with zero residual urine with multiple straight catheterization confirmations.

Conclusion: Sacral neuromodulation may successfully correct traumatic urinary retention in male patients. Additionally, pudendal neuromodulation can be successfully utilized as a salvage method for an infected sacral neuromodulation impulse generator (IPG) and tined lead with a return to proper voiding.

Keywords: Sacral neuromodulation, Male urinary retention, Pudendal neuromodulation, Unilateral ischial fracture

Background

Traumatic urethral injury may result in partial or total urinary retention in male patients. Clean intermittent catheterization or chronic indwelling Foley catheterization are frequently instituted to properly empty the bladder as a temporary or permanent treatment measure. However, after primary healing of 6 months or more, consideration may be given to the surgical treatment of urinary retention [1]. In the literature, sacral neuromodulation has reportedly been utilized following surgical trauma but not blunt or penetrating trauma. We now report the first case in the literature utilizing bilateral sacral neuromodulation followed by bilateral pudendal neuromodulation after an industrial accident left our male patient with a severe pubic symphysis fracture and subsequent urinary retention.

Case presentation

M.E. is a 50-year-old Caucasian male, working as a Drum Dock Manager in a car manufacturing factory. On April 23, 2012, as he was unloading a forklift, the machine automatically engaged itself, speeding toward him and running him over. His quick-thinking co-workers positioned him flat on

* Correspondence: urourogyn@yahoo.com
Department of Urology, Detroit Medical Center, Harper Hospital, Detroit, MI 48202, USA

the floor with his head tilted to the left. M.E. was conscious and complaining of severe chest and pelvic pain. When emergency medical services arrived, he was stable. A decision was made to fly him to a nearby Trauma One Medical Center. He was diagnosed with seven left-sided rib fractures, transection of the pubic symphysis (Fig. 1), and L_1-L_3 transverse process fractures. There was blood at his urethral meatus, and after a retrograde urethrogram (RUG) with live fluoroscopy and without a hard copy print, a guide wire was placed through a cystoscope and into the bladder with fluoroscopic confirmation. M.E. later underwent orthopedic stabilization and repair of his pubis symphysis. His lumbar/sacral MRI redemonstrated the lumbar transverse fractures with moderate degenerative lumbar disc disease without nerve impingement (Fig. 2). The RUG demonstrated bulbar extravasation, but a Council tip catheter was successfully guided into the bladder to determine urethral continuity. At 6 weeks, his RUG demonstrated a well-healed urethra. He was given multiple trials of voids after being able to ambulate well for one month, but in spite of a sensation to void, he could not generate a detrusor pressure, and no voiding occurred. He failed two more trials of void. A urodynamics study was then performed (Fig. 3), demonstrating a first desire to void at 155 mls. Even at 550 mls, he experienced a strong desire to void but no detrusor pressure. The patient had good rectal sphincter tone and could volitionally tighten his rectum, so the pudendal nerve was assumed to be working well. We recommended a minimally invasive approach of sacral neuromodulation, which he successfully underwent 6 months after the accident. His bellows and ipsilateral plantar flexion were arrived at two volts on lead 0,

1 and 2, and at three volts on lead 3. Within six hours of surgery, he was emptying half his bladder, and post void residuals were 300 mls with straight catheterization. After 2 months of follow-up, he continued to urinate at maximum flows of 17.2 mls/sec but with 250–300 residual urines, so another sacral neuromodulation was performed on his contralateral side. He immediately improved to straight catheterization residual urine of 50–100 mls with a max flow of 16.8 mls/sec with 400 mls voided. Unfortunately 6 months later, after M.E. had returned to work, his uniform was irritating both of his implants, and within 3 weeks, he had a bilateral cellulitis with purulent drainage from both lead sites and implantable pulse generators. At surgery to remove each implants each buttock pocket wound culture grew non-methicillin resistant Staph aureus and he was subsequently treated with Ciprofloxin home intravenous therapy for six weeks and the resumption of clean intermittent catheterization. Three months later, re-examination revealed both sites to be well healed. Our next alternative was bilateral pudendal neuromodulation (Table 1), which would avoid placement near or cross over with the two formerly infected sites. Bilateral pudendal neuromodulation was performed with a right and left 0–3 lead result of 1,1,2,4, and 2,2,4,5 volts, and within six hours, the patient began to void without difficulty with a straight catheterization post-void residual urine of 0–50 mls and a max flow of 14.5 mls/sec. We then performed urodynamics, which demonstrated high pressure voiding with Pdet greater than 120 cm H2O. While having been on both tamsulosin

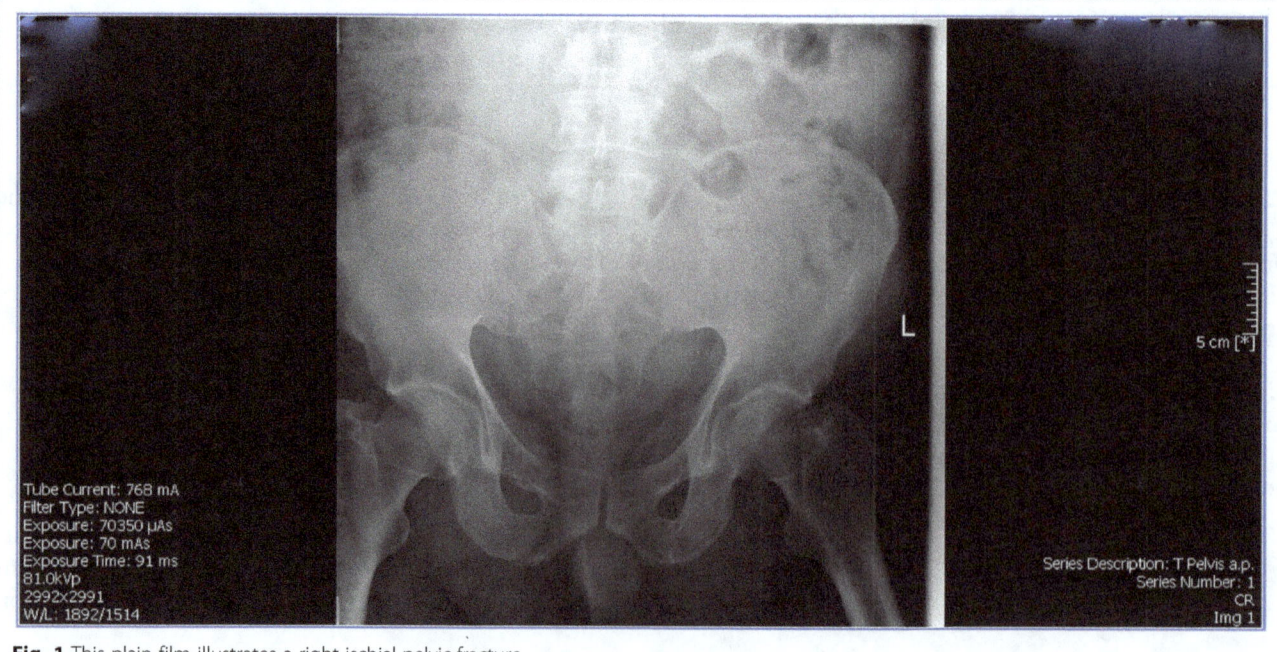

Fig. 1 This plain film illustrates a right ischial pelvic fracture

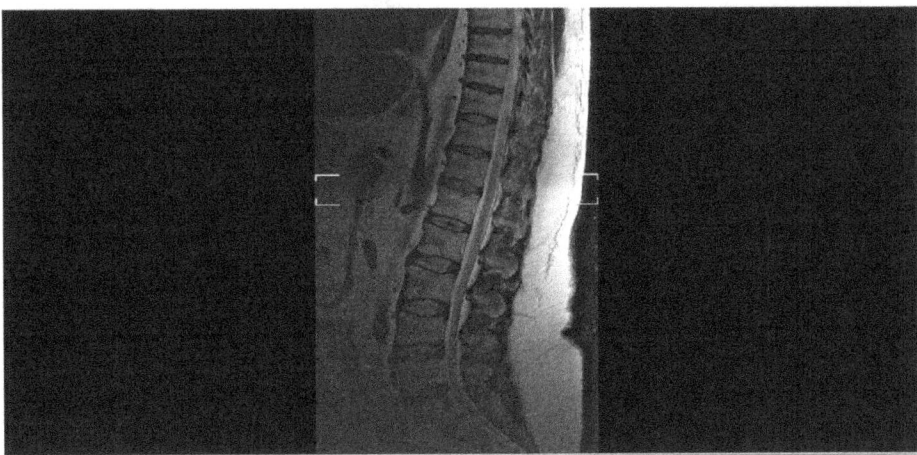

Fig. 2 This lateral lumbar Magnetic Resonance Image demonstrates severe degenerative disc disease with a few bulging intervertebral discs

and finesteride for more than 5 years, M.E. had failed medical therapy and was a high pressure voider. Sustained high pressure is well known to damage the bladder much like hypertension can damage the heart. To protect his bladder, we recommended a Green light transurethral resection of the prostate, which was performed on July 17, 2014. His subsequent straight catheterization post void residual urines had been 0–50 mls and his mean max flow was 22.6 mls/sec. With one-year of follow-up, his voiding parameters remain stable while his treatment power on both implantable pulse generators has been 2.8 volts on the right and 4.2 volts on the left. He feels perineal sensation and is without discomfort. We now follow the patient in 4-month intervals.

Discussion

Treatment of complete detrusor areflexia has included Valsalva voiding, intermittent straight catheterization, chronic Foley catheterization, and most recently sacral neuromodulation. Women achieve higher success rates than men with sacral neuromodulation, but the use of pudendal neuromodulation [2–8], particularly dual pudendal neuromodulation for the treatment of detrusor areflexia, has not been described. Several physicians with whom I have communicated have stated that pudendal neuromodulation for male urinary retention does not work well. How sacral and pudendal neuromodulation work to treat both overactive bladder symptoms and, to a lesser extent, urinary retention has not been clearly

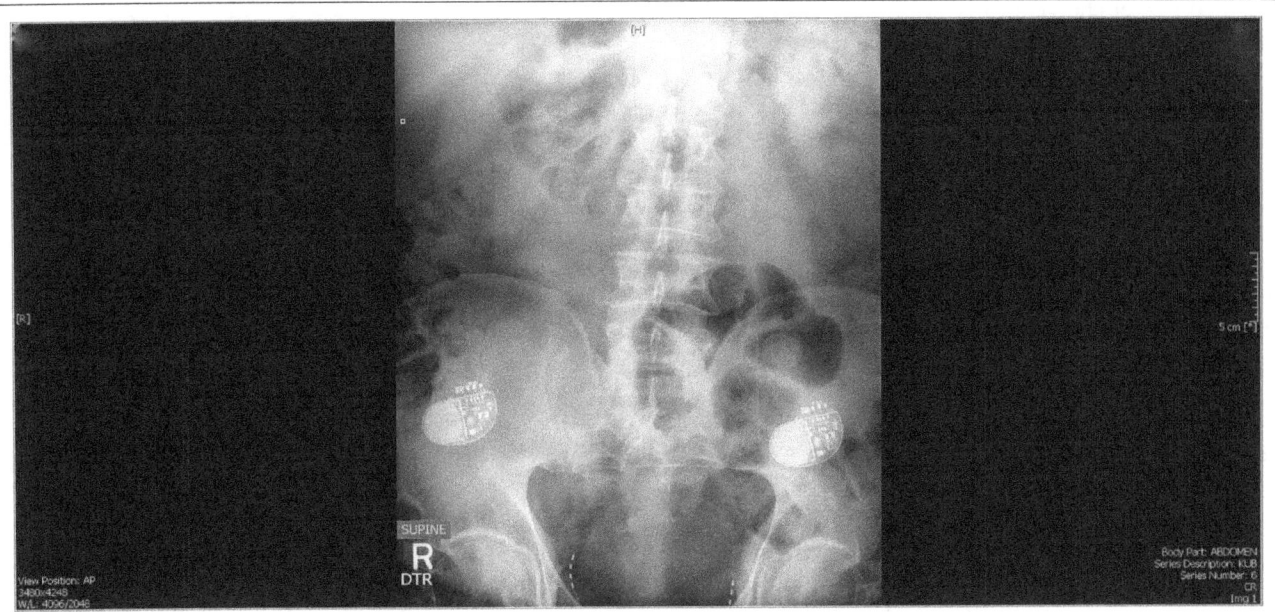

Fig. 3 The written report of this patient's first multichannel urodynamics study

Table 1 Multichannel urodynamics report

1st Sensation	165 mls
1st Desire to Void	389 mls
Strong Desire to Void	510 mls
P$_{abd}$	51 cm H$_2$O
P$_{det}$	0 cm H$_2$O
Max Flow	0 ml/sec
Cough Leak Point Pressure	No leak
Rectal Tone	Contracts external sphincter around a finger in his rectum, indicating that the pudendal nerve is working well

defined. What is important to note is that the lower the voltage level achieved to elicit good motor provocation during sacral neuromodulation (bellows and ipsilateral big toe plantar flexion and potentially pudendal neuromodulation anal wink with an EMG documented EMG tracing at less than or equal to 3 volts at one or more leads) the better the end result for urinary retention and overactive bladder symptoms. Our patient had both bilateral sacral neuromodulation and bilateral pudendal neuromodulation and feels that pudendal neuromodulation has given him the closest sensation and performance to his normal voiding prior to the 2012 accident. He has also noticed an improvement in erections. While he was unable to have any erections without a phosphodiesterase 5 inhibitor for two years prior to the accident, he now can manage an erection without any medication. His voiding max flow and post-void residuals are now normal for his age, and he checks his post void residual via a home ultrasound device provided free of charge for his use. Pudendal neuromodulation is used as a salvage surgical operation for those who, with sacral neuromodulation, experience a decrease in efficacy and now fail to meet treatment expectations. Pudendal neuromodulation has not been described for urinary retention, but with our patient, the procedure appears to have improved his outcome after volitional voiding was not previously possible and his sacral implants became infected. We hope that with this patient's continued success, we can appreciate the potential utilization of pudendal neuromodulation when sacral neuromodulation has failed for urinary retention.

Conclusion

Sacral neuromodulation may successfully correct traumatic urinary retention, in male patients. Additionally, pudendal neuromodulation can be successfully utilized as a salvage method for an infected sacral neuromodulation impulse generator (IPG), and tined lead with a return to proper voiding.

Consent

Written informed consent was obtained from the patient was obtained from the patient for publication of this case report and any accompanying images. A copy of the written consent is available for review by the Editor of this journal.

Competing interests

None of the authors has any competing interests, financial assistance from any of the products utilized in the care of this patient, or in their entire practice of urological surgery.

Authors' contribution

All authors have contributed equally to the preparation and writing of this case report.

References

1. Saber-khalaf M, Abtahi B, Gonzales G, Helai M, Elneil S. Sacral neuromodulation outcome in male patients with chronic urinary retention. Neuromodulation. 2015;18(4):329–34. doi:10.1111/ner.12268.
2. Peters KM. Alternative approaches to sacral nerve stimulation. Int Urogynecol J. 2010;21(12):1559–63. doi:1007/s00192-010-1282-2.
3. Heinze K, van Ophoven A. Neuromodulation: new techniques. Urologe A. 2015;54(3):373–7. doi:10.1007/s00120-014-3686-y.
4. Heinze K, Hoermann R, Fritsch H, Dermietzel R, van Ophoven A. Comparative pilot of implantation techniques for pudendal neuromodulation: technical and clinical outcomes in the first 20 patients with chronic pelvic pain. World J Urol. 2015;33(2):89–294.
5. Possover M. A novel implantation technique for pudendal nerve stimulation for treatment of overactive bladder and urgency incontinence. J Minim Invasive Gynecol. 2014;21(5):888–92.
6. Wang S, Zhang S, Zhao L. Long-term efficacy of electrical pudendal nerve stimulation for urgency-frequency syndrome in women. Int Urogynecol J. 2014;25(3):397–402.
7. Peters KM, Killinger KA, Boguskawski BM, Boura JA. Chronic pudendal neuromodulation: expanding available treatment options for refractory urologic symptoms. Neurourol Urodyn. 2010;29(7):1267–71. doi:10.1002/nau.20823.
8. Spinelli M, Malaguti S, Giardiello G, Lazzeri M, Tarantola J, Den Hombergh H. A new minimally invasive procedure for pudendal nerve stimulation to treat neurogenic bladder: description of the method and preliminary data. Neurourol Urodyn. 2005;24(4):305–9.

20

Xanthogranulomutous pyelonephritis presenting as "Wilms' tumor"

Shakilu Iumanne[1,3*], Aika Shoo[2], Larry Akoko[1] and Patricia Scanlan[2]

Abstract

Background: Xanthogranulomatous pyelonephritis (XGP) is a rare renal tumor that arises as a complication of chronic obstructive pyelonephritis of uncertain etiology. It is primarily an adult tumor seen occasionally in children associated with urinary tract obstruction due to congenital urological anomalies, nephrolithiasis, and recurrent urinary tract infections. Radiologically, it may show neoplastic features such as those seen in common pediatric renal malignancies like wilms' tumor and renal cell carcinoma. This overlap in radiological manifestation frequently leads to misdiagnosis and delay in appropriate intervention. We report a case of a 3 years old boy who presented with history of recurrent urinary tract infections and a left renal mass initially thought to be Wilms' tumor.

Case presentation: We present a case of a 3 years old boy admitted to the Pediatric oncology unit at Muhimbli National Hospital in Dar es Salaam, Tanzania with one year history of recurrent fever and urinary tract infection signs and symptoms refractory to antibiotic therapy. He was eventually found to have a left kidney mass detected at the District hospital by abdominal ultrasound performed to evaluate a flank mass that was felt by his mother. He was then referred to our unit for a suspicion of Wilms' tumor which finally turned out to be a left kidney Xanthogranulomatous pyelonephritis.
He underwent a successful left nephrectomy and was discharged from hospital in a stable clinical condition and remains asymptomatic at the time of submission of this case report.

Conclusion: This case report underscores the need for clinicians attending a febrile child with a renal mass that can be confused with common pediatric renal malignancies such as Wilms' tumor to broaden their differential diagnosis. The case also underlines the significance of individualized patient evaluation because this patient would have otherwise received preoperative chemotherapy under the International Society of Pediatric Oncology (SIOP) guidelines if the diagnosis of Wilms tumor was not ruled out.

Keywords: Xanthogranulomatous pyelonephritis, Wilms' tumor, Pseudotumor

Background

Xanthogranulomatous pyelonephritis is a rare renal tumor of uncertain etiology believed to occur as a complication of chronic obstructive pyelonephritis with bacterial superinfection. It is more of an adult disease with peak age at 5th to 6th decade of life, occasionally seen in children associated with urinary tract obstruction mostly from congenital urological malformations such as posterior urethral valve, nephrolithiasis, and recurrent urinary tract infections [1]. Radiologically, it may display similar neoplastic features as those seen with common renal malignancies such as wilms' tumor and renal cell carcinoma appearing as a flank mass invading neighboring structures [2]. This overlap in radiological characteristics frequently leads to misdiagnosis and delay in appropriate interventions. Surgery and antibiotic therapy are the mainstay of treatment for this rare urological condition with open radical nephrectomy and resection of affected neighbouring structures being the standard of treatment but laparascopic surgery has been used to treat some cases [3]. We report a case of a 3 years old boy presenting with history of recurrent urinary tract infections and a left renal mass that was finally diagnosed as Xanthogranulomatous pyelonephritis.

* Correspondence: shakiluj@gmail.com
[1]Muhimbili University of health and Allied Sciences, P.O. Box 65001, Dar es Salaam, Tanzania
[3]College of Health Sciences, University of Dodoma, Box 339, Dodoma, Tanzania
Full list of author information is available at the end of the article

Table 1 Summarized laboratory investigation results

Total white cell count (/µl)	Neutrophil count (/µl)	Lymphocyte count (/µl)	Monocyte count (/µl)	Hemoglobin (g/dl)
12700	6770	4227	700	6.17
Redblood cell (/µl)	MCV (fl)	MCH (pg/cell)	Plateletcount (/µl)	RDW (%)
2680	57.5	16.7	608	16
Serum Chemistry				
Serum creatinine (µmol/L)	Urea (µmol/L)	LDH (U/L)	Sodium (mmol/L)	Calcium (mmol/L)
41.6 µmol/L	5.4	281	133	1.25
Urine analysis				
Leukocytes/ (hpf)	Nitrites	Protein	pH	Specific gravity
20	1$^+$	2^{++}	6.8	1.005

Case presentation

A 3 years old boy presented with history of recurrent fever, episodes of painful urination, increased frequency and haematuria for one year. He had been treated with several courses of antibiotics for urinary tract infections with temporary relief of symptoms before recurrence. At initial presentations several urine analysis using dipstics were performed at the local dispensary and reported to show features of urinary tract infections but no further work up such as urine culture, voiding cyctourethrogram or abdominal ultrasound was performed. Three months before admission to our unit, his mother had felt a mass on his left flank and an abdominal ultrasound done at the nearby District Hospital suspected Wilms' tumor and the patient was referred to our unit for further evaluation. The patient had otherwise attained his developmental mile stones as per age and had no any dysmorphic features.

On examination; the child was febrile with body temperature of 38.8 °C with tenderness on the left lumber region and had a palpable mass on the same side. Laboratory investigations performed are summarised in the concise table below; Table 1.

A repeat abdominal ultrasound showed a left renal mass 7.4X7.1X5 cm with multiple cystic lesions. The renal pelvis was destroyed with some calcific changes but no extension to the neighboring structures were noted. The right kidney was normal in size and echogenicity.

Abdominal CT Scan (Figs. 1 and 2) showed an enlarged left kidney measuring 7.9X6.7 cm in size with

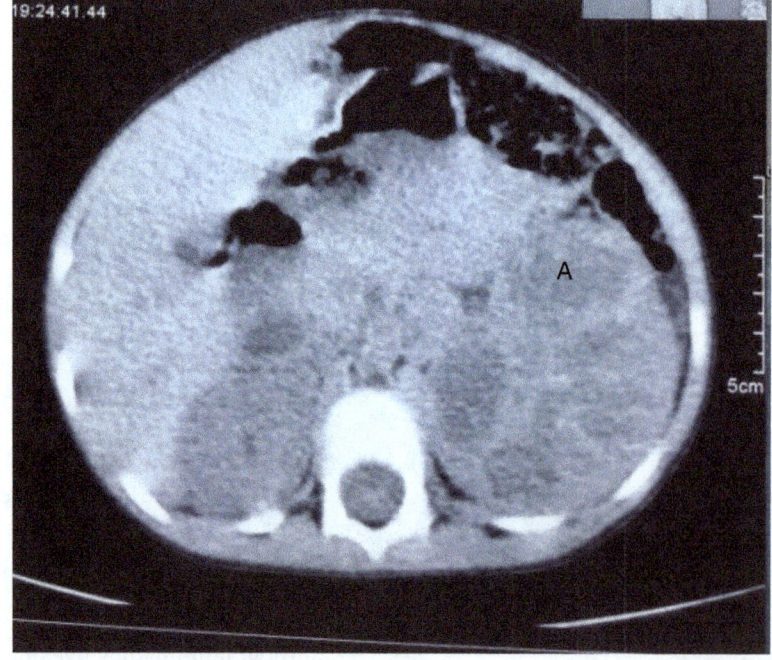

Fig. 1 Plain abdominal CT-scan showing an enlarged left kidney with multiple cystic components (A) and calcifications

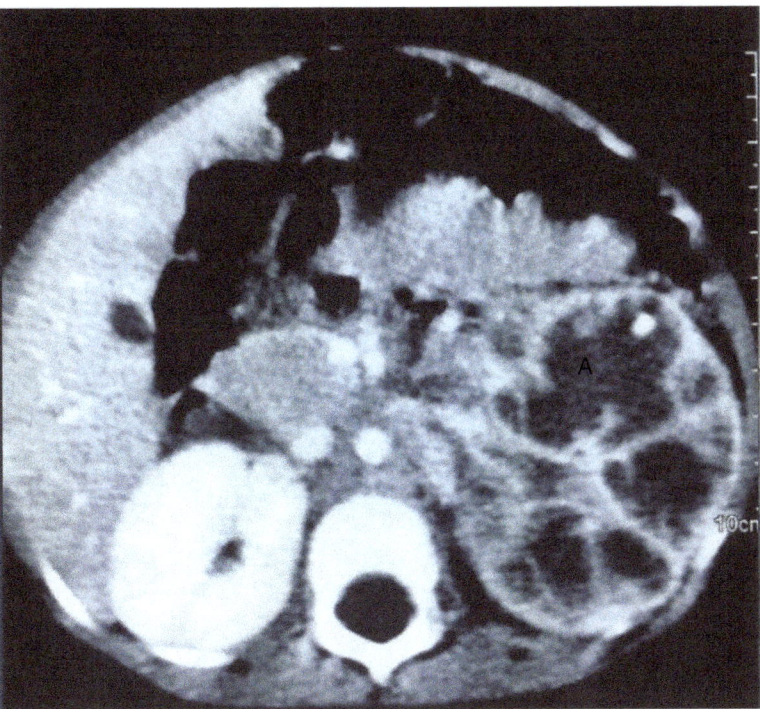

Fig. 2 Contrast enhanced abdominal CT-scan showing multiple cysts in the left kidney (A) with peripheral enhancement of residual normal renal tissues

thinning of the cortices and loss of corticomedullary differentiation, foci of calcifications were also seen and the renal parenchyma was replaced with multiple septations (A). Contrast enhanced CT scans showed areas of peripheral enhancement surrounding non-enhancing cystic foci within the mass. There was no obvious filling defect seen in the renal vein or inferior vena cava. The right kidney was normal in size and shape, urinary bladder displayed normal outline and other abdominal organs were all normal.

Based on the clinical presentation and abdominal CT scan, a clinical diagnosis of Xanthogranulomatous pyelonephritis was made and the patient underwent left radical nephrectomy. Intra-operatively an enlarged yellowish grey left kidney with multiple mesenteric and hilar lymph nodes was seen, radical left nephroureterectomy and hilar lymphnode resection was performed, the right kidney was normal on inspection. The resected tissues were sampled and sent for culture and sensitivity but there was no bacterial growth after 7 days. Histological studies reported macroscopically gross yellowish renal tissues microscopically showing a renal histology infiltrated with foamy lipid laden macrophages in a mixture of chronic inflammatory cells and fibrosis confirming a diagnosis of Xanthogralomatous pyelophritis (Fig. 3).

The patient faired well postoperatively and was kept on a 7 days course of intravenous Tazobactam/piperacillin and discharged home 10 days post nephrectomy.

Discussion

Xanthogranulomatous pyelonephritis is a rare chronic obstructive pyelonephritis characterized by infiltration of the renal parenchyma with lipid laden Macrophages and an enlarged non-functional kidney [4]. It is most commonly associated with superinfections by bacteria such as *E.coli, Proteus mirabilis,* and occasionally *Pseudomonas species* [5]. Renal calculi, diabetes mellitus and immunosuppressive conditions are also reported to predispose an individual to this rare renal tumor [6]. The affected kidney is usually non-functional and can be mistaken with common renal neoplasms because it may locally extend to invade adjacent structures such as the psoas muscle, pancreas, spleen and the duodenum.

In most cases, Xanthogranulomatous pyelonephritis involve one kidney but cases of bilateral renal involvement have been published [7, 8]. XGP is predominantly a disease of adults reported to occur in approximately 1 % of pyelonephritis. It is four times more common in females than males with a peak age at fifth and sixth decades of life [9]. XGP in adults affects both kidneys equally but it involves the left kidney more often than the right kidney in children as it was the case for our patient [10]. XGP in children occur more in boys usually from 8 years of age and it is encountered in approximately 16 % of pediatric nephrectomy specimens [11]. Histologically the disease is characterized by renal

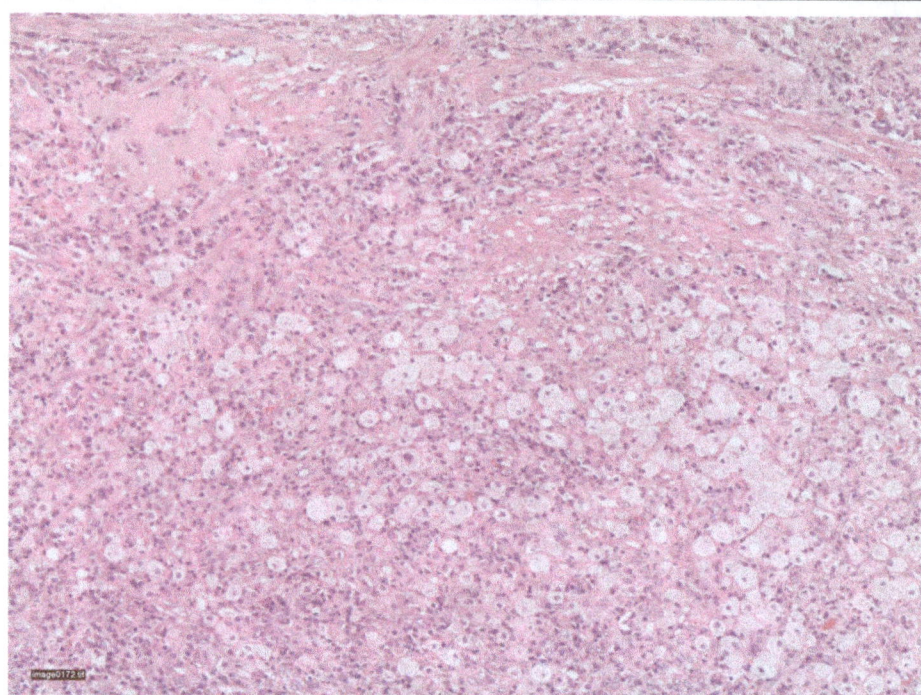

Fig. 3 H&E micrograph of a histological section of the mass showing lipid laden macrophages in a mixture of chronic inflammatory cells

parenchyma infiltration by lipid laden macrophages and chronic inflammatory cells in line with the histological finding for our patient [12]. The exact mechanism of xanthogranulomatous pyelonephritis (XGP) is unclear, but it is generally agreed that the disease process requires a long-term renal obstruction superimposed with infection by *Proteus* species, *Escherichia coli* and *Pseudomonas* species in a setting of impaired ability of the body to clear the infection. Congenital urinary tract malformations are highly linked with development of XGP in children [13]. Ultrasound and other imaging modalities can be used to suspect XGP, but CT-scan and MRI are thought to be more sensitive and usually show an enlarged nonfunctional kidney with or without invasion to neighbouring structures [14].

On abdominal CT scan, our patient showed foci of calcifications with no calculi but renal calculi (frequently of staghorn proportions) are reported in up to 80 % of cases with XGP.

XGP can manifest with malignant features capable of local tissue invasion and destruction explaining the frequent confusion with renal neoplasm hence it is often referred to as a pseudo tumor [15].

Our case presented with one year history of antibiotic refractory urinary tract symptoms and fever, which is a typical presentation of this condition [16]. The obstruction associated with XGP in the pediatric population is frequently linked to congenital urinary tract

malformations than from obstructive calculi but our patient did not have any anomaly or calculi from the imaging performed. Histologically; XGL has a pathognomonic appearance characterized by lipid laden foamy macrophages in a mixture of acute and chronic inflammatory cells [17]. Other laboratory investigations including complete blood count and differential are usually nonspecific but may show leukocytosis and anemia with elevated erythrocyte sedimentation rate.

If XGP is unilateral, serum creatinine and urea are usually normal, except for cases of bilateral extensive disease destroying both kidneys in which case long-term renal replacement therapy is required. Urine analysis reveals leukocytosis, proteins and culture may be positive for bacteria which also helps to ascertain the antibiotic sensitivity pattern [18].

Surgery remains the mainstay for a definitive diagnosis and cure of Xanthogranulomatous pyelonephritis (XGP) requiring extirpation (nephrectomy) as the standard surgical technique but for small tumor, partial nephrectomy can be attempted. In most cases extirpation is necessary because the disease results in an infected, nonfunctioning kidney. Nephron-sparing surgery is an option, especially in cases of bilateral disease with demonstrated significant residual functional renal tissues [19]. Laparoscopic nephrectomy is feasible for some cases of XGP and few cases have been cured by this operative modality and its advantage over radical nephrectomy is being explored. Some pediatric case series of laparascopic resection of XGP have reported promising success with this apporach [20]. The technical difficulty and complications of the procedure raise concern on its wide spread use especially in limited resource settings [21].

Medical therapy with antibitics only has been effective for treatment of XGP in a handful of cases but may be appropriate as a temporary measure for patients requiring workup before nephrectomy and prophylactic antibiotics should be administered before and after surgical intervention. The choice of antibiotic has to be tailored toward the identity and sensitivity of the offending organism. *Proteus* species and *E coli* are usually sensitive to several antibiotics, including first-generation cephalosporins which can be started empirically pending sensitivity results [22]. *Pseudomonas* species has a narrow spectrum of sensitivity and usually require the use of aminoglycosides, third-generation cephalosporins, or fluoroquinolones. For non-septic patients and those evaluated on an outpatient basis, some authors recommend use of oral antibiotics until surgery, at which point intravenous antibiotics should be administered [23]. There is no clear recommendation regarding the duration of antibiotic therapy but data from published case series favor a continuation of oral antibiotics at least for one week post nephrectomy [24, 25]. Our patient underwent left radical nephrectomy and was kept on intravenous Piperacillin-tazobactam for 7 days post nephrectomy and remains asymptomatic at the time of submission of this manuscript.

Conclusion

This case report highlights the importance of clinicians attending children presenting with fever and renal mass to broaden the differential diagnosis for Wims' tumor the commonest childhood renal neoplasm to exclude benign tumors, which can be cured by surgical resection and avoid exposure to chemotherapy especially if treatment is to be given using the European (SIOP) guidelines.

Abbreviations
XGP, Xanthogranulomatous pyelonephritis; CT, computed tomography; WBC, white cell count; RBC, red blood cell; MCV, mean corpuscular volume; MCH, mean corpuscular hemoglobin

Acknowledgements
We thank the guardian for giving us the permission to use the child's information for this publication. We also thank the whole medical, nursing and psychosocial team at the Oncology unit who were involved in the care of this patient.
We also thank the Pathologists at Our Ladys children's hospital Crumlin in Dublin Ireland (Dr. Michael McDermott and Professor Maureen O'Sullivan) and the Pathology team at this laboratory for reviewing and confirming the histological diagnosis for our patient.

Authors' contributions
SJ Participated in the case diagnosis and management, preparation of the case report and literature review, draft of the manuscript. *AS* Participated in the case management, preparation of the case details and review of the manuscript draft *LA* Participated in the in case management, performed the surgery and review of the manuscript draft *PS* Participated in case diagnosis, management and review of the manuscript draft. All authors read and approved the final manuscript.

Competing interests
The authors declare that they have no competing interests.

Consent for publication
Written informed consent was obtained from the guardian of this child for publication of this Case Report and any accompanying images. A copy of the written consent is available for review by the Editorial team of this journal.

Author details
[1]Muhimbili University of health and Allied Sciences, P.O. Box 65001, Dar es Salaam, Tanzania. [2]Muhimbli National Hospital, P.O. Box 65000, Dar es Salaam, Tanzania. [3]College of Health Sciences, University of Dodoma, Box 339, Dodoma, Tanzania.

References
1. Al-Ghazo MA, Ghalayini IF, Matalka II, Al-Kaisi NS, Khader YS. Xanthogranulomatous pyelonephritis: Analysis of 18 cases. Asian J Surg. 2006;29(4):257–61.
2. Rao AG, Eberts PT. Xanthogranulomatous pyelonephritis: an uncommon pediatric renal mass. Pediatr Radiol. 2011;41(5):671–2. author reply 673–4.
3. Shinde S, Kandpal DK, Chowdhary SK. Focal xanthogranulomatous pyelonephritis presenting as renal tumor. Indian J Nephrol. 2013;23(1):76–7.
4. Addison B, Zargar H, Lilic N, Merrilees D, Rice M. Analysis of 35 cases of Xanthogranulomatous pyelonephritis. ANZ J Surg. 2015;85(3):150–3.
5. Aurégan C, Berteloot L, Pierrepont S, Chéron G. Xanthogranulomatous pyelonephritis with pyonephrosis in a 4-year-old child. Arch Pédiatrie Organe Off la Sociéte Fr Pédiatrie. 2015;22(3):287–91.
6. Chalmers D, Marietti S, Kim C. Xanthogranulomatous pyelonephritis in an adolescent. Urology. 2010;76(6):1472–4.
7. Shah K, Parikh M, Pal B, Modi P. Bilateral focal xanthogranulomatous pyelonephritis in a child presenting as complex cystic renal mass: a report on non-surgical treatment. Eur J Pediatr Surg. 2011;21(3):207–8.
8. Tsai K-H, Lai M-Y, Shen S-H, Yang A-H, Su N-W, Ng Y-Y. Bilateral xanthogranulomatous pyelonephritis. J Chin Med Assoc. 2008;71(6):310–4.
9. Kim SW, Yoon BI, Ha US, Sohn DW, Cho YH. Xanthogranulomatous pyelonephritis: clinical experience with 21 cases. J Infect Chemother. 2013; 19(6):1221–4.
10. Siddappa S, Ramprasad K, Muddegowda MK. Xanthogranulomatous pyelonephritis: a retrospective review of 16 cases. Korean J Urol. 2011;52(6):421–4.
11. Nandedkar SS, Malukani K, Sakhi P. Xanthogranulomatous pyelonephritis masquerading as a tumor in an infant. Indian J Urol. 2014;30(3):354–6.
12. Richardson K, Henderson SO. Xanthogranulomatous pyelonephritis presentation in the ED: a case report. Am J Emerg Med. 2009;27(9):1175. e1–3.
13. Hammadeh MY, Nicholls G, Calder CJ, Buick RG, Gornall P, Corkery JJ. Xanthogranulomatous pyelonephritis in childhood: pre-operative diagnosis is possible. Br J Urol. 1994;73(1):83–6.
14. Verswijvel G, Oyen R, Van Poppel H, Roskams T. Xanthogranulomatous pyelonephritis: MRI findings in the diffuse and the focal type. Eur Radiol. 2000;10(4):586–9.
15. Samuel M, Duffy P, Capps S, Mouriquand P, Williams D, Ransley P. Xanthogranulomatous pyelonephritis in childhood. J Pediatr Surg. 2001; 36(4):598–601.
16. Gramage Tormo J, Gavilán Martín C, Atienza Almarcha T. Xanthogranulomatous pyelonephritis in a child with severe malnutrition and recurrent fever. An Pediatr (Barc). 2015;82(1):e184–8.
17. Li L, Parwani AV. Xanthogranulomatous pyelonephritis. Arch Pathol Lab Med. 2011;135(5):671–4.
18. Chen T-Y, Yu T-J, Ko S-F, Huang C-C, Tain Y-L. Diffuse xanthogranulomatous pyelonephritis and staghorn calculus: report of one case. Acta Paediatr Taiwan. 2004;45(1):45–7.

19. Hyla-Klekot L, Paradysz A, Kucharska G, Lipka K, Zajecki W. Successfully treated bilateral xanthogranulomatous pyelonephritis in a child. Pediatr Nephrol. 2008;23(10):1895–6.

20. Pastore V, Niglio F, Basile A, Cocomazzi R, Faticato MG, Aceto G, et al. Laparascopic-assisted nephroureterectomy for shaped urolithiasis and xanthogranulomatous pyelonephritis: case report and review of literature. Afr J Paediatr Surg. 2013; 10(3):285–8.

21. Bercowsky E, Shalhav AL, Portis A, Elbahnasy AM, McDougall EM, Clayman RV. Is the laparoscopic approach justified in patients with xanthogranulomatous pyelonephritis? Urology. 1999;54(3):437–42. discussion 442–3.

22. Ergun T, Akin A, Lakadamyali H. Stage III xanthogranulomatous pyelonephritis treated with antibiotherapy and percutaneous drainage. JBR-BTR. 2011;94(4):209–11.

23. Fritsch S, Gomes WF, Hirt CG, Carvalho M. A distorted yellowish kidney occupied by foamy macrophages. QJM. 2010;103(6):425–6.

24. Mehrotra A, Khanna P, Kumar S, Abraham G. Renal abscess after the Fontan procedure: a case report. J Med Case Rep. 2011;5:50.

25. Oostergo T, Rietbergen JBW, Schrama YC. Refractory urinary tract infections: diagnosis and treatment of xanthogranulomatous pyelonephritis. Ned Tijdschr Geneeskd. 2013;157(11):A5328.

21

Coffee and caffeine intake and risk of urinary incontinence

Shenyou Sun[1], Dongbin Liu[1] and Ziyao Jiao[2]*

Abstract

Background: Previous results from studies on the relationship between coffee/caffeine consumption and risk of urinary incontinence (UI) are inconclusive. We aim to assess this association using a meta-analysis of observational studies.

Methods: Pertinent studies were identified by searching electronic database (Embase, PubMed and Web of Science) and carefully reviewing the reference lists of pertinent articles until July 2015. Random-effects models were used to derive the summary ORs and corresponding 95 % CIs.

Results: Seven studies (one case-control, two cohort and four cross-sectional) were included in our meta-analysis. The summary ORs for any versus non-consumption were 0.75 (95 % CI 0.54–1.04) for coffee and 1.29 (95 % CI 0. 94–1.76) for caffeine consumption. Compared with individuals who never drink coffee, the pooled OR of UI was 0.99 (95 % CI 0.83–1.18) for regular coffee/caffeine drinkers. Coffee/caffeine consumption was not associated with moderate to severe UI (OR 1.18, 95 % CI 0.88–1.58). In stratified analyses by gender, no significant association was found between UI risk and coffee/caffeine consumption in both men (OR 0.99, 95 % CI 0.42–2.32) and women (OR 0.92, 95 % CI 0.80–1.06). By subtype, the pooled ORs were 1.01 (95 % CI 0.86–1.19) for stress UI, 0.99 (95 % CI 0.84–1.16) for urge UI and 0.93 (95 % CI 0.79–1.10) for mixed UI.

Conclusions: This meta-analysis found no evidence for an association between coffee/caffeine consumption and the risk of UI.

Keywords: Coffee, Caffeine, Urinary incontinence, Risk, Meta-analysis

Background

Urinary incontinence (UI) is a common condition with significant impact on overall health and quality of life. It has been estimated that UI prevalence ranged from 5 to 21 % among community dwelling United States men [1–4]. However, UI prevalence estimates differ considerably due to the definition adopted and ranges between 10 % and 40 % among community-dwelling women [5–8]. Although UI is only a symptom of several conditions, ascertaining risk factors would be helpful for identifying high-risk persons and avoidable environmental causes. As for initial UI treatment, lifestyle changes such as fluid modification are strongly recommended.

Coffee and caffeine (coffee/caffeine) are one of the most common beverages worldwide, especially among western countries; thus, investigating its association with various diseases has important public health implications. The relationships between coffee/caffeine and risk of UI have been reported in many studies. However, present epidemiological evidence is inconsistent considering the relationships between coffee/caffeine consumption and the risk of stress, urge and mixed UI. Bortolotti et al. observed no association between coffee and risk of UI in 2000 [9]. Since then, several other studies have been published with inconclusive results [10–12]. For instance, Tettamanti reported that women who often drank coffee had a lower risk of any UI compared to women who did not drink coffee [13]. However, Davis noticed that caffeine consumption was associated with moderate to severe UI in United States men [12].

* Correspondence: jiaoziyao66@sina.com
[2]Department of Anesthesiology, Linyi People's Hospital, Shandong 276000, People's Republic of China
Full list of author information is available at the end of the article

In order to define the possible associations between coffee/caffeine intake and the risk of UI, we performed a meta-analysis of relevant cohort, case-control and cross-sectional studies.

Methods

Search strategy

In performing this meta-analysis, we abided by the Meta-Analysis of Observational Studies in Epidemiology (MOOSE) [14] and preferred reporting items for systematic reviews and meta-analyses (PRISMA) [15] guidelines. Three electronic databases (Medline, Embase and Web of Science) until July 2015 were used for systematic literature search, and search terms included coffee, caffeine, drink, beverage, risk and urinary incontinence. We did not set language or other restrictions in the literature search. As this manuscript is a meta-analysis of available studies, it does not involve ethics and require written informed consent from participants.

Inclusion criteria

The present meta-analysis only included studies which met the following inclusion criteria: (1) the exposure of interest was coffee or caffeine intake; (2) the outcome of interest was UI; (3) the study design was observational; (4) the study reported adjusted risk estimates with corresponding 95 % CIs for the relationship between coffee/caffeine consumption and risk of UI.

Data extraction

According to the guidelines for meta-analysis [14], two reviewers independently carried out eligibility evaluation and data extraction. We collected detailed information including year of publication, the name of first author, study design, age and gender of participants, number of cases, exposure, sample size and multivariate adjusted ORs and 95 % CIs for each category of coffee/caffeine intake.

Statistical analysis

It has been stated that when the outcome was rare, relative risks and ORs could provide similar estimates of risk [16]. In this present meta-analysis, ORs were adopted as a common measure of the association between coffee or caffeine intake and UI risk. In all included studies, the highest level of coffee or caffeine intake was defined as 'regularly drink coffee', and the lowest level of coffee or caffeine intake was defined as 'never drink coffee'. Notably, we only adopted the adjusted OR for this meta-analysis. We derived summary OR estimates with 95 % CIs using the method of DerSimonian and Laird.

To assess heterogeneity among studies, we used the Cochran Q and I^2 statistics. Subgroup analyses stratified by gender, extent and type of UI were also carried out to explore potential sources of heterogeneity. We evaluated publication bias using a funnel plot and the test proposed by the Begg's adjusted rank correlation test and by the Egger's regression test [17, 18]. We carried out statistical analyses using STATA, version 11.0 (STATA, College Station, TX, USA). A p value of less than 0.05 was considered statistically significant.

Results

Identification of studies

The workflow of the study review is summarized in Fig. 1. A total of 259 studies were retrieved from the initial literature search (61 from the Medline, 167 from the EMBASE, and 31 from the Web of Science). After excluding 249 studies based on title and abstract reading, we reviewed the full texts of the remaining 10 potentially pertinent articles. Finally, seven studies [9–13, 19, 20] which stated the relationship between coffee/caffeine intake and risk UI were included in our meta-analysis. The characteristics of the included studies are shown in Table 1. Among the seven included studies, three reported the data of coffee consumption and four reported caffeine consumption.

Coffee/caffeine consumption and UI risk

The results combining the ORs for the risk of UI associated with coffee/caffeine consumption was summarized in Fig. 2. The summary OR for any versus non-consumption were 0.75 (95 % CI 0.54–1.04) for coffee and 1.29 (95 % CI 0.94–1.76) for caffeine consumption. When combining coffee and caffeine, the summary OR was 0.99 (95 % CI 0.85–1.16) with statistically significant heterogeneity among studies ($I^2 = 89.1$ %, $p = 0.000$). Additionally,

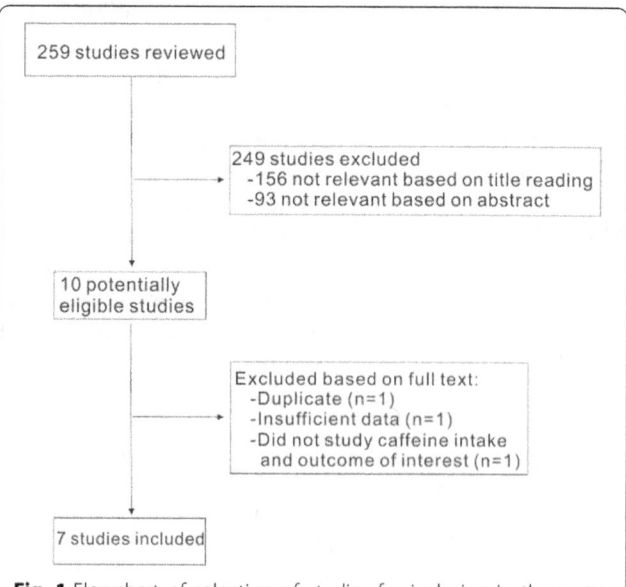

Fig. 1 Flowchart of selection of studies for inclusion in the meta-analysis on coffee/caffeine consumption and UI risk

Table 1 Main characteristics of included studies

First author, year	Country	Study design	Age	Gender	Number of cases	Number of participants	Exposure	Adjustments
Bortolotti, 2000	Italy	Cross-sectional	≥50 (M) ≥40 (F)	Both	408	2721 (M) / 2767 (F)	Coffee	Age
Hannestad, 2003	Norway	Cross-sectional	≥20	Female	6876	27,936	Coffee	Age, BMI and smoking
Jura, 2011	USA	Cohort	37 to 79	Female	15,683	65,176	Caffeine	Age, cohort, parity, BMI, cigarette smoking, race, diabetes, total fluid intake and physical activity
Tettamanti, 2011	Sweden	Cohort	19 to 47	Female	/	14,094	Coffee	Age, parity, BMI, smoking and educational level
Hirayama, 2012	Japan	Case-control	40 to 75	Both	131	683 (M)/298 (F)	caffeine	Age, BMI, smoking status, alcohol drinking, physical activity level, total fluid intake and presence of co-morbidity
Gleason, 2013	USA	Cross-sectional	≥20	Female	1767	4309	Caffeine	Age, race/ethnicity, poverty income ratio, BMI, self-rated health status, major depression, chronic diseases, alcohol use, water intake, total dietary moisture intake and reproductive factors in women including vaginal deliveries
Davis, 2013	USA	Cross-sectional	≥20	Male	511	3960	Caffeine	Age, race/ethnicity, education, BMI, vigorous activity, poverty-to income ratio, chronic disease, health status, depression, alcohol intake, water intake and total moisture intake

compared with individuals who never drink coffee, the pooled OR of UI was 0.99 (95 % CI 0.83–1.18) for regular coffee/caffeine drinkers (Fig. 3).

Coffee /caffeine consumption and incidence of moderate/ severe UI

Three studies provided results on risk of moderate/ severe UI [10, 12, 20], and one study reported the risk of frequent UI among women with daily caffeine intakes [11]. In this subgroup meta-analysis, frequent

UI was also regarded as moderate/severe UI. The summary OR was 1.18 (95 % CI 0.88 to 1.58) with statistically significant heterogeneity among studies ($I^2 = 86.9$ %, $p = 0.000$) (Fig. 4).

Coffee /caffeine consumption and incidence of UI by sex

Two articles reported data on risk of UI specific for gender [9, 19]; one article consisted entirely of men [12] and four articles consisted entirely of women [10, 11, 13, 20]. In stratified analyses by gender, we did not observe any

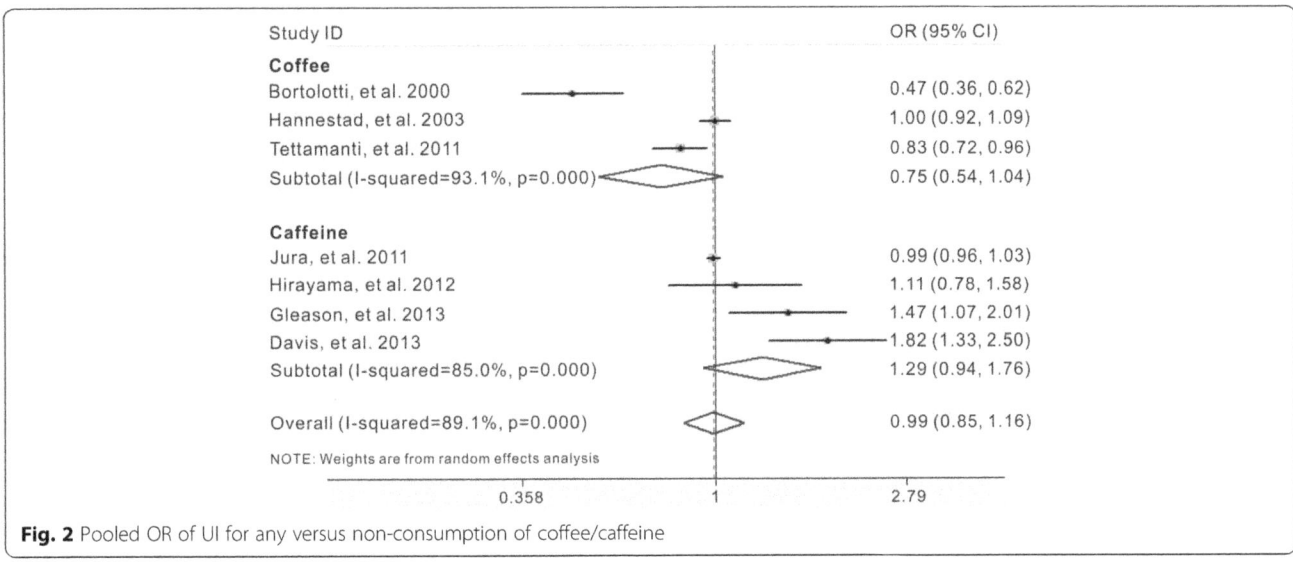

Fig. 2 Pooled OR of UI for any versus non-consumption of coffee/caffeine

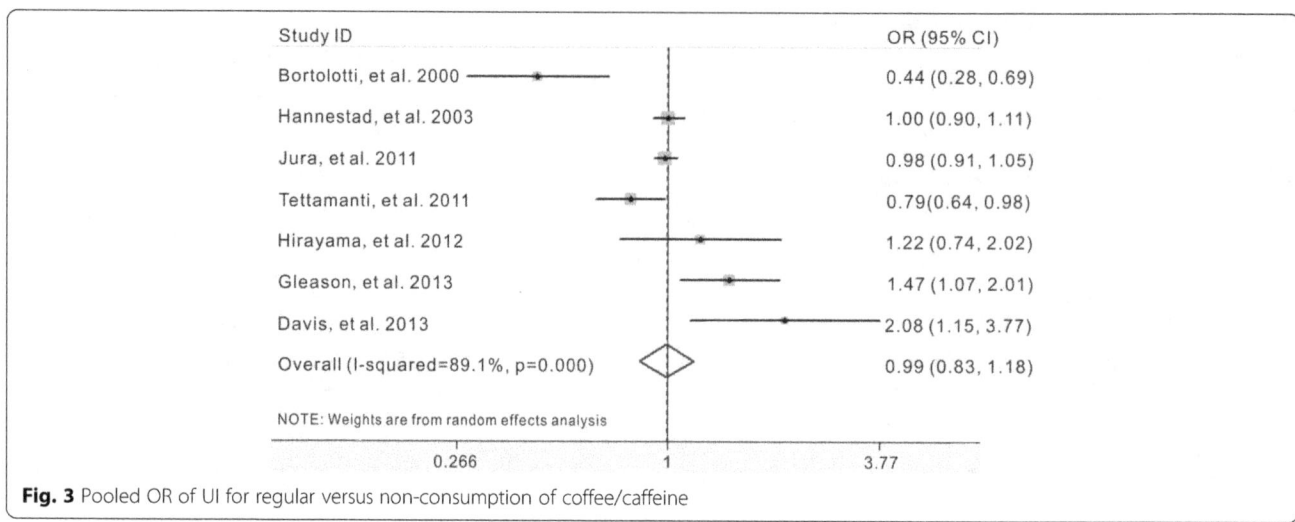

Fig. 3 Pooled OR of UI for regular versus non-consumption of coffee/caffeine

association between coffee/caffeine intake and risk of UI in both men (summary ORs, 0.99; 95 % CI, 0.42–2.32) and women (summary ORs, 0.92; 95 % CI, 0.80–1.06) (Fig. 5).

Coffee /caffeine consumption and risk of UI by subtype

For stress UI, the combined OR was 1.01 (95 % CI 0.86–1.19) (Fig. 6). For urge UI, the summary OR was 0.99 (95 % CI 0.84–1.16). For mixed UI, the pooled OR was 0.93 (95 % CI 0.79 to 1.10). For the different subtypes of incontinence, we did not observe significant association between coffee/caffeine intake and risk of UI.

Sensitivity analysis

As for sensitivity analysis, we removed one study at a time and analyzed the rest. After excluding the study which carried the most weight [11], the OR was 1.01 (95 % CI 0.77–1.32). After excluding the study which carried the least weight [19], the OR was 0.98 (95 % CI 0.83–1.16).

Publication bias

No funnel plot asymmetry was observed for the relationship between coffee/caffeine and UI. *P* values for Egger's regression asymmetry test was 0.998 and the Begg's adjusted rank correlation test was 0.764, indicating a low probability of publication bias (Fig. 7).

Discussion

To our knowledge, this is the first meta-analysis to explore the association between coffee/caffeine intake and UI. We observed that coffee/caffeine consumption was not significantly associated with risk of overall UI. After deleting one study at a time and analyzing the rest, the summary OR ranged from 1.01 (95 % CI 0.77–1.32) to 0.98 (95 % CI 0.83–1.16). When evaluating the severity of UI symptoms, we found no relationship between coffee/caffeine consumption and moderate/severe UI. Moreover, coffee/caffeine consumption was not associated with types of UI (stress, urge, and mixed UI) when controlling for other UI risk factors.

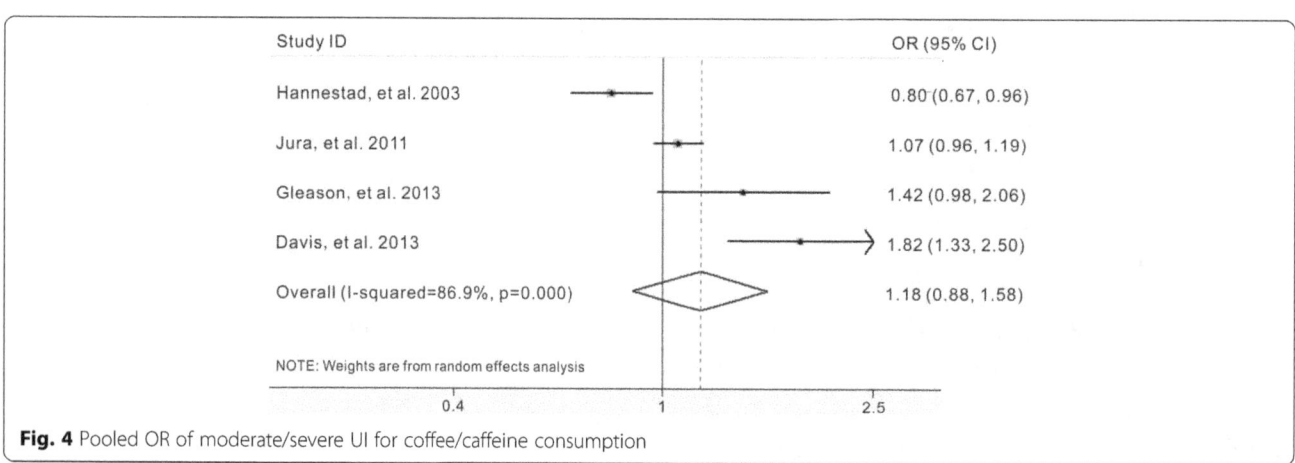

Fig. 4 Pooled OR of moderate/severe UI for coffee/caffeine consumption

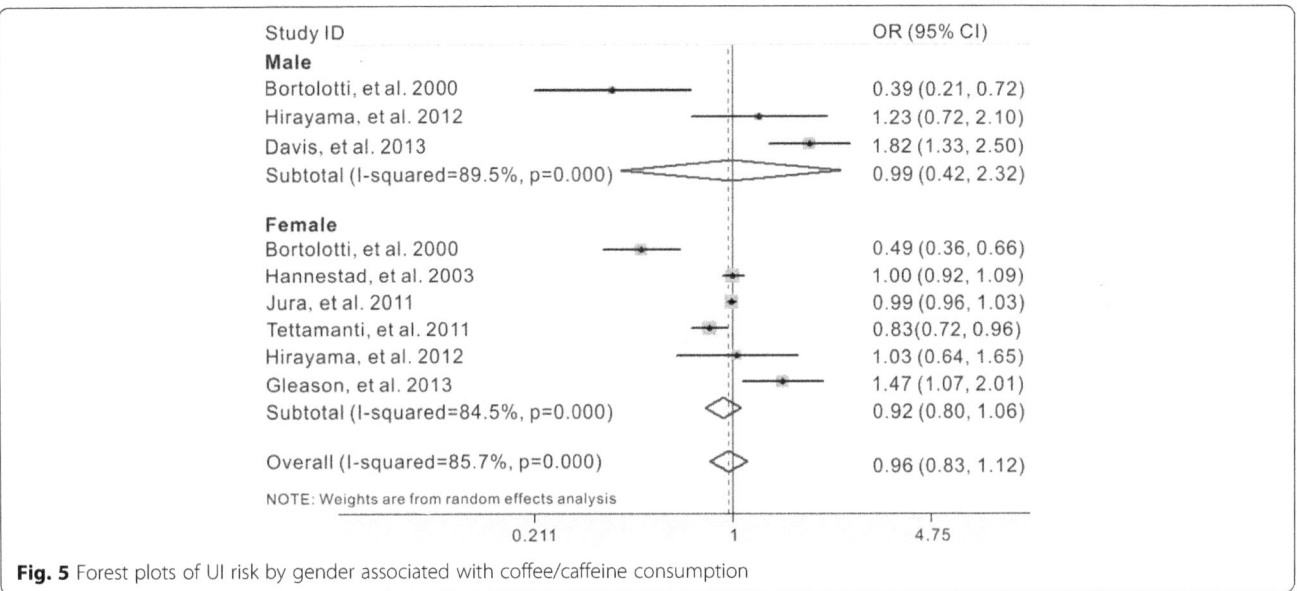

Fig. 5 Forest plots of UI risk by gender associated with coffee/caffeine consumption

Creighton and Stanton observed a statistically significant increase in detrusor pressure on bladder filling following administration of caffeine in women with detrusor instability [21]. Tomlinson et al. reported that the relationship between a decrease in the amount of dietary caffeine consumed and fewer daytime episodes of involuntary urine loss approached significance [22]. Thus, the relationship between lower urinary tract dysfunction and coffee/caffeine intake might be plausible. Considering that coffee/caffeine may exacerbate urinary incontinence, physicians often recommend a reduction in coffee/caffeine intake for individuals with incontinence symptoms.

To ascertain the impact of cumulative dose of coffee/caffeine intake on the risk of UI, we used a meta-analytic approach to estimate overall OR and 95 % CIs for regular coffee/caffeine drinkers versus individuals who seldom drank coffee/caffeine. In the seven studies, the lowest level of coffee/caffeine intake was defined as 'never drink coffee', whereas the highest level of coffee/caffeine intake was defined as 'regularly drink coffee'. Of note, regular coffee/caffeine drinkers experienced an

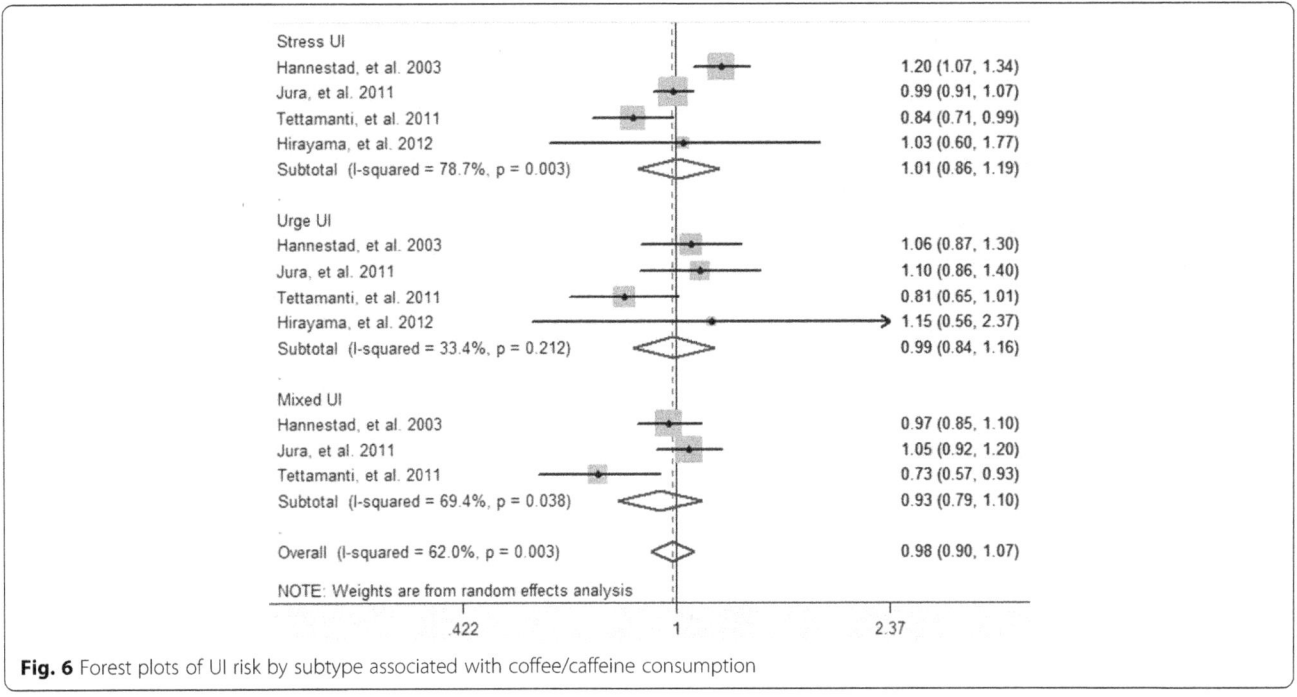

Fig. 6 Forest plots of UI risk by subtype associated with coffee/caffeine consumption

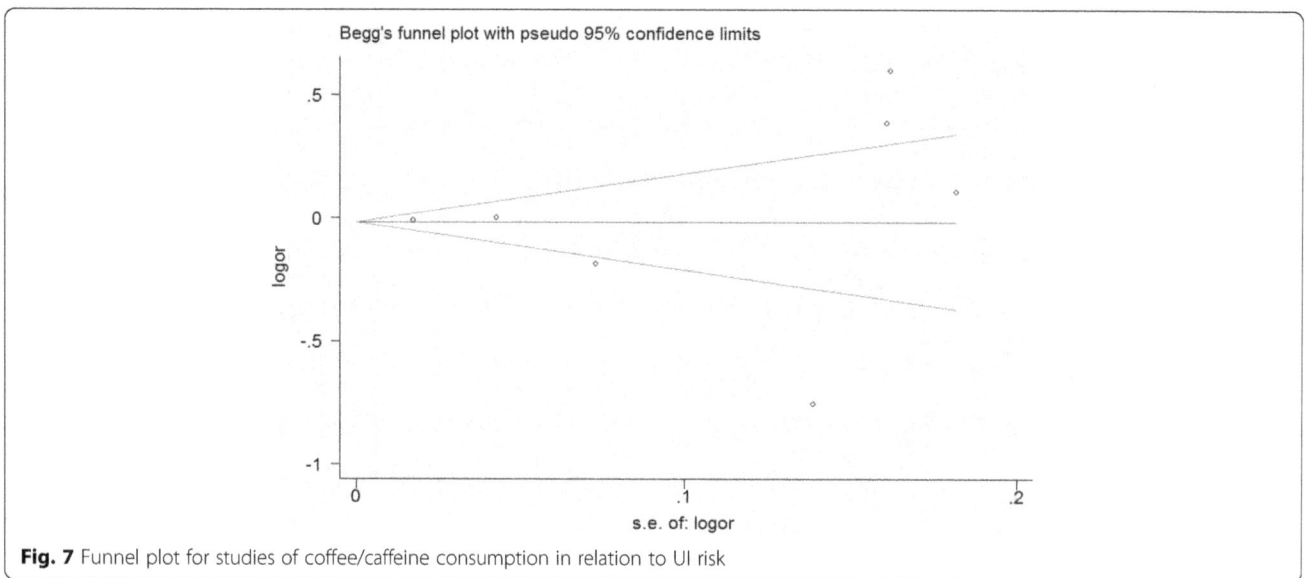

Fig. 7 Funnel plot for studies of coffee/caffeine consumption in relation to UI risk

increased risk of 18 % for UI. However, no significant difference was found between the two groups.

According to the Incontinence Severity Index or other items, UI was categorized as "any" or "moderate/severe". Three studies provided results on risk of moderate/severe UI [10, 11, 20], and one study reported the risk of frequent UI among women with daily caffeine intakes [12]. Jura stated that frequent incontinence was UI at least once per week among incident cases. Thus, frequent UI was also regarded as moderate/severe UI in the subgroup meta-analysis.

We also explored the association between coffee/caffeine consumption and incidence of UI by gender. Tettamanti and colleagues reported that women with a high coffee intake were at lower risk of any urinary incontinence compared with women not drinking coffee [13]. Gleason et al. found that caffeine intake ≥ 204 mg/day was associated with any UI in United States women [20]. A case-control study of Japanese adults failed to find an association between coffee/caffeine intake and incidence of UI [19]. Davis et al. demonstrated that caffeine consumption was significantly associated with moderate to severe urinary incontinence in United States men [12]. However, in stratified analyses by gender, no significant association was found between coffee/caffeine consumption and UI risk in both men and women.

We also analyzed type of incontinence as outcome. Four studies provided results on risk of UI specific for type (stress, urge, and mixed UI). To the best of our knowledge, the present study is the first meta-analysis that summarized the association between coffee consumption and risk of UI by type. Hannestad and colleagues stated that coffee intake was associated with an increased risk of stress UI [10]. However, we did not

observe any significant (positive or negative) relations with UI subtypes in our study.

There are several strengths in the present meta-analysis. First of all, when different ORs were provided according to the different levels of coffee/caffeine consumption, we could combine the results of subgroups and calculated a common OR. Secondly, through visual inspection of a funnel plot and Begg's and Egger's tests, we observed no evidence of publication bias. Moreover, our findings were robust and reliable based on the consistent results from sensitivity analysis.

Some limitations in our study should be of concern. Firstly, adjusted confounding factors varied among different studies. Several potential confounding factors such as parity, BMI, smoking and water intake were not considered in several articles. Secondly, although no significant evidence of publication bias was observed, publication bias might be inevitable due to unpublished studies or original data. Thirdly, categories of coffee/caffeine intake varied from articles, which might lead to significant heterogeneity. Fourthly, due to the lack of relevant studies, crucial influences of coffee/caffeine consumption, including duration of coffee/caffeine intake and type of coffee/caffeine, had not been studied enough. Furthermore, a dose-response analysis could not be carried out due to the limited data provided by the included studies.

Conclusion

In summary, to our knowledge, this is the first meta-analysis to date on the association between coffee/caffeine intake and risk of UI. The results from this meta-analysis of observational studies demonstrated that coffee/caffeine consumption was not associated with overall UI risk. Nevertheless, because of the potential limitations of this meta-analysis, conclusions must be drawn with caution, and more well-designed studies with large sample sizes should be conducted for further validation.

Acknowledgements
None.

Funding
No funding was obtained for this study.

Authors' contributions
Systematic review and meta-analysis SY S. Identification of studies, critical evaluation and discussion DB L and JZ Y. All authors read and approved the final manuscript.

Competing interest
The authors declare that they have no competing interests.

Author details
[1]Department of General surgery, Linyi People's Hospital, Shandong 276000, People's Republic of China. [2]Department of Anesthesiology, Linyi People's Hospital, Shandong 276000, People's Republic of China.

References

1. Markland AD, Richter HE, Fwu CW, et al. Prevalence and trends of urinary incontinence in adults in the United States, 2001 to 2008. J Urol. 2011;186: 589–93.
2. Abrams P, Andersson KE, Birder L, et al. Fourth International Consultation on Incontinence Recommendations of the International Scientific Committee: Evaluation and treatment of urinary incontinence, pelvic organ prolapse, and fecal incontinence. Neurourol Urodyn. 2010;29:213–40.
3. Landefeld CS, Bowers BJ, Feld AD, et al. National Institutes of Health state-of-the-science conference statement: prevention of fecal and urinary incontinence in adults. Ann Intern Med. 2008;148:449–58.
4. Anger JT, Saigal CS, Stothers L, et al. The prevalence of urinary incontinence among community dwelling men: results from the National Health and Nutrition Examination survey. J Urol. 2006;176:2103–8. discussion 2108.
5. Coyne KS, Sexton CC, Thompson CL, et al. The prevalence of lower urinary tract symptoms (LUTS) in the USA, the UK and Sweden: results from the Epidemiology of LUTS (EpiLUTS) study. BJU Int. 2009;104:352–60.
6. Nygaard I, Barber MD, Burgio KL, et al. Prevalence of symptomatic pelvic floor disorders in US women. JAMA. 2008;300:1311–6.
7. Tennstedt SL, Link CL, Steers WD, McKinlay JB. Prevalence of and risk factors for urine leakage in a racially and ethnically diverse population of adults: the Boston Area Community Health (BACH) Survey. Am J Epidemiol. 2008; 167:390–9.
8. Hunskaar S, Burgio K, Diokno A, et al. Epidemiology and natural history of urinary incontinence in women. Urology. 2003;62:16–23.
9. Bortolotti A, Bernardini B, Colli E, et al. Prevalence and risk factors for urinary incontinence in Italy. Eur Urol. 2000;37:30–5.
10. Hannestad YS, Rortveit G, Daltveit AK, Hunskaar S. Are smoking and other lifestyle factors associated with female urinary incontinence? The Norwegian EPINCONT Study. BJOG. 2003;110:247–54.
11. Jura YH, Townsend MK, Curhan GC, et al. Caffeine intake, and the risk of stress, urgency and mixed urinary incontinence. J Urol. 2011;185:1775–80.
12. Davis NJ, Vaughan CP, Johnson 2nd TM, et al. Caffeine intake and its association with urinary incontinence in United States men: results from National Health and Nutrition Examination Surveys 2005-2006 and 2007-2008. J Urol. 2013;189:2170–4.
13. Tettamanti G, Altman D, Pedersen NL, et al. Effects of coffee and tea consumption on urinary incontinence in female twins. BJOG. 2011;118:806–13.
14. Stroup DF, Berlin JA, Morton SC, et al. Meta-analysis of observational studies in epidemiology: a proposal for reporting. Meta-analysis Of Observational Studies in Epidemiology (MOOSE) group. JAMA. 2000;283:2008–12.
15. Moher D, Liberati A, Tetzlaff J, Altman DG. Preferred reporting items for systematic reviews and meta-analyses: the PRISMA statement. J Clin Epidemiol. 2009;62:1006–12.
16. Greenland S. Quantitative methods in the review of epidemiologic literature. Epidemiol Rev. 1987;9:1–30.
17. Begg CB, Mazumdar M. Operating characteristics of a rank correlation test for publication bias. Biometrics. 1994;50:1088–101.
18. Egger M, Davey SG, Schneider M, Minder C. Bias in meta-analysis detected by a simple, graphical test. BMJ. 1997;315:629–34.
19. Hirayama F, Lee AH. Is caffeine intake associated with urinary incontinence in Japanese adults. J Prev Med Public Health. 2012;45:204–8.
20. Gleason JL, Richter HE, Redden DT, et al. Caffeine and urinary incontinence in US women. Int Urogynecol J. 2013;24:295–302.
21. Creighton SM, Stanton SL. Caffeine: does it affect your bladder. Br J Urol. 1990;66:613–4.
22. Tomlinson BU, Dougherty MC, Pendergast JF, et al. Dietary caffeine, fluid intake and urinary incontinence in older rural women. Int Urogynecol J Pelvic Floor Dysfunct. 1999;10:22–8.

22

Prevalence, risk factors and severity of symptoms of pelvic organ prolapse among Emirati women

Hassan M. Elbiss[1], Nawal Osman[1] and Fayez T. Hammad[2*]

Abstract

Background: Similar to other Gulf countries, the society in United Arab Emirates is pro-natal with high parity and high prevalence of macrosomic babies. Therefore, it is possible to have a high prevalence of pelvic organ prolapse (POP). Thus, the aim of this study was to determine the prevalence of POP symptoms in one of the UAE cities.

Methods: A cross-sectional study of all women who attended the three family development centres was conducted in Al-Ain from January 2010 to January 2011. Non-Emirati, pregnant and nulliparous women younger than 30 years were excluded.

Results: Out of 482 women who met the inclusion criteria, 429 (89.0 %) agreed to fully participate in the study. 127 women (29.6 %) reported symptoms of POP (mean age: 38.2 years, range: 18–71).
Out of the 127 affected women, a dragging lump was felt occasionally in 68 %, sometimes in 19 %, most of times in 9 % and all the times in 4 %. 73 % of affected women experienced soreness in the vagina. Around one third had to insert their fingers in the vagina to either start or complete emptying of the bladder or to empty the bowel.
Using multivariate analysis, the independent risk factors were history of constipation, level of education, chronic chest disease, nature of occupation, birth weight and body mass index (Odds ratio; 95 % Confidence interval): (4.1; 2.3-7.3), (1.7; 1.2-2.3), (2.9; 1.6-5.5), (0.5; 0.4-0.8), (1.7; 1.1-2.5), (1.1; 1.0-1.1), respectively (P < 0.05 for all).

Conclusion: Symptoms of POP are prevalent among Emirati women. Independent risk factors included history of chronic constipation and chest disease, level of education, job type, birth weight and body mass index. Additional healthcare campaigns are required to educate the public regarding these risk factors.

Keywords: Genital organ prolapse, Prevalence, Risk factors, Emirati women

Brief summary

Symptoms of POP are common among Emirati women. Several risk factors were identified. Healthcare campaigns are required to educate the public regarding these risk factors.

Background

Female pelvic floor organ prolapse (POP) is a relatively common condition which might result in bothering symptoms. The prevalence of POP and associated symptoms vary among different studies depending on the population studied and research methodology. On examination, 32-41 % of women were found to have some degree of

POP [1, 2]. However, among women with POP, 3–8.3 % have prolapse-related symptoms [3–8].

POP is associated with several risk factors such as multiparity and macrosomia [2, 3, 9]. In this regards the communities in the Gulf countries including UAE are generally pro-natal and hence, women tend to have high parity and short inter-pregnancy intervals. Moreover, these countries also report a high prevalence of macrosomic neonates due to increased prevalence of gestational diabetes [10]. Therefore, the prevalence of POP in UAE may be higher than those reported from the West.

No study has been conducted previously to investigate the prevalence of POP and associated risk factors among women in this part of the world. Therefore, the aim of the present study was to evaluate the prevalence, risk factors and severity of POP symptoms among women in UAE.

* Correspondence: fayez@mail2doctor.com
[2]Department of Surgery, College of Medicine and Health Sciences, United Arab Emirates University, Al AinPO Box 17666United Arab Emirates
Full list of author information is available at the end of the article

Methods

A cross-sectional study of all Emirati women attending all the three family development centres in Al Ain, UAE was conducted from January 2010 to January 2011. These centres are the main and the only governmental facilities in the city and are visited by large number of Emirati women with different ages and backgrounds. Non-Emirati, pregnant and nulliparous women younger than 30 years were excluded. Approval was obtained from the Research Ethical Committee at the College of Medicine and Health Sciences, UAE University. Written consent was obtained from all eligible participants.

The initial phase of the study included developing the required questionnaire for data collection (Additional file 1), testing it to suite our population's attitudes to discuss issues related to POP symptoms. To achieve this, a pilot study was performed on 20 randomly-selected female staff working at the College of Medicine and Health Sciences, UAE University who met the selection criteria of the study. Subsequent modifications were made to the questionnaire based on the results of this pilot study and the questionnaire was then retested on the same group to ensure its suitability in identifying the issues to be addressed in the present study.

The second phase included interviewing all the eligible subjects in the family development centres face to face by well-trained healthcare providers. After explaining the survey to the eligible subjects, all women who agreed to participate were asked to sign a consent form. This was followed by administering the pre-tested questionnaire. The questionnaire consisted of items related to socio-demographic, obstetrics, medical and surgical history. The woman was then asked if she had a dragging lump coming down in the vagina, lump coming out of vagina or lump felt or seen outside vagina; the presence of any of these symptoms were considered to indicate the presence of POP in this study. This was followed by other questions to determine the severity of the condition, other vaginal symptoms and if the women had to insert her finger into the vagina to reduce the lump in order to be able to empty the bladder or bowel.

Data was analysed using SPSS version 19.0 (IBM, Armonk, NY, USA). The subjects were classified into two groups: those with and those without POP symptoms. Inter-group comparisons were performed initially using univariate analysis for all potential risk factors. Student-t test was performed for continuous variables and chi-square or Fisher exact tests for categorical variables. Multivariate direct binary logistic regression analysis was, then, performed on all variables which showed significance on univariate analysis, to determine independent risk factors for POP. A P value of <0.05 was considered statistically significant.

Results

Out of 482 women approached and met the inclusion criteria, 429 (89.0 %) agreed to fully participate in the study. Out of these, there were 127 women (29.6 %) who reported symptoms of POP with a mean age of mean age of 38.2 years (range: 18–71). There was no significant difference in the age between the group with and the group without POP symptoms as shown in Table 1.

The socio-demographic characteristics are shown in Table 1. Several socio-demographic factors were significantly associated with POP symptoms. These included body mass index (BMI) (women with POP symptoms were more obese than those with no symptoms, $P =$ 0.004). As shown in Table 1, it appears that women with university degree had a lower incidence of POP symptoms compared to those with lower degree of education or illiterate women (9 % of women with POP symptoms were university graduates compared to 20 % of those without POP symptoms) ($P = 0.009$).

There was a tendency for women with higher income to have more prevalence of POP symptoms compared to women with lower income although this did not reach statistical significance. The type of occupation also affected the prevalence of POP symptoms which was more prevalent among housewives and women with office jobs compared to those who had jobs which required physical effort (only 13 % of women with POP symptoms had physical jobs compared to 24 % of those without POP symptoms). Marital status, however, did not affect the prevalence of POP symptoms.

Table 2 summarizes the medical, surgical, and obstetrics data in relation to POP symptoms. Some medical diseases or conditions were significantly associated with POP symptoms. These included chronic chest disease, constipation and Diabetes Mellitus. History of smoking was not associated with an increased prevalence of POP symptoms.

Some of the features in the previous obstetric history affected the prevalence of POP symptoms whereas others did not. For instance, parity and the previous history of elective or emergency caesarean sections did not affect whereas the history of previous instrumental delivery and high birth weight significantly increased the prevalence of POP symptoms. As might be expected, women with POP symptoms had a significantly higher incidence of urinary incontinence and previous history of POP or urinary incontinence surgery.

Despite the fact that several factors were significantly associated with the symptoms of POP on univariate analysis, multivariate logistic regression of these factors (BMI, level of education, nature of occupation, history of chronic chest disease, constipation, diabetes mellitus, previous instrumental delivery, maximum birth weight, history of urinary incontinence and previous surgery for

Table 1 Socio-demographic characteristics of women with and without POP symptoms. All variables are expressed as number and percentage from the total number of patients from the respective group (with or without POP symptoms) except age and body mass index which were expressed as mean ± standard error of the mean

	No POP Symptoms (n = 302)	POP Symptoms (n = 127)	P-value
Age (in years)	37.4 ± 0.6	38.2 ± 0.9	0.45
Body Mass Index (BMI)	28.2 ± 0.3	29.9 ± 0.5	0.004
Monthly income (AED)			
<5000	36 (12 %)	4 (3 %)	
5000-10000	161 (53 %)	55 (43 %)	0.07
>10000	105 (35 %)	70 (55 %)	
Education			
Illiterate	82 (27 %)	29 (23 %)	
Primary School	98 (32 %)	54 (43 %)	0.009
Secondary School	61 (20 %)	33 (26 %)	
University	61 (20 %)	11 (9 %)	
Occupation			
Housewife	198 (66 %)	91 (72 %)	
Office Job	32 (11 %)	19 (15 %)	0.036
Physical Job	72 (24 %)	17 (13 %)	
Marital Status			
Never married	11 (3 %)	2 (0.5 %)	
Married/ previously married	291 (68 %)	125 (29 %)	0.3

Table 2 Medical and Obstetric history of women with and without POP symptoms. All variables are expressed as number and percentage from the total number of patients from the respective group (with or without POP symptoms) parity and maximum birth weight which were expressed as mean ± standard error of the mean

	No POP Symptoms (n = 302)	POP Symptoms (n = 127)	P-value
Chronic Chest disease	33 (11 %)	35 (28 %)	0.0001
Constipation	32 (11 %)	48 (38 %)	0.0001
Diabetes Mellitus	45 (15 %)	29 (23 %)	0.047
Smoking	25 (8 %)	12 (9 %)	0.7
Parity	4.6 ± 0.2	4.5 ± 0.3	0.7
Previous instrumental delivery	23 (8 %)	20 (16 %)	0.01
Previous emergency LSCS	49 (16 %)	20 (16 %)	0.6
Previous elective LSCS	13 (4 %)	4 (3 %)	0.3
Maximum birth weight	3.3 ± 0.04	3.49 ± 0.06	0.005
History of urinary incontinence	94 (31 %)	88 (69 %)	0.0001
Previous surgery for urinary incontinence	11 (4 %)	11 (9 %)	0.03
Previous surgery for POP	2 (1 %)	20 (16 %)	0.0001

urinary incontinence) revealed that there were only few independent risk factors. These include the history of constipation, level of education, chronic chest disease, nature of occupation, maximum birth weight and BMI (Table 3).

In regard to the severity of POP symptoms, out of the 127 patients with symptoms of POP, the dragging lump was felt occasionally in 68 % of the women, sometimes in 19 %, most of times in 9 % and all the times in 4 %. In addition to the dragging sensation, the majority of affected women had soreness in the vagina as demonstrated in Table 4. Similarly, around one third of them had to insert their fingers in the vagina to either start or complete emptying of the bladder or to empty the bowel (Table 4).

Discussion

The findings of the present study indicated that symptoms of POP are highly prevalent among women in UAE. Prevalence of POP symptoms in our study appears to be higher than what was previously reported from the western countries [3–8]. The exact reason for

this difference is difficult to ascertain without performing a comparative study; however, it could potentially reflect the difference in study populations and or risk factors. High prevalence of increased BMI, and high birth weight in our society may attribute to higher prevalence of POP in the current study [10]. Indeed, both these factors were found to be independent risk factor for having POP symptoms, similar to other studies some of which had used multivariate analysis [2, 9, 11].

In the present study, several factors were shown to be significantly associated with POP on univariate analysis. These findings were similar to other studies in which the data was analysed using univariate analysis only [1, 7, 11–13]. Age, however, was not found to be associated with POP in our population. This finding was in agreement with previous studies [11, 12].

In the current study, the nature of occupation was found to be significantly and independently associated with the prevalence of POP symptoms in such a way that women with physical jobs such as nurses, for instance, were associated with less POP symptoms. This could possibly be explained by the fact that these types of jobs would improve the pelvic musculature in women and hence decreases the pelvic organ descent. Women with other types of jobs or housewives in our population tend to do minimal exercise due to cultural reasons and the widespread employment of several housemaids per household which would leave women with minimal

Table 3 The independent risk factors for POP symptoms in women using multivariate logistic regression analysis

	Odds ratio	95 % CI	P value
Constipation	4.1	2.3-7.3	0.0001
Education	1.7	1.2-2.3	0.001
Chronic Chest Disease	2.9	1.6-5.5	0.001
Occupation	0.5	0.4-0.8	0.002
Maximum Birth Weight	1.7	1.1-2.5	0.016
Body Mass Index	1.1	1.0-1.1	0.046

exercise to do unless they go to work or get involved in some form of gymnastic activities which is not common in this society.

In addition to the type of occupation, the level of education independently determined the prevalence of POP symptoms. Surprisingly, women with university degree had less prevalence of POP symptoms compared to women with lower level of education or illiterate women. This could be due to the fact that university graduates are more aware of healthy life style techniques including pelvic floor exercise compared to other women. Alternatively, these women tend to be more open in discussing their health issues. Certainly, more research is required to clarify this issue.

In the current study, we also investigated the relationship of POP symptoms with some underlining medical conditions. With this regard, both chronic chest disease and chronic constipation have been found to be independent risk factors for developing POP symptoms. Both conditions are associated with chronic straining and increased intra-abdominal pressure and this finding is consistent with previous reports [2, 11, 12]. So although constipation could be a consequence of POP, some studies has shown that constipation in the early age before the onset of POP was significantly more common in women who subsequently developed POP (61 %) compared to women who did not (4 %) [14].

To the best of our knowledge, this is the first study which assessed the prevalence of POP symptoms among women from this part of the world. One of the limitations of the study is the exclusion of nulliparous women younger than 30 years of age. This was based on the previously published data which showed a low incidence of POP in nulliparous women [7].

Due to the conservative nature of this society, it was difficult to carry out vaginal examination to identify women who had anatomical POP. However, a good correlation has been shown to exist between POP symptoms and the present of POP on vaginal examination [15]. In the current study, such symptoms were

Table 4 Severity of vaginal soreness and the need to insert the finger into the vaginal to complete bladder or bowel emptying. The percentages are out of the 127 women who complaint of a dragging lump in the vagina

	Not at all	Occasionally	Sometimes	Most of times	All the times
Are you aware of soreness of your vagina?	27 %	50 %	13 %	5 %	5 %
Do you have to insert finger into your vagina to start or complete emptying your bladder?	66 %	19 %	9 %	3 %	3 %
Do you have to insert finger into your vagina to empty your bowel?	62 %	24 %	9 %	3 %	2 %

identified using a pre-tested questionnaire which included questions used in many previous studies [7, 12, 16, 17]. The use of healthcare providers to question the participants and fill the questionnaire eliminated the potential misunderstanding of the questions by the participants, which may have been interpreted differently otherwise.

In the current report, all women from the three family development centres who met the inclusion criteria were enrolled in the study. These centres are used for social, cultural and educational activities and are visited by women from different social and cultural backgrounds and hence more representative of the general population compared to subjects from hospitals or primary healthcare centres. The fact that the women included in the current study came from only one city makes it difficult to generalise the results to the whole country. However, the fact that this city (Al Ain) is the home for approximately 20 % of the whole national Emirati population [18, 19] indicates that the results obtained might provide a reasonable estimate of the prevalence of the POP in the whole country.

Conclusion

In conclusion, symptoms of pelvic organ prolapse appear to be prevalent among Emirati women. History of chronic constipation and chest disease, level of education, job type, birth weight and body mass index were independent risk factors for having symptoms of pelvic organ prolapse. Additional healthcare programs and campaigns are required to educate the public regarding these risk factors to decrease the prevalence of this potentially bothersome condition.

Abbreviations
UAE: United Arab Emirates; POP: Pelvic organ prolapse; BMI: Body mass index.

Competing interests

The authors declare that they have no competing interests.

Authors' contributions

HME: Project development, Data management, Manuscript writing. NO: Protocol development, Data collection, approval of final version of manuscript. FTH: Project development, Data management & analysis, Manuscript writing & editing. All authors read and approved the final manuscript.

Acknowledgment

The authors would like to acknowledge Prof. N. Nagelkerke for statistical input and Dr F. Radi, R. Z. Al Mazroei, F. Al Ahbabi, K. Al Ameri, N. Al Bloushi and E. NUR for technical assistance in data collection.

Author details

[1]Department of Obstetrics and Gynaecology, College of Medicine and Health Sciences, United Arab Emirates University, Al Ain, United Arab Emirates. [2]Department of Surgery, College of Medicine and Health Sciences, United Arab Emirates University, Al AinPO Box 17666United Arab Emirates.

References

1. Handa VL, Garrett E, Hendrix S, Gold E, Robbins J. Progression and remission of pelvic organ prolapse: a longitudinal study of menopausal women. Am J Obstet Gynecol. 2004;190(1):27–32.
2. Hendrix SL, Clark A, Nygaard I, Aragaki A, Barnabei V, McTiernan A. Pelvic organ prolapse in the Women's Health Initiative: gravity and gravidity. Am J Obstet Gynecol. 2002;186(6):1160–6.
3. Nygaard I, Barber MD, Burgio KL, Kenton K, Meikle S, Schaffer J, et al. Prevalence of symptomatic pelvic floor disorders in US women. JAMA. 2008;300(11):1311–6.
4. Tegerstedt G, Maehle-Schmidt M, Nyren O, Hammarstrom M. Prevalence of symptomatic pelvic organ prolapse in a Swedish population. Int Urogynecol J Pelvic Floor Dysfunct. 2005;16(6):497–503.
5. Wu JM, Vaughan CP, Goode PS, Redden DT, Burgio KL, Richter HE, et al. Prevalence and trends of symptomatic pelvic floor disorders in U.S. women. Obstet Gynecol. 2014;123(1):141–8.
6. Barber MD, Maher C. Epidemiology and outcome assessment of pelvic organ prolapse. Int Urogynecol J. 2013;24(11):1783–90.
7. Slieker-ten Hove MC, Pool-Goudzwaard AL, Eijkemans MJ, Steegers-Theunissen RP, Burger CW, Vierhout ME. The prevalence of pelvic organ prolapse symptoms and signs and their relation with bladder and bowel disorders in a general female population. Int Urogynecol J Pelvic Floor Dysfunct. 2009;20(9):1037–45.
8. Bradley CS, Nygaard IE. Vaginal wall descensus and pelvic floor symptoms in older women. Obstet Gynecol. 2005;106(4):759–66.
9. Samuelsson EC, Victor FT, Tibblin G, Svardsudd KF. Signs of genital prolapse in a Swedish population of women 20 to 59 years of age and possible related factors. Am J Obstet Gynecol. 1999;180(2 Pt 1):299–305.
10. Alshami HA, Kadasne AR, Khalfan M, Iqbal SZ, Mirghani HM. Pregnancy outcome in late maternal age in a high-income developing country. Arch Gynecol Obstet. 2012;284(5):1113–6.
11. Rortveit G, Brown JS, Thom DH, Van Den Eeden SK, Creasman JM, Subak LL. Symptomatic pelvic organ prolapse: prevalence and risk factors in a population-based, racially diverse cohort. Obstet Gynecol. 2007;109(6):1396–403.
12. McLennan MT, Harris JK, Kariuki B, Meyer S. Family history as a risk factor for pelvic organ prolapse. Int Urogynecol J Pelvic Floor Dysfunct. 2008;19(8):1063–9.
13. Swift SE, Pound T, Dias JK. Case–control study of etiologic factors in the development of severe pelvic organ prolapse. Int Urogynecol J Pelvic Floor Dysfunct. 2001;12(3):187–92.
14. Spence-Jones C, Kamm MA, Henry MM, Hudson CN. Bowel dysfunction: a pathogenic factor in uterovaginal prolapse and urinary stress incontinence. Br J Obstet Gynaecol. 1994;101(2):147–52.
15. Swift SE, Tate SB, Nicholas J. Correlation of symptoms with degree of pelvic organ support in a general population of women: what is pelvic organ prolapse? Am J Obstet Gynecol. 2003;189(2):372–7. discussion 7–9.
16. Gonzalez-Argente FX, Jain A, Nogueras JJ, Davila GW, Weiss EG, Wexner SD. Prevalence and severity of urinary incontinence and pelvic genital prolapse in females with anal incontinence or rectal prolapse. Dis Colon Rectum. 2001;44(7):920–6.
17. World Health Organization G. Measuring Reproductive Morbidity: Report of Technical Working Group. Geneva: World Health Organization: Division of Family Planning; 1989. WHO/MCH/90.4.
18. National Bureau of Statistics UAE. Methodoloy of Estimating the population in UAE 2011 [cited 2013 Accessed February 15, 2013]. 1st Edition:[Available from: http://www.uaestatistics.gov.ae/ReportDetailsEnglish/tabid/121/Default.aspx?ItemId=1914&PTID=104&MenuId=1.
19. Statistics Centre AD. Statistical Yearbook of Abu Dhabi 2011 [updated 2011; cited 2013 Accessed February 15, 2113]. 1st Edition:[Available from: http://www.scad.ae/SCADDocuments/EBOOK%20English%20SYB%202011.pdf.

23

Urinary incontinence, mental health and loneliness among community-dwelling older adults in Ireland

Andrew Stickley[1*], Ziggi Ivan Santini [2] and Ai Koyanagi[3]

Abstract

Background: Urinary incontinence (UI) is associated with worse health among older adults. Little is known however, about its relation with loneliness or the role of mental health in this association. This study examined these factors among older adults in Ireland.

Methods: Data were analyzed from 6903 community-dwelling adults aged ≥ 50 collected in the first wave of The Irish Longitudinal Study on Ageing (TILDA) in 2009–11. Information was obtained on the self-reported occurrence (yes/no) and severity (frequency/activity limitations) of UI in the past 12 months. Loneliness was measured using the UCLA Loneliness Scale short form. Information was also obtained on depression (CES-D), anxiety (HADS-A) and other sociodemographic variables. Logistic regression analysis was used to examine the association between variables.

Results: In a model adjusted for all potential confounders except mental disorders, compared to no UI, any UI was associated with significantly higher odds for loneliness (odds ratio: 1.51). When depression was included in the analysis, the association was attenuated and became non-significant while the inclusion of anxiety had a much smaller effect. Similarly, although frequency of UI and activity limitations due to UI were both significantly associated with loneliness prior to adjustment for mental disorders, neither association remained significant after adjustment for both depression and anxiety.

Conclusion: UI is associated with higher odds for loneliness among older community-dwelling adults but this association is largely explained by comorbid mental health problems, in particular, depression.

Keywords: Urinary incontinence, Lonely, Anxiety, Depression

Background

Urinary incontinence (UI), which is defined as the involuntary leakage of urine [1] is highly prevalent in the general population and can severely affect many aspects of daily life [2, 3]. Although this condition can exist in adults of all ages [3], a large body of research has shown that the prevalence of UI increases with age [4, 5] and that the elderly are especially vulnerable to this condition [6] particularly in a severe form [7, 8]. While previously reported prevalence figures vary due to the different operational definitions of UI employed (type,

severity etc.), an earlier review article presented figures which showed that the prevalence of UI ranges between 9 and 59% in those aged 50 and above [9].

Studies have indicated that UI can have a significant negative effect on the lives of older people [10]. For example, it has been associated with troublesome symptoms such as aches, pain, weakness, and shortness of breath [11], as well as with an increased risk for outcomes such as falls and fractures [12, 13]. The avoidance of physical activity in an attempt to manage/control the condition may also have an effect on overall health by increasing the risk of conditions such as hypertension [14, 15]. In addition, UI is also associated with poorer mental health among older persons including anxiety disorders [16] and depression [16, 17].

* Correspondence: amstick66@gmail.com
[1]The Stockholm Center for Health and Social Change (SCOHOST), Södertörn University, Huddinge 141 89, Sweden
Full list of author information is available at the end of the article

Despite the large number of studies on UI and its associated adverse health outcomes, one condition which has been little studied to date in relation to UI is loneliness. This is an important research gap given that: (a) incontinent individuals can experience feelings of frustration, embarrassment and shame [18, 19] as a result of their condition and will sometimes reduce/avoid social contacts and activities in order to control UI and its effects [18], which may lead to increased social isolation and feelings of loneliness; and (b) loneliness has itself been linked to an increased risk for morbidity and mortality among older persons [20, 21]. To the best of our knowledge, to date, there have been only three studies which have investigated this association. Specifically, two recent studies have shown that older adults (≥57 years old) with UI in Canada and the United States have an increased risk of feeling lonely compared to those who are continent [22] or who have no/less severe UI symptoms (no/weekly/monthly/yearly vs. daily) [23], respectively. An earlier study from the United States also found similar results where UI and UI severity (measured by the quantity of urine loss) were both associated with loneliness among middle-aged and older adults (≥ 40 years old) [24].

Although these studies have advanced understanding of the psychological consequences of UI, there are aspects of the association between UI and loneliness among older adults that are yet to be elucidated. In particular, there has been an absence of research on the role of common mental disorders (CMDs) in this association. This is an important gap in the research as not only are anxiety and depression linked to UI in older persons [16, 17], but other research has highlighted their close link with loneliness in older adults [25–27] and that in middle-aged and older adults, depressive symptoms and loneliness may be reciprocally related [28]. Therefore, there is a need to assess the extent to which CMDs explain the association between UI and loneliness. In addition, until now, there has been no research on whether the specific consequences of UI, such as activity limitations, are important for loneliness in older adults.

Thus, using data from a nationally representative sample of community-dwelling older adults (aged 50 and above) in Ireland, the current study had three aims: (1) to determine if UI is associated with an increased risk of feeling lonely; (2) to examine if the severity of UI, as measured by the frequency of urine loss and activity limitations, is associated with loneliness; and (3) to assess the role of CMDs in the association between UI, UI severity and loneliness.

Methods

Study design and sample

The data used in this study came from the first wave of The Irish Longitudinal Study on Ageing (TILDA) which was conducted by Trinity College Dublin between October 2009 and February 2011. Details of the survey and its sampling procedure have been published previously [29, 30]. In brief, TILDA was a nationally representative survey of community-based adults aged 50 and above living in Ireland. The target sample included every household resident meeting this age criterion. Clustered random sampling was used to obtain a nationally representative sample. Individuals who were institutionalized and those who had doctor-diagnosed dementia were excluded. If severe cognitive impairment (judged at the interviewer's discretion) prevented individuals from providing written informed consent to participate in the survey, they were also excluded [31]. The data was collected by trained interviewers using computer-assisted personal interviewing (CAPI), and with the use of self-completion questionnaires (SCQs). All individuals that underwent a CAPI interview were also asked to complete the SCQ. The overall response rate was 62%, while 84% of those who participated in the survey returned the SCQ [29, 30].

In total, 8504 people aged ≥50 years ($n = 8175$) and their spouses or partners younger than 50 years ($n = 329$) comprised the survey sample. In the current study, the analysis was restricted to participants aged 50 years and above and those who completed the SCQ. These conditions were necessary as information on certain variables (e.g., loneliness, anxiety etc.) was obtained from the SCQ. Following these restrictions, the analytic sample comprised 6903 individuals. The Faculty of Health Sciences Ethics Committee of Trinity College Dublin provided ethical approval for TILDA, with written informed consent being obtained from all participants.

Measures

Loneliness (Dependent variable)

The short form of the University of California, Los Angeles (UCLA) Loneliness Scale was used to assess feelings of loneliness [32, 33]. The short form UCLA Loneliness Scale, which assesses subjective feelings of social isolation, is a commonly used measure in loneliness research. The dominant factor underlying the UCLA Loneliness scale is 'perceived social isolation' [34, 35]. The UCLA three-item scale is comprised of three negatively-worded questions relating to feelings of isolation, feeling left out and companionship. The three response options are coded as 1 (hardly ever), 2 (some of the time), and 3 (often). Scores are summed to create a total score that runs from 3 to 9, with higher scores indicating a greater degree of loneliness (Cronbach's alpha = 0.81). Previous research has indicated that this scale has an acceptable degree of reliability and has both concurrent and discriminant validity [33]. As the distribution of the loneliness variable was right-skewed, in this study we used a dichotomous loneliness variable for the regression analyses. Specifically, in accordance with a recent study, a score of 4–9 was categorized as feeling lonely while a score of 3 (i.e., replying 'hardly ever' to all of the questions) was classified as not feeling lonely [22].

Urinary incontinence (UI) (Independent variable)

Any UI was assessed by the question 'During the last 12 months, have you lost any amount of urine beyond your control?' with the answer options 'yes' or 'no'. For those who responded affirmatively to this question, follow-up questions on the frequency of UI and limitations in activity due to UI were asked. Frequency was assessed by the question 'Did this happen more than once during a 1 month period?' and activity limitations were examined by the question 'Do you ever limit your activities, for example, what you do or where you go, because of UI?' Both of these questions had 'yes' or 'no' as answer options.

Depression

Depressive symptoms were measured with the 20-item Center for Epidemiologic Studies Depression (CES-D) scale [36], which assesses symptoms experienced in the preceding week. Its 20 items are scored on a scale from 0 (rarely or none of the time, less than one day in the week) to 3 (most or all of the time, five to seven days in the week). In order to avoid an overlap with the outcome (loneliness), and following the lead of an earlier study [37], we excluded the item on loneliness ('I felt lonely') that is included in the CES-D scale. Thus, scores from the remaining 19 items were summed to create a scale with values ranging from 0 to 57 where higher scores signified more depressive symptoms (Cronbach's alpha = 0.87). Previous studies have highlighted the validity of the CES-D scale as a measure of depression in community-dwelling older adults [38, 39].

Anxiety

The Hospital Anxiety and Depression Scale (HADS-A) [40] was used to assess anxiety symptoms. This scale measures the presence of anxiety symptoms without reference to a specific time frame. The scale consists of seven items rated on a four-point scale from 0 (not at all) to 3 (very often indeed), five of which are reverse coded. The scores from the individual items were summed to create a total score that ranged from 0 to 21, with higher scores indicating more anxiety (Cronbach's alpha = 0.65). Previous research has indicated that the HADS is a reliable measure in both younger and older persons [41].

Control variables

Social network index

The Berkman-Syme Social Network Index (SNI) was used to assess social networks. The SNI is a validated self-report questionnaire [42] that assesses the degree to which a person is socially integrated. Information is elicited on marital/partnership status (married/with partner versus not), sociability (number of children, close relatives, and close friends and the frequency of contact with them), and church group or community organization membership. A composite score is calculated that ranges from 0 to 4. In this study, we used what is regarded as the standard categorization [i.e., 0–1 (most isolated), 2 (moderately isolated), 3 (moderately integrated), and 4 (most integrated)] [42]. Further information on the psychometric properties of the SNI and evidence relating to its predictive validity has been provided elsewhere [43].

Chronic medical conditions

To assess chronic health conditions, participants were presented with a list of 17 medical conditions and asked, "has a doctor ever told you that you have any of the conditions on this card?" These conditions were: high blood pressure or hypertension; angina; heart attack (including myocardial or coronary thrombosis); congestive heart failure; diabetes or high blood sugar; stroke (cerebral vascular disease); ministroke or transient ischemic attack; high cholesterol; heart murmur; abnormal heart rhythm; any other heart trouble; chronic lung disease such as chronic bronchitis or emphysema; asthma; arthritis (including osteoarthritis, or rheumatism); osteoporosis; cancer or a malignant tumor (including leukemia or lymphoma but excluding minor skin cancers); cirrhosis or serious liver damage. The total number of chronic medical conditions was calculated and divided into three categories: 0 (none), 1, or ≥2.

Activities of daily living (ADL) disability

To assess ADL disability participants were asked to indicate whether they had difficulty performing six activities (dressing, walking, bathing, eating, getting in or out of bed, and using the toilet) [44]. Participants having difficulty with one or more ADLs were categorized as having an ADL disability.

Sociodemographic variables

Sociodemographic characteristics included age (50–59, 60–69, 70–79, and ≥80 years), sex, education, and wealth. Education was divided into three categories: primary (some primary/not complete; primary or equivalent); secondary (intermediate/junior/group certificate or equivalent; leaving certificate or equivalent); and tertiary (diploma/certificate; primary degree; postgraduate/higher degree). As more than 50% of the income values were missing, a proxy measure (financial strain) was used to assess wealth. Participants were thus asked to respond to the statement that a 'shortage of money stops me from doing the things I want to do' using one of the answer options, 'never', 'rarely', 'sometimes', and 'often'.

Statistical analysis

Stata version 14.1 (Stata Corp LP, College Station, Texas) was used to perform the analysis. In the first stage, descriptive statistics are presented of the study sample. The difference in sample characteristics by the presence of UI was tested by using Chi-square and Student's t-tests for categorical and continuous variables, respectively. Logistic regression analysis was then used to firstly assess the association between any UI (independent variable) and loneliness (dependent variable) based on the question 'During the last 12 months, have you lost any amount of urine beyond your control?'. A hierarchical analysis was conducted by including different variables sequentially in different models to assess how these variables influenced the

association between UI and loneliness. Six different models were thus constructed: Model 1: unadjusted; Model 2: adjusted for age, sex, education, financial strain, number of chronic conditions, and ADL disability; Model 3: adjusted for the variables in Model 2 and the SNI; Model 4: adjusted for the variables in Model 3 and depression; Model 5: adjusted for the variables in Model 3 and anxiety; Model 6: adjusted for the variables in Model 3, depression, and anxiety. The selection of the variables used for adjustment was based on past literature.

To assess the association between UI severity and loneliness, we repeated the analytic method described above but replaced the any UI variable with a three-category UI variable which incorporates the frequency of urinary inconsistence [UI (-); UI (+) once a month or less; UI (+) more than once a month], or activity limitations due to UI [UI (-); UI (+) but no activity limitations; UI (+) with

Table 1 Sample characteristics (overall and by urinary incontinence)

Characteristic	Categories	Overall	Urinary incontinence		P-value[a]
			No	Yes	
Age (years)	50–59	40.5	41.9	30.3	<0.001
	60–69	30.7	30.9	29.8	
	70–79	20.0	19.2	25.1	
	≥80	8.8	7.9	14.9	
Sex	Male	47.9	51.4	23.8	<0.001
	Female	52.1	48.6	76.2	
Education	Primary	38.1	37.2	44.0	<0.001
	Secondary	43.3	44.1	38.3	
	Tertiary	18.6	18.8	17.6	
Financial strain	Never	23.1	23.4	20.7	<0.001
	Rarely	21.6	21.7	21.5	
	Sometimes	36.4	36.8	33.3	
	Often	18.9	18.1	24.6	
Number of	None	23.4	25.2	11.5	<0.001
chronic conditions	One	28.1	28.8	22.9	
	Two or more	48.5	46.0	65.6	
ADL disability	No	90.9	92.7	78.7	<0.001
	Yes	9.1	7.3	21.3	
Social Network Index	Most isolated	7.5	7.0	10.5	0.011
	Moderately isolated	28.8	28.9	27.4	
	Moderately integrated	41.0	41.1	40.3	
	Most integrated	22.7	22.9	21.9	
Depression	Mean (SD)	5.7 (6.8)	5.2 (6.4)	9.1 (8.6)	<0.001
Anxiety	Mean (SD)	5.5 (3.7)	5.3 (3.6)	6.7 (4.1)	<0.001

The data are column percentages unless otherwise stated
Estimates are based on weighted sample
Abbreviation: ADL Activities of daily living, *SD* Standard deviation
[a]The difference in sample characteristics by urinary incontinence was tested by Chi-square tests and Student's t-tests for categorical and continuous variables, respectively

activity limitations]. This analysis used 'no UI' as the reference category. Finally, we also performed this analysis while restricting it to those with UI to assess whether the frequency of UI or activity limitations due to UI confers an increased risk for loneliness among those with UI. All variables included in the models were categorical variables apart from depression and anxiety which were continuous variables. The dataset also included sampling weights that were created based on the age, sex and educational attainment values in the Quarterly National Household Survey 2010. In order to obtain nationally representative estimates, the sample weighting and the complex study design, including within household clustering, was taken into account in all analyses. Results are expressed as odds ratios (OR) and 95% confidence intervals (95% CIs). A *p*-value <0.05 was considered to be statistically significant.

Results

The mean age (standard deviation) of the sample was 63.6 (9.2) years and 52.1% were women. Overall, the prevalence of any UI was 12.4% (95% CI = 11.5–13.4%). Among those with UI, it occurred more than once a month in 76.6%, and 26.4% had activity limitations due to UI. The sample characteristics are shown in Table 1. Older age, female sex, lower education, financial strain, a higher number of chronic conditions, ADL disability, less social network integration, depression, and anxiety were all significantly associated with UI. The prevalence of any UI by the level of loneliness is illustrated in Fig. 1. Greater loneliness was associated with a higher prevalence of UI with the prevalence of UI ranging from 9.2%

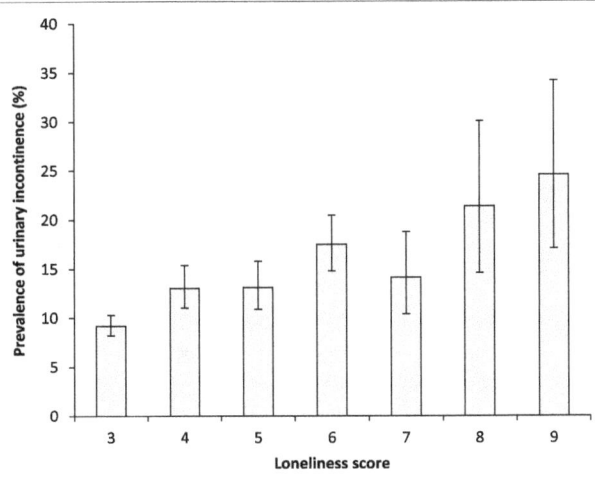

Fig. 1 Prevalence of urinary incontinence by loneliness score. Bars denote 95% confidence intervals. Estimates are based on the weighted sample. Urinary incontinence was assessed by the question 'During the last 12 months, have you lost any amount of urine beyond your control?' with answer options 'yes' or 'no'. The loneliness score was based on the short form UCLA loneliness scale with higher scores indicating greater levels of loneliness

(lowest level of loneliness) to 24.6% (highest level of loneliness). The results of the logistic regression analysis assessing the association between any UI and loneliness are shown in Table 2. In the unadjusted model, the OR (95% CI) was 1.74 (1.49-2.05) (Model 1). This was attenuated when the model was adjusted for sociodemographic factors, chronic conditions, and ADL disability but remained statistically significant (Model 2). Further adjustment for the SNI had little effect on the association (Model 3). The OR became non-significant when depression was included in the model (Model 4) but not when anxiety was included (Model 5). In the final model adjusting for all potential confounders the OR (95% CI) was 1.14 (0.94–1.37) (Model 6).

When the frequency of UI or activity limitations due to UI were taken into account, compared to no UI, having activity limitations due to UI was associated with particularly high odds for loneliness even in models adjusted for either depression or anxiety (Model 4 and 5) although the OR was no longer significant when depression and anxiety were included simultaneously in the model (Model 6). Frequency of UI was not as strongly associated with loneliness as activity limitations due to UI and became non-significant in the models where depression and anxiety were included (Table 3). Finally, in the analysis restricted to those with UI, a higher frequency of UI was not associated with elevated odds for loneliness, but activity limitations due to UI were associated with significantly higher odds for loneliness in all models except those which adjusted for depression (Table 4).

Discussion

Using data from a nationally representative sample of community-dwelling older Irish adults, this study showed that having any UI was associated with an increased risk for loneliness. When depression or anxiety was included in the analysis ORs were attenuated, particularly for depression, which suggests that this association is mainly explained by depression. Worse mental health was also important in the relation between UI severity and loneliness as depression fully attenuated the significant association between an increased frequency of UI and loneliness, while an association between activity limitations and loneliness became non-significant when both depression and anxiety were included in the fully adjusted model. When the analysis was restricted to those with UI, depression alone fully attenuated the significant association that was observed between activity limitations and loneliness.

The finding that UI was associated with loneliness when not adjusting for mental health conditions, accords with the results of earlier studies in Canada and the United States [22–24]. This result seems plausible given that UI has been linked to a range of 'safety-seeking

Table 2 Association between urinary incontinence (independent variable) and loneliness (dependent variable) estimated by logistic regression

Characteristic	Categories	Model 1	Model 2	Model 3	Model 4	Model 5	Model 6
Urinary incontinence	No	Ref	Ref	Ref	Ref	Ref	Ref
	Yes	1.74***	1.50***	1.51***	1.20	1.27*	1.14
		[1.49,2.05]	[1.27,1.78]	[1.27,1.80]	[1.00,1.43]	[1.06,1.53]	[0.94,1.37]
Age (years)	50–59		Ref	Ref	Ref	Ref	Ref
	60–69		0.95	1.03	1.13	1.22**	1.27**
			[0.83,1.08]	[0.90,1.17]	[0.99,1.30]	[1.06,1.41]	[1.10,1.46]
	70–79		1.19*	1.30**	1.43***	1.74***	1.76***
			[1.01,1.40]	[1.10,1.53]	[1.20,1.70]	[1.46,2.07]	[1.47,2.10]
	≥80		1.46**	1.36*	1.53**	2.05***	2.06***
			[1.13,1.88]	[1.05,1.77]	[1.17,1.99]	[1.56,2.70]	[1.56,2.72]
Sex	Male		Ref	Ref	Ref	Ref	Ref
	Female		1.12*	1.10	0.98	0.92	0.87*
			[1.01,1.24]	[1.00,1.22]	[0.88,1.08]	[0.83,1.03]	[0.78,0.98]
Education	Primary		Ref	Ref	Ref	Ref	Ref
	Secondary		0.95	1.03	1.07	1.07	1.08
			[0.82,1.09]	[0.89,1.19]	[0.92,1.24]	[0.92,1.25]	[0.93,1.27]
	Tertiary		0.92	1.04	1.11	1.13	1.15
			[0.80,1.07]	[0.90,1.21]	[0.95,1.29]	[0.96,1.32]	[0.98,1.35]
Financial strain	Never		Ref	Ref	Ref	Ref	Ref
	Rarely		1.38***	1.41***	1.44***	1.21*	1.24*
			[1.18,1.62]	[1.20,1.66]	[1.21,1.70]	[1.02,1.43]	[1.04,1.48]
	Sometimes		1.87***	1.88***	1.80***	1.53***	1.54***
			[1.63,2.16]	[1.63,2.17]	[1.55,2.09]	[1.32,1.79]	[1.32,1.81]
	Often		3.66***	3.35***	2.66***	2.14***	1.99***
			[3.03,4.42]	[2.77,4.06]	[2.17,3.26]	[1.75,2.61]	[1.61,2.45]
Number of Chronic conditions	None		Ref	Ref	Ref	Ref	Ref
	One		1.01	1.04	1.02	1.03	1.02
			[0.86,1.18]	[0.89,1.22]	[0.87,1.20]	[0.87,1.22]	[0.87,1.21]
	Two or more		1.24**	1.25**	1.15	1.12	1.08
			[1.07,1.43]	[1.07,1.44]	[0.99,1.34]	[0.96,1.31]	[0.93,1.27]
ADL disability	No		Ref	Ref	Ref	Ref	Ref
	Yes		1.14	1.06	0.74**	0.94	0.76*
			[0.93,1.39]	[0.87,1.31]	[0.59,0.92]	[0.75,1.18]	[0.60,0.97]
Social Network Index	Mostly isolated			Ref	Ref	Ref	Ref
	Moderately isolated			0.59***	0.63**	0.60***	0.63**
				[0.45,0.77]	[0.47,0.83]	[0.45,0.80]	[0.46,0.84]
	Moderately integrated			0.40***	0.46***	0.40***	0.43***
				[0.31,0.52]	[0.35,0.60]	[0.30,0.52]	[0.32,0.57]
	Most integrated			0.26***	0.30***	0.25***	0.28***
				[0.20,0.34]	[0.23,0.40]	[0.19,0.33]	[0.21,0.37]
Depression	(per one-unit increase)				1.10***		1.06***
					[1.09,1.11]		[1.05,1.07]
Anxiety	(per one-unit increase)					1.24***	1.20***
						[1.21,1.26]	[1.17,1.22]

Data are odds ratio [95% confidence interval]
Models are adjusted for all the variables in the respective columns
Abbreviation: Ref Reference category, *ADL* Activities of daily living
*p < 0.05, **p < 0.01, ***p < 0.001

Table 3 Association between frequency of urinary incontinence or activity limitations due to urinary incontinence (independent variables) and loneliness (dependent variable) estimated by logistic regression with no urinary incontinence as the reference category

Characteristic	Categories	Model 1	Model 2	Model 3	Model 4	Model 5	Model 6
Frequency of	No urinary incontinence	Ref	Ref	Ref	Ref	Ref	Ref
Urinary incontinence	Once a month or less	1.62**	1.50*	1.53*	1.33	1.25	1.21
		[1.20,2.20]	[1.08,2.07]	[1.09,2.14]	[0.94,1.90]	[0.88,1.78]	[0.85,1.74]
	More than once a month	1.79***	1.51***	1.52***	1.16	1.29*	1.11
		[1.49,2.15]	[1.24,1.83]	[1.25,1.84]	[0.94,1.42]	[1.04,1.59]	[0.90,1.38]
Activity limitations	No urinary incontinence	Ref	Ref	Ref	Ref	Ref	Ref
Due to urinary	No activity limitations	1.53***	1.36**	1.37**	1.13	1.16	1.06
Incontinence		[1.28,1.84]	[1.12,1.64]	[1.12,1.67]	[0.92,1.39]	[0.94,1.43]	[0.86,1.32]
	Activity limitations	2.60***	2.07***	2.08***	1.46*	1.71**	1.41
		[1.91,3.55]	[1.51,2.84]	[1.50,2.88]	[1.03,2.05]	[1.20,2.45]	[0.98,2.04]

Data are odds ratio [95% confidence interval]
Model 1: Unadjusted
Model 2: Adjusted for age, sex, education, financial strain, number of chronic conditions, and ADL disability
Model 3: Adjusted for variables in Model 2 and the Social Network Index
Model 4: Adjusted for variables in Model 3 and depression
Model 5: Adjusted for variables in Model 3 and anxiety
Model 6: Adjusted for variables in Model 3, depression, and anxiety
Abbreviation: Ref Reference category
*p < 0.05, **p < 0.01, ***p < 0.001

behaviors' that are used to manage the condition and its effects, such as avoiding contact with others, intimacy and activities outside the home [45] that might all lead to social isolation among those with UI and give rise to feelings of loneliness. Moreover, the results from the analyses examining UI severity also seem to support this idea as activity limitations were strongly associated with loneliness in the whole sample and when the analysis was restricted to those with UI. Being treated differently by other people because of their condition [18] might also act to isolate those with UI and lead to feelings of loneliness, especially as a recent study from the United States has indicated that older women with daily UI often feel left out and that they lack companionship [23].

When the common mental disorder variables, in particular, depression, were entered into the analysis, however, the association between UI, UI severity and loneliness became non-significant. Together with our finding that those with UI are more likely to experience greater anxiety and depression, this suggests that poorer mental health might be an intervening variable between UI and loneliness. It can only be speculated what underlies the association between depression and loneliness among those with UI, as even though earlier research has indicated that they can both influence each other over time [28], as yet, there has been comparatively little research on the specific mechanisms linking depression to loneliness [27]. It is possible, for example, that certain psychological resources might be

Table 4 Association between frequency of urinary incontinence or activity limitations due to urinary incontinence (independent variables) and loneliness (dependent variable) restricted to individuals with urinary incontinence estimated by logistic regression

Characteristic	Categories	Model 1	Model 2	Model 3	Model 4	Model 5	Model 6
Frequency of	Once a month or less	Ref	Ref	Ref	Ref	Ref	Ref
Urinary incontinence	More than once a month	1.10	0.99	0.99	0.87	1.04	0.91
		[0.78,1.56]	[0.69,1.43]	[0.68,1.44]	[0.59,1.29]	[0.71,1.54]	[0.61,1.36]
Activity limitations	No activity limitations	Ref	Ref	Ref	Ref	Ref	Ref
Due to urinary	Activity limitations	1.70**	1.52*	1.54*	1.30	1.51*	1.34
Incontinence		[1.20,2.41]	[1.05,2.20]	[1.06,2.24]	[0.87,1.93]	[1.00,2.28]	[0.88,2.04]

Data are odds ratio [95% confidence interval]
Model 1: Unadjusted
Model 2: Adjusted for age, sex, education, financial strain, number of chronic conditions, and ADL disability
Model 3: Adjusted for variables in Model 2 and the Social Network Index
Model 4: Adjusted for variables in Model 3 and depression
Model 5: Adjusted for variables in Model 3 and anxiety
Model 6: Adjusted for variables in Model 3, depression, and anxiety
Abbreviation: Ref Reference category
*p < 0.05, **p < 0.01

important in this context. Specifically, a recent study has reported that a lower sense of mastery significantly contributes to the association between depression and (emotional) loneliness [27] while other research has indicated that UI is associated with a lower sense of mastery [46] and that there is an association between a poor sense of mastery and depression in those with UI [47]. One of the safety-seeking behaviors among those with UI – inquiring frequently if he or she smells [45] – might also be a factor that links depression and loneliness, as a more general connection has been shown to exist between seeking reassurance excessively and both depression and interpersonal rejection [48].

There are several limitations that should be borne in mind when considering this study's findings. UI data were self-reported in this study. Given the stigma and embarrassment that is associated with UI, it is possible that underreporting may have been an issue [4], although the prevalence estimate obtained fell within the range of those reported in other studies. We also lacked information on the type of UI that was experienced. This might be an important omission as there is some evidence that urge incontinence may affect well-being more than stress incontinence [11] and have a stronger association with worse mental health [49]. There may have also been a problem with one of the instruments used in this study. Specifically, a recent systematic review has questioned the ability of HADS to clearly differentiate between anxiety and depression and indicated that it might be better regarded as a measure of 'emotional distress' [50]. In addition, since individuals with cognitive impairment that was severe enough to preclude participation in the survey, and the institutionalized were not included in our study sample, the study results cannot be generalized to this population. Finally, as this study was cross-sectional, it was not possible to determine causality or the temporality of the observed associations.

Conclusion

This study, which used data from a nationally representative sample of almost 7000 community dwelling adults aged ≥ 50, has shown that UI and UI severity are linked to loneliness but that this association is largely dependent on the presence of comorbid depression. The results of this study and the detrimental (psychological/mental health) outcomes that have been reported in earlier studies, together with the fact that at least one-third of older adults with UI do not seek help [14], suggest that more effort is required to educate older respondents about this condition and its effects, as well as about the wide variety of

treatment options that are available for it [51]. For patients, clinician screening for loneliness and then referral to agencies that run social programs (e.g. group meals) that might help alleviate this phenomenon [52] may be one way to improve the quality of life in those individuals with UI. In addition, as poorer mental health is more prevalent among people with UI, and can affect the course and outcome of UI [49, 53], routine mental health screening and close collaboration with mental health professionals may also prove efficacious for patients with UI.

Abbreviations

95% CI: 95% confidence interval; ADL disability: Activities of daily living disability; CAPI: Computer-assisted personal interviewing; CES-D: Center for Epidemiologic Studies Depression scale; CMDs: Common mental disorders; HADS-A: The Hospital Anxiety and Depression Scale; OR: Odds ratio; SCQ: Self-completion questionnaire; SNI: The Berkman-Syme Social Network Index; TILDA: The Irish Longitudinal Study on Ageing; UCLA Loneliness Scale: University of California, Los Angeles Loneliness Scale; UI: Urinary incontinence

Acknowledgements

N/A.

Funding

ZIS's work has received funding from the People Programme (Marie Curie Actions) of the European Union's Seventh Framework Programme FP7/2007 _ 2013 under REA grant agreement n° 316795. AK's work was supported by the Miguel Servet contract financed by the CP13/00150 and PI15/00862 projects, integrated into the National R + D + I and funded by the ISCIII - General Branch Evaluation and Promotion of Health Research - and the European Regional Development Fund (ERDF-FEDER).

Authors' contributions

AS had the study idea, designed the study and wrote the main text. AK and ZIS analyzed the data and commented on and wrote parts of the manuscript. All authors read and approved the final manuscript.

Competing interests

The authors declare that they have no competing interests.

Author details

₁The Stockholm Center for Health and Social Change (SCOHOST), Södertörn University, Huddinge 141 89, Sweden. ²The Danish National Institute of Public Health, University of Southern Denmark, Oester Farimagsgade 5A, 1353 Copenhagen, Denmark. ³Parc Sanitari Sant Joan de Déu, Universitat de Barcelona, Fundació Sant Joan de Déu/CIBERSAM, Barcelona, Spain.

References

1. Abrams P, Cardozo L, Fall M, Griffiths D, Rosier P, Ulmsten U, van Kerrebroeck P, Victor A, Wein A. The standardization of terminology of lower urinary tract function: report from the standardization sub-committee of the International Continence Society. Neurourol Urodyn. 2002;21:167–78.
2. Bartoli S, Aguzzi G, Tarricone R. Impact on quality of life of urinary incontinence and overactive bladder: a systematic literature review. Urology. 2010;75:491–500.

3. Minassian VA, Drutz HP, Al-Badr A. Urinary incontinence as a worldwide problem. Int J Gynaecol Obstet. 2003;82:327–38.

4. Chang CH, Gonzalez CM, Lau DT, Sier HC. Urinary incontinence and self-reported health among the U.S. Medicare managed care beneficiaries. J Aging Health. 2008;20:405–19.

5. Van Oyen H, Van Oyen P. Urinary incontinence in Belgium; prevalence, correlates and psychosocial consequences. Acta Clin Belg. 2002;57:207–18.

6. Chapple CR, Manassero F. Urinary incontinence in adults. Surgery. 2005; 23:101–7.

7. Hannestad YS, Rortveit G, Sandvik H, Hunskaar S. A community-based epidemiological survey of female urinary incontinence: the Norwegian EPINCONT study. J Clin Epidemiol. 2000;53:1150–7.

8. Melville JL, Katon W, Delaney K, Newton K. Urinary incontinence in US women: a population-based study. Arch Intern Med. 2005;165:537–42.

9. Hunskaar S, Arnold EP, Burgio K, Diokno AC, Herzog AR, Mallett VT. Epidemiology and natural history of urinary incontinence. Int Urogynecol J Pelvic Floor Dysfunct. 2000;11:301–19.

10. Gavira Iglesias FJ, Caridad y Ocerín JM, Pérez del Molino Martín J, Valderrama Gama E, López Pérez M, Romero López M, Pavón Aranguren MV, Guerrero Muñoz JB. Prevalence and psychosocial impact of urinary incontinence in older people of a Spanish rural population. J Gerontol A Biol Sci Med Sci. 2000;55:M207–14.

11. Heidrich SM, Wells TJ. Effects of urinary incontinence: psychological well-being and distress in older community-dwelling women. J Gerontol Nurs. 2004;30:47–54.

12. Coyne KS, Wein A, Nicholson S, Kvasz M, Chen CI, Milsom I. Comorbidities and personal burden of urgency urinary incontinence: a systematic review. Int J Clin Pract. 2013;67:1015–33.

13. Gibson W, Wagg A. New horizons: urinary incontinence in older people. Age Ageing. 2014;43:157–63.

14. Farage MA, Miller KW, Berardesca E, Maibach HI. Psychosocial and societal burden of incontinence in the aged population: a review. Arch Gynecol Obstet. 2008;277:285–90.

15. Reigota RB, Pedro AO, de Souza Santos Machado V, Costa-Paiva L, Pinto-Neto AM. Prevalence of urinary incontinence and its association with multimorbidity in women aged 50 years or older: a population-based study. Neurourol Urodyn. 2016;35:62–8.

16. Felde G, Ebbesen MH, Hunskaar S. Anxiety and depression associated with urinary incontinence. A 10-year follow-up study from the Norwegian HUNT study (EPINCONT). Neurourol Urodyn. 2015. doi:10.1002/nau22921.

17. Kwak Y, Kwon H, Kim Y. Health-related quality of life and mental health in older women with urinary incontinence. Aging Ment Health. 2016;20:719–26.

18. Heintz PA, DeMucha CM, Deguzman MM, Softa R. Stigma and microaggressions experienced by older women with urinary incontinence: a literature review. Urol Nurs. 2013;33:299–305.

19. Teunissen D, Van Den Bosch W, Van Weel C, Lagro-Janssen T. "It can always happen": the impact of urinary incontinence on elderly men and women. Scand J Prim Health Care. 2006;24:166–73.

20. Luanaigh CO, Lawlor BA. Loneliness and the health of older people. Int J Geriatr Psychiatry. 2008;23:1213–21.

21. Luo Y, Hawkley LC, Waite LJ, Cacioppo JT. Loneliness, health, and mortality in old age: a national longitudinal study. Soc Sci Med. 2012;74:907–14.

22. Ramage-Morin PL, Gilmour H. Urinary incontinence and loneliness in Canadian seniors. Health Rep. 2013;24:3–10.

23. Yip SO, Dick MA, McPencow AM, Martin DK, Ciarleglio MM, Erekson EA. The association between urinary and fecal incontinence and social isolation in older women. Am J Obstet Gynecol. 2013;208:146e. 1-7.

24. Fultz NH, Herzog AR. Self-reported social and emotional impact of urinary incontinence. J Am Geriatr Soc. 2001;49:892–9.

25. Drageset J, Espehaug B, Kirkevold M. The impact of depression and sense of coherence on emotional and social loneliness among nursing home residents without cognitive impairment - a questionnaire survey. J Clin Nurs. 2012;21:965–74.

26. Losada A, Márquez-González M, Pachana NA, Wetherell JL, Fernández-Fernández V, Nogales-González C, Ruiz-Díaz M. Behavioral correlates of anxiety in well-functioning older adults. Int Psychogeriatr. 2015;27:1135–46.

27. Peerenboom L, Collard RM, Naarding P, Comijs HC. The association between depression and emotional and social loneliness in older persons and the influence of social support, cognitive functioning and personality: a cross-sectional study. J Affect Disord. 2015;182:26–31.

28. Cacioppo JT, Hughes ME, Waite LJ, Hawkley LC, Thisted RA. Loneliness as a specific risk factor for depressive symptoms: cross-sectional and longitudinal analyses. Psychol Aging. 2006;21:140–51.

29. Kearney PM, Cronin H, O'Regan C, Kamiya Y, Savva GM, Whelan B, Kenny R. Cohort profile: the Irish Longitudinal Study on Ageing. Int J Epidemiol. 2011; 40:877–84.

30. Whelan BJ, Savva GM. Design and methodology of the Irish Longitudinal Study on Ageing. J Am Geriatr Soc. 2013;61 Suppl 2:S265–8.

31. Richardson K, Kenny RA, Peklar J, Bennett K. Agreement between patient interview data on prescription medication use and pharmacy records in those aged older than 50 years varied by therapeutic group and reporting of indicated health conditions. J Clin Epidemiol. 2013;66:1308–16.

32. Russell D, Peplau LA, Cutrona CE. The revised UCLA Loneliness Scale: concurrent and discriminant validity evidence. J Pers Soc Psychol. 1980;39:472–80.

33. Hughes ME, Waite LJ, Hawkley LC, Cacioppo JT. A short scale for measuring loneliness in large surveys: results from two population-based studies. Res Aging. 2004;26:655–72.

34. Austin BA. Factorial structure of the UCLA Loneliness Scale. Psychol Rep. 1983;53:883–9.

35. Russell DW. UCLA Loneliness Scale (Version 3): reliability, validity, and factor structure. J Pers Assess. 1996;66:20–40.

36. Radloff LS. The CES-D scale: a self-report depression scale for research in the general population. Appl Psychol Meas. 1977;1:385–401.

37. Hawkley LC, Thisted RA, Cacioppo JT. Loneliness predicts reduced physical activity: cross-sectional & longitudinal analyses. Health Psychol. 2009;28:354–63.

38. Hertzog C, Van Alstine J, Usala PD, Hultsch DF, Dixon R. Measurement properties of the Center for Epidemiological Studies Depression Scale (CES-D) in older populations. Psychol Assess J Consult Clin Psychol. 1990;2:64–72.

39. Lewinsohn PM, Seeley JR, Roberts RE, Allen NB. Center for Epidemiologic Studies Depression Scale (CES-D) as a screening instrument for depression among community-residing older adults. Psychol Aging. 1997;12:277–87.

40. Zigmond AS, Snaith RP. The hospital anxiety and depression scale. Acta Psychiatr Scand. 1983;67:361–70.

41. Spinhoven P, Ormel J, Sloekers PPA, Kempen GI, Speckens AE, Van Hemert AM. A validation study of the Hospital Anxiety and Depression Scale (HADS) in different groups of Dutch subjects. Psychol Med. 1997;27:363–70.

42. Berkman LF, Syme SL. Social networks, host resistance, and mortality: a nine-year follow-up study of Alameda County residents. Am J Epidemiol. 1979; 109:186–204.

43. Berkman LF, Breslow L. Health and ways of living: the Alameda County study. New York: Oxford University Press; 1983.

44. Katz S, Ford AB, Moskowitz RW, Jackson BA, Jaffe MW. Studies of illness in the aged. The index of ADL: a standardized measure of biological and psychosocial function. JAMA. 1963;185:914–9.

45. Molinuevo B, Batista-Miranda JE. Under the tip of the iceberg: psychological factors in incontinence. Neurourol Urodyn. 2012;31:669–71.

46. Woods NF, Mitchell ES. Consequences of incontinence for women during the menopausal transition and early postmenopause: observations from the Seattle Midlife Women's Health Study. Menopause. 2013;20:915–21.

47. Chiverton PA, Wells TJ, Brink CA, Mayer R. Psychological factors associated with urinary incontinence. Clin Nurse Spec. 1996;10:229–33.

48. Starr LR, Davila J. Excessive reassurance seeking, depression, and interpersonal rejection: a meta-analytic review. J Abnorm Psychol. 2008;117:762–75.

49. Melville JL, Walker E, Katon W, Lentz G, Miller J, Fenner D. Prevalence of comorbid psychiatric illness and its impact on symptom perception, quality of life, and functional status in women with urinary incontinence. Am J Obstet Gynecol. 2002;187:80–7.

50. Cosco TD, Doyle F, Ward M, McGee H. Latent structure of the Hospital Anxiety And Depression Scale: a 10-year systematic review. J Psychosom Res. 2012;72:180–4.

51. Norton P, Brubaker L. Urinary incontinence in women. Lancet. 2006;367:57–67.

52. Perissinotto CM, Stijacic Cenzer I, Covinsky KE. Loneliness in older persons: a predictor of functional decline and death. Arch Intern Med. 2012;172:1078–83.

53. Stach-Lempinen B, Hakala AL, Laippala P, Lehtinen K, Metsänoja R, Kujansuu E. Severe depression determines quality of life in urinary incontinent women. Neurourol Urodyn. 2003;22:563–8.

24

The efficacy of mirabegron additional therapy for lower urinary tract symptoms after treatment with α1-adrenergic receptor blocker monotherapy

Tomohiro Matsuo, Yasuyoshi Miyata[*], Katsura Kakoki, Miki Yuzuriha, Akihiro Asai, Kojiro Ohba and Hideki Sakai

Abstract

Background: Mirabegron is a β3-adrenoreceptor agonist developed for treatment of overactive bladder (OAB). α1-Adrenergic receptor blockers are effective for lower urinary tract symptoms (LUTS) in male patients. However, the efficacy of mirabegron additional treatment in elderly male patients with persistent male LUTS, especially in OAB after monotherapy with α1-adrenergic blockers, is not fully understood.

Methods: This study was conducted in male LUTS patients who were ≥ 65 years of age and had persistent OAB symptoms, regardless of whether they took an α1-adrenergic receptor blocker orally. Before and 12 weeks after mirabegron additional therapy (50 mg once daily), we evaluated the efficacy of this treatment using the Overactive Bladder Symptom Score (OABSS) and International Prostate Symptom Score (IPSS), and changes in the maximum flow rate (Qmax) and post-void residual urine volume (PVR). We evaluated patients overall and divided into two groups by age: young-old (from 65 to 74 years old) and old-old (from 75 to 84 years old).

Results: Fifty men were enrolled in this study. Mirabegron additional therapy improved the total OABSS, total IPSS, and IPSS-quality of life (QOL) score. The voided volume (VV) and Qmax improved after treatment in patients overall. However, there was no significant change in PVR. The total OABSS, total IPSS, and IPSS-QOL score significantly improved in both of the young-old and old-old groups. However, a significant increasing of VV was detected in the young-old group. There were no significant differences in the Qmax or PVR in either group.

Conclusions: Mirabegron additional therapy was effective for male patients whose persistent LUTS and particularly OAB was not controlled with α1-adrenergic receptor blocker monotherapy, and mirabegron did not have negative effects on voiding function. Additionally, mirabegron additional therapy was considered effective regardless of patient age.

Keywords: Mirabegron, Elderly male, Overactive bladder, α1-adrenergic blockers

* Correspondence: int.doc.miya@m3.dion.ne.jp
Department of Urology, Nagasaki University Graduate School of Biochemical Sciences, 1-7-1 Sakamoto, Nagasaki 852-8501, Japan

Background

Overactive bladder (OAB) is defined as a condition with characteristic symptoms of urinary urgency that is usually accompanied by frequency and nocturia, with or without urgency incontinence [1]. It is particularly burdensome to older people because of its higher prevalence, and because the impact of its symptoms may be more pronounced due to the increased burden of chronic comorbidities [2, 3]. The symptoms caused by OAB decrease patients' quality of life (QOL), and OAB can lead to various pathological conditions such as increases in the fracture rate, sleep disturbances, and depressive feelings) [4, 5]. Anti-muscarinic agents are often used as first-line therapy for patients with OAB. However, unfortunately, about a third quarter of patients cannot continue taking these drugs due to unsatisfactory efficacy and various adverse events [6, 7].

In addition, mainly due to the adverse effects of anti-muscarinic drugs, Japanese clinical guidelines for both male lower urinary tract symptoms (LUTS) and benign prostatic hyperplasia recommend physicians to use α1-adrenergic blockers as the first choice drug for male LUTS patients regardless of the presence or absence of OAB symptoms [8, 9].

Mirabegron is a β3-adrenoceptor agonist approved for treating OAB in Europe, the United States, Canada, Japan, and Australia [10]. Mirabegron is a specific agonist, acting on β3-adrenoceptors in the human detrusor, the stimulation of which leads to active relaxation of the human detrusor in the storage phase, which increases bladder capacity without exerting an effect on voiding [11]. The efficacy and safety of mirabegron have been studied in several randomized trials. For example, SCORPIO, a large, randomized, placebo-controlled phase III study, evaluated the efficacy, safety, and tolerability of mirabegron over 12 weeks in patients with OAB [12], and TAURUS, a 1-year, randomized, double-blind, safety study, evaluated the safety, tolerability, and efficacy of mirabegron [13]. Both studies mainly improved storage symptoms, including urgency incontinence and increased voiding volume, and demonstrated that the efficacy of mirabegron lasted 4 weeks later and continued until the end of the observation periods. Furthermore, the rate of adverse events due to 50 mg mirabegron was similar to that of a placebo, and significantly lower than that of the anti-muscarinic drug tolterodine (4 mg) [12, 13]. In addition, other researchers have reported that mirabegron add-on therapy combined with α1-adrenergic receptor blockers is very effective for storage symptoms, even in male patients with OAB [14–16]. However, no studies have focused on elderly male patients aged 65 years old and over.

To our knowledge, the present study is the first to focus on the efficacy of mirabegron additional therapy in elderly male patients with OAB after treatment with α1-adrenergic receptor blocker monotherapy.

Methods

This prospective study was conducted in male patients who were 65 years or older in age, had persistent LUTS and particularly OAB symptoms, and had been taking a regular dose of α1-adrenergic receptor blockers for more than 12 weeks. OAB was diagnosed using the Overactive Bladder Symptom Score (OABSS), and persistent OAB symptoms were defined as a total OABSS of 3 or more points with urinary urgency at least once per week [17]. Exclusion criteria were a post-void urine volume (PVR) of 50 mL, history of urinary retention, prior diagnosis of neurogenic bladder, urethral stricture, severe hypertension (systolic blood pressure ≥ 180 mmHg and/or diastolic blood pressure ≥ 110 mmHg) not well controlled by medication, renal insufficiency (glomerular filtration rate < 30 mL/min/1.73 m^2), liver impairment, intention to have a child, urological malignancy, patients taking any anti-muscarinic drugs, or those considered unsuitable for the trial by the treating physicians.

The patients continued all of their prescribed drugs during this study period. Before and 12 weeks after mirabegron (Betanis®, Astellas Pharma Inc., Tokyo, Japan; 50 mg once daily) treatment was added to a previous α1-adrenergic receptor blocker for urinary symptoms, we evaluated the efficacy of the treatment using the OABSS and International Prostate Symptom Score (IPSS) to assess subjective symptoms, and we used uroflowmetry and PVR to assess objective symptoms. We measured the maximum flow rate (Qmax) using the Duet® Logic G2 system (Mediwatch UK Ltd., Rugby, UK) on free uroflowmetry and PVR using transabdominal ultrasound sonography (HI VISION Avius®, Hitachi-Aloka Medical, Ltd, Tokyo, Japan). Moreover, before mirabegron add-on treatment was administered, we evaluated the prostate volume (PV) using transabdominal ultrasound sonography.

The primary endpoint was the change in total OABSS. The secondary endpoints evaluated were the change in the subscale scores of the OABSS, total IPSS, each subscale score of the IPSS and IPSS-QOL, voided volume (VV) on free uroflowmetry, Qmax, and PVR. In this study, we compared these subjective and objective parameters between two groups defined according to the patients' age: young-old (from 65 to 74 years old) and old-old (from 75 to 84 years old).

During the clinical study, the current α1-adrenergic receptor blocker that the patients had been taking orally was not changed to a different one. Additionally, no patients were taking multiple α1-adrenergic receptor blockers. The safety assessment included a change in adverse events. We observed patients' complaints of adverse effects, and information on the adverse events was recorded throughout the study period.

All statistical analyses were performed using computer software (JMP 10; SAS Institute Inc., Cary, NC, USA). Differences in the changes in patients' parameters from baseline to 12 weeks were examined using the Wilcoxon signed-rank test. $P < 0.05$ was considered statistically significant.

Results

Fifty men were enrolled in this study. As shown in Table 1, overall, the mean ± standard deviation (SD) of patients' age was 75.7 ± 7.6 years, and the mean ± SD PV was 33.7 ± 8.6 mL. All patients had taken a previous α1-adrenergic receptor blocker, including silodosin (26 patients), naftopidil (15), tamsulosin (8), and urapidil (1). Among the 50 patents, 22 (44.0 %) and 28 (56.0 %) were classified into the young-old group and old-old group, respectively. No other demographic or clinical parameters significantly differed between the young-old and old-old groups.

Figure 1a shows the change in the OABSS before and after mirabegron add-on treatment was administered to patients overall. Mirabegron add-on treatment improved the total OABSS (from 6.0 ± 2.1 to 4.4 ± 1.4, $P < 0.001$), and the nighttime frequency (OABSS Q2, $P < 0.001$) and urgency (OABSS Q3, $P < 0.001$) subscale scores of the OABSS after the 12-week treatment period. Although the urgency incontinence subscale score (OABSS Q4) improved after 12 weeks compared to that before treatment, the difference did not reach statistical significance ($P < 0.05$). Similarly, mirabegron add-on treatment significantly improved the total IPSS (before 15.1 ± 4.2 to 11.8 ± 4.6, $P < 0.001$); frequency (IPSS Q2, $P < 0.001$), urgency (IPSS Q4, $P < 0.001$), and nocturia subscales (IPSS Q7, $P < 0.001$); and IPSS-QOL score ($P < 0.001$) after treatment (Fig. 1b). There were no significant differences in voiding symptoms, including incomplete emptying, intermittency, weak stream, and straining before and after 12-week mirabegron add-on treatment.

In the entire patient, changes in the objective parameters of VV, Qmax, and PVR are shown in Fig. 2. VV on free uroflowmetry increased from 137.3 ± 62.9 mL to 154.1 ± 64.1 mL after treatment ($P = 0.005$). Similarly, Qmax improved from 9.1 ± 3.7 mL/s to 11.1 ± 3.6 mL/s ($P = 0.036$). However, no significant change was detected in PVR (from 23.1 ± 15.6 mL to 27.3 ± 21.5 mL, $P = 0.349$).

Next, changes of these parameters on subjective symptoms and objective measurements depending on age (young-old and old-old group) were showed in Table 2. The total OABSS and nighttime frequency (OABSS Q2), and urgency (OABSS Q3) subscales were improved in both groups. However, urgency incontinence (OABSS Q4) was improved only in the young-old group (*P = 0.021*; old-old group, *P = 0.686*). Significant improvements were also observed in the total IPSS; IPSS-QOL; and frequency (IPSS Q2), urgency (IPSS Q4), and nocturia (IPSS Q7) subscales in both groups. No IPSS-related parameter significantly differed between the young-old group and the old-old group. However, although all IPSS parameters were unchanged or decreased in the young-old group after treatment, incomplete emptying (Q1), intermittency (Q3), weak stream (Q5), and straining (Q6) had a tendency to increase after treatment in the old-old group.

Among the objective symptoms, VV on free uroflowmetry increased after treatment in the young-old group ($P = 0.012$) but not in the old-old group ($P = 0.113$). There were no significant changes in the Qmax and PVR after treatment in either group.

A safety analysis was performed on all patients during the clinical trial. Two patients (4 %) complained of dry mouth. One patient (2 %) complained of constipation. However, since these adverse effects were very mild, the patients did not need to stop taking mirabegron. In addition, none of the patients with hypertension experienced worsening of their blood pressure levels. Hence, all patients completed this clinical study, including all scheduled examinations during the study period.

Table 1 Patients' characteristics

	Overall	Young-old group	Old-old group	P value[a]
Number of patients (N/%)	50	22 (44.0)	28 (56.0)	-
Age (years)	75.7 ± 7.6	68.7 (2.7)	81.1 (5.3)	< 0.001
Prostate volume (mL)	33.7 ± 8.6	33.5 (7.6)	33.7 (9.5)	0.961
α1-adrenergic receptor blocker				
Silodosin (N/%)	26 (52.0)	13 (59.1)	13 (46.4)	
Naftopidil	15 (30.0)	5 (22.7)	10 (35.7)	
Tamsulosin	8 (16.0)	3 (13.6)	5 (17.9)	
Urapidil	1 (2.0)	1 (4.5)	0 (0)	

Data are shown as mean ± standard deviation
[a]Difference between the young-old group and old-old group

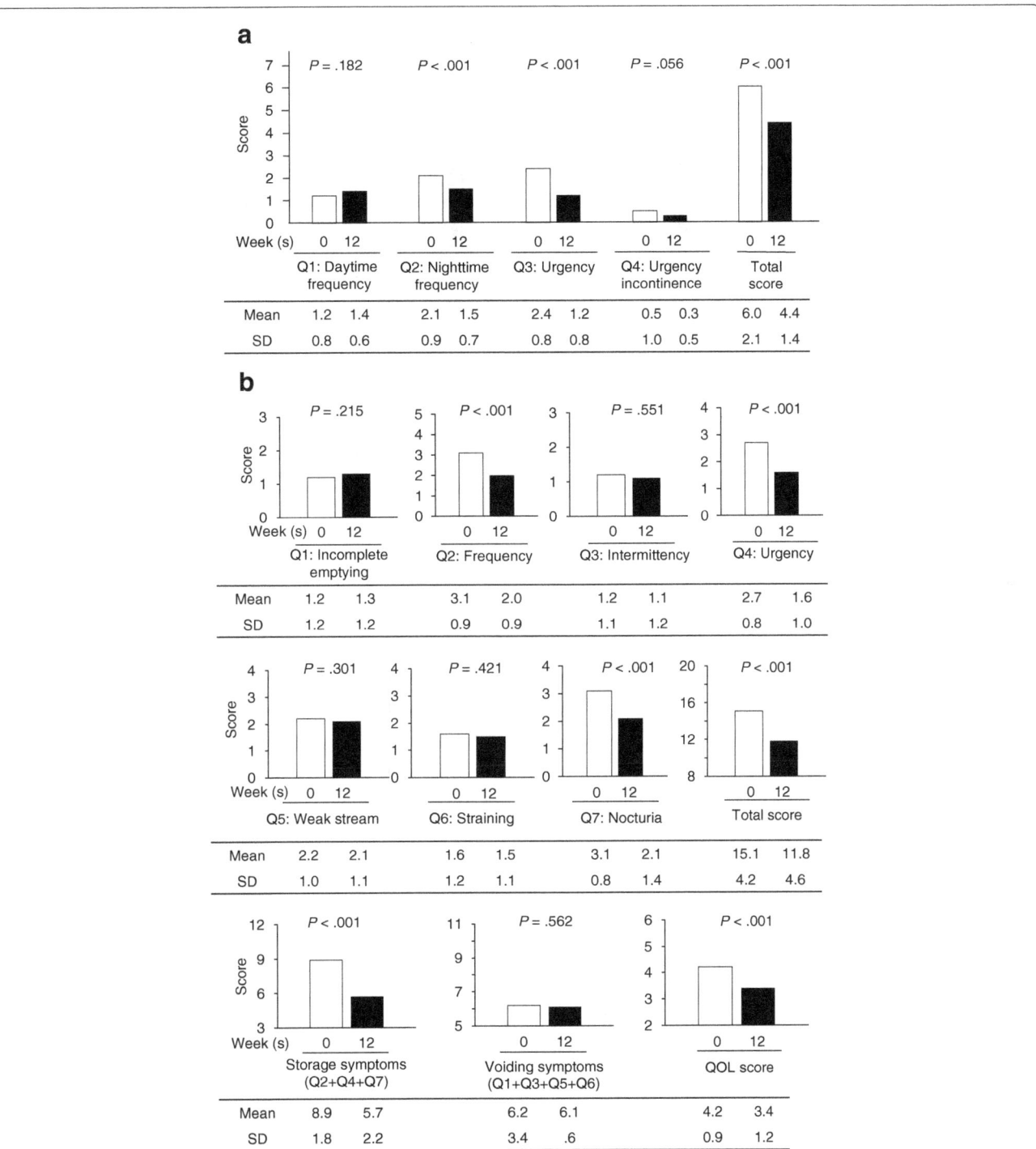

Fig. 1 Changes in subjective symptoms. **a** shows changes in the Overactive Bladder Symptom Score (OABSS). Combination therapy with α-1 adrenergic receptor blocker and mirabegron for 12 weeks significantly improved the total OABSS, nighttime frequency (Q2), and urgency (Q3). **b** shows the change in the International Prostate Symptom Score (IPSS). Combination therapy significantly improved the IPSS total score, IPSS-quality of life, and storage symptoms (frequency [Q2], urgency [Q4], nocturia [Q7], and IPSS-storage symptoms [Q2 + Q4 + Q7]). However, combination therapy did not affect voiding symptoms (incomplete emptying [Q1], intermittency [Q3], weak stream [Q5], straining [Q6], and IPSS-voiding symptoms [Q1 + Q3 + Q5 + Q6]). The *white columns* show the scores at 0 weeks, and the *black columns* show scores at 12 weeks. SD, standard deviation

Discussion

To the best of our knowledge, the present study is the first to focus on the efficacy of mirabegron additional therapy in elderly male patients with OAB after monotherapy with α1-adrenergic receptor blockers. Our findings indicated that mirabegron additional therapy was

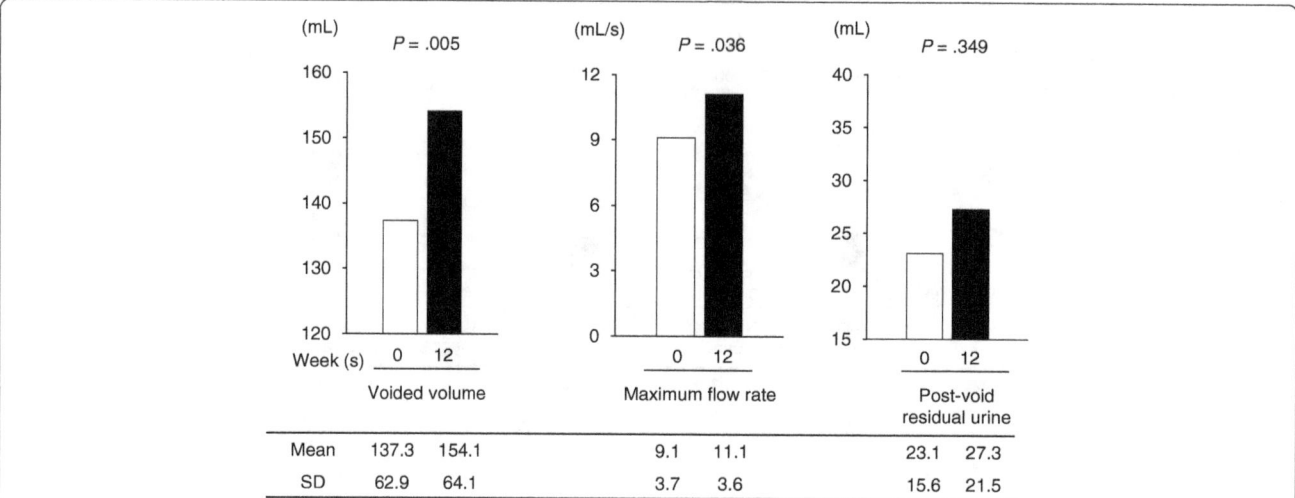

Fig. 2 Changes in the measurements of objective symptoms in patients overall. The *white columns* show the values at 0 weeks, and the *black columns* show those at 12 weeks. After 12 weeks of α1-adrenergic receptor blocker and mirabegron combination therapy, the voided volume and maximum flow rate improved significantly. Post-void residual urine increased at the end of the period; however, this change was not statistically significant. SD, standard deviation

Table 2 Changes in the values of the subjective and objective symptoms in each group of elderly male patients with overactive bladder

	Young-old group (N = 22)			Old-old group (N = 28)		
	0 W	12 W	P Value	0 W	12 W	P Value
OABSS						
Q1 Daytime frequency	1.1 ± 0.7	1.4 ± 0.8	0.307	1.1 ± 0.8	1.4 ± 0.5	0.148
Q2 Nighttime frequency	2.1 ± 1.0	1.5 ± 0.9	0.034	2.0 ± 0.8	1.5 ± 0.6	0.005
Q3 Urgency	2.7 ± 1.1	1.2 ± 1.1	< 0.001	2.2 ± 0.4	1.3 ± 0.6	< 0.001
Q4 Urgency incontinence	0.9 ± 1.3	0.3 ± 0.6	0.021	0.2 ± 0.4	0.3 ± 0.4	0.686
Total score	6.5 ± 2.7	4.4 ± 1.6	0.004	5.6 ± 1.3	4.2 ± 1.2	< 0.001
IPSS						
Q1 Incomplete emptying	1.2 ± 1.4	1.2 ± 1.3	1.000	1.2 ± 1.0	1.4 ± 1.2	0.093
Q2 Frequency	3.0 ± 1.1	2.0 ± 1.0	0.001	3.1 ± 0.7	2.1 ± 0.9	< 0.001
Q3 Intermittency	1.4 ± 1.3	1.2 ± 1.3	0.205	1.0 ± 1.0	1.1 ± 1.2	0.529
Q4 Urgency	2.8 ± 0.8	1.7 ± 0.9	< 0.001	2.6 ± 0.8	1.5 ± 1.0	< 0.001
Q5 Weak stream	2.2 ± 1.1	2.0 ± 1.2	0.142	2.2 ± 1.0	2.3 ± 1.0	0.689
Q6 Straining	2.0 ± 1.5	1.7 ± 1.4	0.110	1.3 ± 0.8	1.4 ± 0.9	0.529
Q7 Nocturia	3.3 ± 0.8	2.3 ± 1.4	0.001	2.9 ± 0.8	1.9 ± 0.9	< 0.001
Total score	16.0 ± 5.1	12.0 ± 5.3	< 0.001	14.5 ± 3.3	11.7 ± 4.1	< 0.001
Storage symptoms (Q2 + Q4 + Q7)	9.1 ± 1.9	6.0 ± 2.5	< 0.001	8.7 ± 5.6	5.6 ± 2.0	< 0.001
Voiding symptoms (Q1 + Q3 + Q5 + Q6)	6.8 ± 4.4	6.0 ± 4.4	0.029	5.8 ± 2.5	6.1 ± 3.0	0.102
QOL score	4.3 ± 1.0	3.5 ± 1.4	0.006	4.1 ± 0.8	3.2 ± 1.0	< 0.001
Urodynamic study						
VV (mL)	141.0 ± 78.1	169.5 ± 74.0	0.012	134.4 ± 49.2	142.0 ± 53.4	0.133
Qmax (mL/s)	9.1 ± 3.0	9.9 ± 2.7	0.159	9.1 ± 2.2	12.0 ± 12.4	0.116
PVR (mL)	27.4 ± 41.8	22.1 ± 22.7	0.879	26.5 ± 17.3	30.4 ± 25.9	0.190

OABSS overactive bladder symptom score, *IPSS* international prostate symptom score, *w* week, *VV* voided volume, *Qmax* maximum flow rate, *PVR* post-void residual urine

effective for those whose OAB was not controlled with α1-adrenergic receptor blockers, according to the OABSS and IPSS. Our results also demonstrated that mirabegron had no suppressive effects on voiding function on uroflowmetry and PVR. In addition, regardless of the patient's age, mirabegron add-on therapy was considered effective and safe to take orally.

In elderly patients with benign prostatic hyperplasia, an α1-adrenergic receptor blocker significantly improved LUTS, especially voiding dysfunction. However, some patients may continue to suffer from storage symptoms such as urgency and frequency. For these patients, some studies have suggested that combination therapy with an α1-adrenergic receptor blocker and anti-muscarinic drug is effective [18, 19]. However, because of the impaired physiological function of elderly people, anti-muscarinic drugs carry the risk for adverse events. In fact, there is a significant incidence of peripheral anti-muscarinic adverse events such as dry mouth, constipation, tachycardia, cognitive dysfunction, and voiding dysfunction in elderly patients [20, 21]. Voiding dysfunction, in particular, due to male LUTS, might lead to excessive residual urine, urinary tract infection, and post-renal renal failure.

Mirabegron, a β3-adrenergic receptor agonist, is a new type of agent for OAB, with a reported adverse effect rate almost as low as that of a placebo [15, 22]. However, recently, concerns have been raised regarding the use of mirabegron to treat OAB patients with severe hypertension (systolic blood pressure ≥ 180 mmHg and/or diastolic blood pressure ≥ 110 mmHg) [23]. In addition, no studies have targeted elderly male patients 65 years old and over, who are more prone to experiencing complications than younger patients.

According to the present study, mirabegron additional therapy improved storage symptoms on the OABSS and IPSS regardless of age. In addition, mirabegron additional therapy improved storage symptoms and voiding symptoms on the IPSS in the young-old patient group. Previous studies have reported that mirabegron improved the OABSS and the total and storage symptoms on the IPSS in male patients with OAB [15, 16, 24]. Moreover, Wada et al. suggested that mirabegron add-on treatment with tamsulosin improved storage symptoms and voiding symptoms [16]. However, these previous studies were complex, as they included patients of various ages and they had small sample sizes; no study has focused only on older male patients. Ichihara et al. reported that combination therapy with tamsulosin and mirabegron was effective for persistent OAB symptoms with benign prostatic obstruction after tamsulosin monotherapy [15]. They divided the patients into two groups, tamsulosin monotherapy ($N = 38$) and combination therapy with tamsulosin and mirabegron ($N = 38$).

Although average age of their study cohort was very similar to that of the present study (74.5 ± 8.2 vs. 75.7 ± 7.6 years), they included male patients aged 50 years or older. Hence they did not target only elderly male LUTS patients. In addition, the number of patients receiving combination therapy with tamsulosin and mirabegron was lower in the previous study compared to ours.

Upon further stratifying our study subjects according to age, our results suggested that voiding symptoms worsened slightly after treatment in the old-old patient group, but this difference was not statistically significant. These findings indicate that the use of mirabegron in elderly patients should be carefully monitored, especially in older patients .

The objective symptoms VV and Qmax on uroflowmetry were improved after treatment in patients overall. VV was particularly improved after treatment in young-old patients. However, objective symptoms did not change significantly in the old-old patient group. A previous pressure-flow study reported that mirabegron did not affect urinary bladder contraction even if older male patients were included in the analysis [16, 25]. However, these studies indicated that mirabegron therapy possibility increased PVR, although the change was not statistically significant. In our study, we obtained similar results for PVR. The older patients' voiding functions declined physiologically, and their initial PVR volume was higher than that of the younger patients [26]. Although many clinicians think that mirabegron is associated with fewer problems in terms of voiding function than anticholinergic agents, it is necessary to consider changes in both the subjective and objective symptoms after treatment with mirabegron, especially in old-old patients.

In the present study, only three patients (6 %) had mild adverse effects (2 patients, thirst; 1 patient, constipation), and all patients continued to take mirabegron during the study period. None of the patients with hypertension experienced worsening of their blood pressure level, although hypertension was well-controlled by medication or not severe in all cases in the present study. Hence, it appears that mirabegron can be used safely, and it has good tolerability. Previous studies have reported that typical adverse events such as dry mouth and constipation occurred at a similar incidence between mirabegron and placebo treatment [10, 12, 27]. The incidence of dry mouth with mirabegron, in particular, is three- to four-fold lower than that with tolterodine. As noted in a meta-analysis, anti-muscarinic drugs are associated with a 29.6 % incidence of dry mouth [27]. As dry mouth is reported to be an important factor determining persistence, the favorable tolerability profile of mirabegron may result in improved treatment adherence compared with anti-muscarinic drugs, which has important implications for patient outcome [10]. Many elderly people suffer from constipation and dry mouth; thus mirabegron may be convenient to administer in the elderly with OAB [28, 29].

The present study has several limitations, the major one being that the number of patients included was very small. The observation period was also limited to only 12 weeks. In addition, this study was open label, not placebo controlled. Moreover, patients with relatively mild voiding symptoms prior to mirabegron treatment (with IPSS subscale scores for voiding symptoms of 6.8 ± 1.4, and PVR of 27.4 ± 41.8 mL) and with low prostate volume (33.7 ± 8.6 mL) unlikely to conducting the urinary dysfunction were mainly included in this study. These factors may have contributed to the low complication rate observed in this study. However, despite these limitations, this is the first prospective study that specifically evaluated elderly male patients with OAB who were administered mirabegron additional therapy after treatment with α1-adrenergic receptor blockers. In recent years, there has been growing interest in the efficacy and safety of mirabegron for elderly patients [30]. We believe that in spite of its small sample size, this investigation contributes important information to the selection of treatment strategies in elderly patients with lower urinary tract symptoms.

Conclusions

Our results indicate that mirabegron additional treatment is effective, safe, and tolerable therapy for persistent OAB in elderly male patients after monotherapy with α1-adrenergic receptor blockers. In addition, mirabegron additional therapy was considered effective regardless of the patient's age.

Abbreviations

IPSS, international prostate symptom score; LUTS, lower urinary tract symptoms; OAB, overactive bladder; OABSS, overactive bladder symptom; PVR, post-void residual urine volume; Qmax, maximum flow rate; QOL, quality of life; VV, voided volume

Acknowledgements

The authors are grateful to Mr. Takumi Shimogama for their outstanding support.

Funding

The work was not supported by any grants.

Authors' contributions

TM and YM performed the design of the study and drafted the manuscript. KK and MY contributed experiments and data analysis, KO and AA helped the experiments and data analysis. HS conceived of and supervised the work. All authors read and approved the final manuscript.

Competing interests

The authors declare that they have no competing interests.

References

1. Abrams P, Cardozo L, Fall M, Griffiths D, Rosier P, Ulmsten U, et al. The standardisation of terminology of lower urinary tract function: report from the Standardisation Sub-committee of the International Continence Society. Neurourol Urodyn. 2002;21(2):167–78.
2. Wagg A, Cardozo L, Nitti VW, Castro-Diaz D, Auerbach S, Blauwet MB, et al. The efficacy and tolerability of the β3-adrenoceptor agonist mirabegron for the treatment of symptoms of overactive bladder in older patients. Age Ageing. 2014;43(5):666–75.
3. Stewart WF, Van Rooyen JB, Cundiff GW, Abrams P, Herzog AR, Corey R, et al. Prevalence and burden of overactive bladder in the United States. World J Urol. 2003;20(6):327–36.
4. Brown JS, McGhan WF, Chokroverty S. Comorbidities associated with overactive bladder. Am J Manag Care. 2000;6(11 Suppl):S574–9.
5. McGhan WF. Cost effectiveness and quality of life considerations in the treatment of patients with overactive bladder. Am J Manag Care. 2001;7(2 Suppl):S62–75.
6. D'Souza AO, Smith MJ, Miller LA, Doyle J, Ariely R. Persistence, adherence, and switch rates among extended-release and immediate-release overactive bladder medications in a regional managed care plan. J Manag Care Pharm. 2008;14(3):291–301.
7. Benner JS, Nichol MB, Rovner ES, Jumadilova Z, Alvir J, Hussein M, et al. Patient-reported reasons for discontinuing overactive bladder medication. BJU Int. 2010;105(9):1276–82.
8. Homma Y, Araki I, Igawa Y, Ozono S, Gotoh M, Yamanishi T, Yokoyama O, Yoshida M. Japanese Society of Neurogenic Bladder. Clinical guideline for male lower urinary tract symptoms. Int J Urol. 2009;16(10):775–90.
9. Homma Y, Gotoh M, Yokoyama O, Masumori N, Kawauchi A, Yamanishi T, Ishizuka O, Seki N, Kamoto T, Nagai A, Ozono S. Japanese Urological Association. Outline of JUA clinical guidelines for benign prostatic hyperplasia. Int J Urol. 2011;18(11):741–56.
10. Chapple CR, Kaplan SA, Mitcheson D, Blauwet MB, Huang M, Siddiqui E, et al. Mirabegron 50 mg once-daily for the treatment of symptoms of overactive bladder: an overview of efficacy and tolerability over 12 weeks and 1 year. Int J Urol. 2014;21(10):960–7.
11. Imran M, Najmi AK, Tabrez S. Mirabegron for overactive bladder: a novel, first-in-class β3-agonist therapy. Urol J. 2013;10(3):935–40.
12. Khullar V, Amarenco G, Angulo JC, Cambronero J, Høye K, Milsom I, et al. Efficacy and tolerability of mirabegron, a β(3)-adrenoceptor agonist, in patients with overactive bladder: results from a randomised European-Australian phase 3 trial. Eur Urol. 2013;63(2):283–95.
13. Chapple CR, Kaplan SA, Mitcheson D, Klecka J, Cummings J, Drogendijk T, et al. Randomized double-blind, active-controlled phase 3 study to assess 12-month safety and efficacy of mirabegron, a β(3)-adrenoceptor agonist, in overactive bladder. Eur Urol. 2013;63(2):296–305.
14. Otsuki H, Kosaka T, Nakamura K, Mishima J, Kuwahara Y, Tsukamoto T. β3-Adrenoceptor agonist mirabegron is effective for overactive bladder that is unresponsive to antimuscarinic treatment or is related to benign prostatic hyperplasia in men. Int Urol Nephrol. 2013;45(1):53–60.
15. Ichihara K, Masumori N, Fukuta F, Tsukamoto T, Iwasawa A, Tanaka Y. A randomized controlled study of the efficacy of tamsulosin monotherapy and its combination with mirabegron for overactive bladder induced by benign prostatic obstruction. J Urol. 2015;193(3):921–6.
16. Wada N, Iuchi H, Kita M, Hashizume K, Matsumoto S, Kakizaki H. Urodynamic Efficacy and safety of mirabegron add-on treatment with tamsulosin for Japanese male patients with overactive bladder. LUTS Low Urin Tract Symptoms. 2015:n/a-n/a. doi:10.1111/luts.12091.
17. Homma Y, Yoshida M, Seki N, Yokoyama O, Kakizaki H, Gotoh M, et al. Symptom assessment tool for overactive bladder syndrome–overactive bladder symptom score. Urology. 2006;68(2):318–23.
21. Gacci M, Novara G, De Nunzio C, Tubaro A, Schiavina R, Brunocilla E, et al. Tolterodine extended release in the treatment of male OAB/storage LUTS: a systematic review. BMC Urol. 2014;14:84. doi:10.1186/1471-2490-14-84.
22. Yamaguchi O, Marui E, Kakizaki H, Homma Y, Igawa Y, Takeda M, et al. Phase III, randomised, double-blind, placebo-controlled study of the β3-adrenoceptor agonist mirabegron, 50 mg once daily, in Japanese patients with overactive bladder. BJU Int. 2014;113(6):951–60.
23. Drug Safety Update Mirabegron (Betmiga®): risk of severe hypertension and associated cerebrovascular and cardiac events. Medicines and Healthcare Products Regulatory Agency. https://www.gov.uk/drug-safety-update/. Accessed 27 July 2016.

The efficacy of mirabegron additional therapy for lower urinary tract symptoms after treatment...

159

24. Maeda T, Kikuchi E, Hasegawa M, Ishioka K, Hagiwara M, Miyazaki Y, et al. Solifenacin or mirabegron could improve persistent overactive bladder symptoms after dutasteride treatment in patients with benign prostatic hyperplasia. Urology. 2015;85(5):1151–5.

25. Nitti VW, Rosenberg S, Mitcheson DH, He W, Fakhoury A, Martin NE. Urodynamics and safety of the β3-adrenoceptor agonist mirabegron in males with lower urinary tract symptoms and bladder outlet obstruction. J Urol. 2013;190(4):1320–7.

26. Matsuo T, Oba K, Miyata Y, Igawa T, Sakai H. Four cases of urinary dysfunction associated with sacral herpes zoster. Hinyokika Kiyo. 2014;60(2):87–90.

27. Chapple CR, Khullar V, Gabriel Z, Muston D, Bitoun CE, Weinstein D. The effects of antimuscarinic treatments in overactive bladder: an update of a systematic review and meta-analysis. Eur Urol. 2008;54(3):543–62.

28. Bouras EP, Tangalos EG. Chronic constipation in the elderly. Gastroenterol Clin North Am. 2009;38(3):463–80.

29. Tanida T, Ueta E, Tobiume A, Hamada T, Rao F, Osaki T. Influence of aging on candidal growth and adhesion regulatory agents in saliva. J Oral Pathol Med. 2001;30(6):328–35.

30. Wagg A, Nitti VW, Kelleher C, Castro-Diaz D, Siddiqui E, Berner T. Oral pharmacotherapy for overactive bladder in older patients: mirabegron as a potential alternative to antimuscarinics. Curr Med Res Opin. 2016;32(4):621–38.

25

Rare adrenal gland incidentaloma: an unusual Ewing's sarcoma family of tumor presentation

Hui Guo[1†], Shuaiqi Chen[2†], Shukun Liu[1], Kaixuan Wang[1], Erpeng Liu[1], Faping Li[1] and Yuchuan Hou[1*]

Abstract

Background: Members of the Ewing's sarcoma family of tumor (ESFT) are malignant neoplasms and rarely observed in the adrenal gland.

Case presentation: We report an extremely exceptional case of ESFT rising from the adrenal gland in a 57-year-old Chinese man. The patient was hospitalized with abdominal swelling for 2 months. Computed tomography (CT) scan revealed a nearly-circular mass measuring about 8.1 × 10.6 cm in the right adrenal region. The patient underwent right adrenal resection. Histopathologic examination found the tumor was composed of small round blue cells forming typical Homer-Wright rosettes in focal area. The immunohistochemical analysis confirmed the case to be ESFT, which was positive for membranous CD99 and nuclear FLI-1. The patient was scheduled for four courses of large doses of chemotherapy and died for cancer metastasis one year later after surgery.

Conclusions: Histopathological evidence of Homer-Wright rosettes and immunohistochemical markers positivity, such as CD99 and FLI-1, are valuable factors for ESFT diagnosis, although cytogenetic analysis is considered as the gold standard. Complete surgery is the treatment of choice for ESFT and adjuvant radiotherapy and combination chemotherapy can significantly improve the survival rate of postoperative patients.

Keywords: Ewing's sarcoma family of tumor, Adrenal gland, Diagnosis, Treatment

Background

The Ewing's sarcoma family of tumor (ESFT) are rare aggressive malignancies and consist of Ewing's sarcoma (ES) of bone, extraosseous Ewing's, primitive neuroectodermal tumor (PNET), and Askin's tumor [1, 2]. These distinct entities are characterized by common histopathological and immunohistochemical features, including a primitive undifferentiated small round blue cell associated to a variable level of palisading and rosette formation, as well as strongly positive for the cell surface glycoprotein CD99 [3–5]. The defining feature of the ESFT is a nonrandom chromosomal translocation and the most frequent is EWS-FLI1 fusion [6, 7]. These highly aggressive malignancies most commonly arise in the soft tissue or bone in adolescents and young adults [8]. Reports of cases arising from the adrenal gland are extremely rare. To the best of our knowledge, there are 32 cases in the English literatures [5, 9–30]. We report an additional ESFT case arising from the adrenal gland and discuss its clinical and histopathological characteristics, as well as unusual therapeutic strategies.

Case presentation

A 57-year-old man presented to the First Hospital of Jilin University (Changchun, China) with the main complaint of abdominal swelling for 2 months. In addition to the mild percussion pain in the right kidney region, no other symptoms were noted during a physical examination. His past medical history was unremarkable. Computed tomography (CT) scan of the abdomen revealed a nearly-circular mass measuring about 8.1 × 10.6 cm arising from the right adrenal gland (Fig. 1a). The CT also showed heterogeneous density, both solid and cystic components and calcification of the mass. The lesion showed heterogeneous enhancement and relatively sharp margination on Contrast-enhanced CT

* Correspondence: hou63@163.com

†Equal contributors

[1]Department of Urology, First Hospital of Jilin University, Changchun, Jilin 130021, China

Full list of author information is available at the end of the article

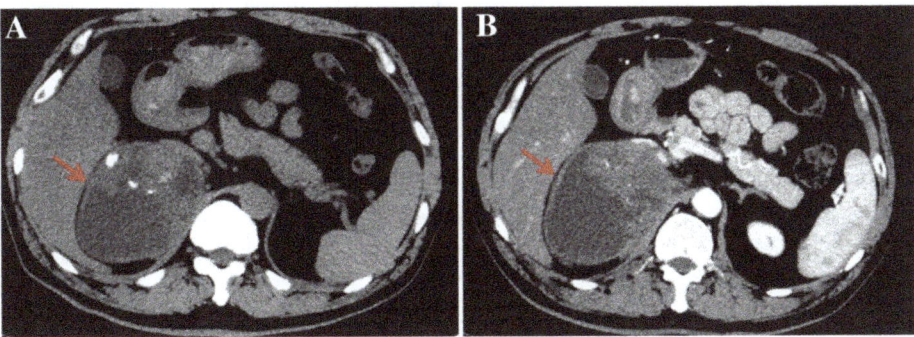

Fig. 1 Abdominal computed tomography (CT) scan revealed a large mass (*arrow*) arising from the right adrenal gland (**a**). The lesion showed heterogeneous enhancement and relatively sharp margination (*arrow*) on Contrast-enhanced CT (**b**)

(Fig. 1b). Contrast-enhanced CT scan further defined the large mass was located between the liver and kidney with characteristics consistent with the soft tissue. Vena cava, right renal vein were compressed and displaced. No obvious metastasis was apparent.

The patient underwent open surgery under general anesthesia. A 10.0 cm × 8.0 cm × 6.0 cm mass was found during laparotomy. The tumor was located above the left renal vein and the right renal vein without venous involvement. Due to firmly adhesion with the surrounding tissue, tumor dissection was difficult. Intraoperative blood loss was 800 mL and the tumor was completely removed eventually. Postoperative histopathology showed a monotonous population of small round blue cells with occasional Homer-Wright-type rosettes (Fig. 2). The results confirmed the diagnosis of PNET. The immunohistochemical staining was performed supporting the previous diagnosis, which was positive for CD99, FLI-1, NeuN, CGA and VIMENTIN (Fig. 2), while negative for EMA, SYN and LCA.

The patient was scheduled for adjuvant chemotherapy with adriamycin, cyclophosphamide, ifosfamide and etoposide. At his follow-up, 5 months after surgery, CT scan results demonstrated a metastatic lesion arising from the right abdominal wall. Unfortunately, the patient died for cancer metastasis one year later after surgery.

Discussion

ESFT rising from the adrenal gland is extremely exceptional but malignant. Patients often present with tumor compression, flank pain or mass. However, its preoperative imaging diagnosis is difficult and histopathological and genetic tools are required for an accurate diagnosis.

Histopathologically, ESFT appear as immature or primitive small round blue cell tumors infiltrating the soft tissue or bone in a diffuse or lobular pattern. The tumor cells have round to oval nuclei with coarsely stippled chromatin and indistinct nucleoli. The scanty cytoplasm is pale or clear. In addition, these cells are often accompanied by

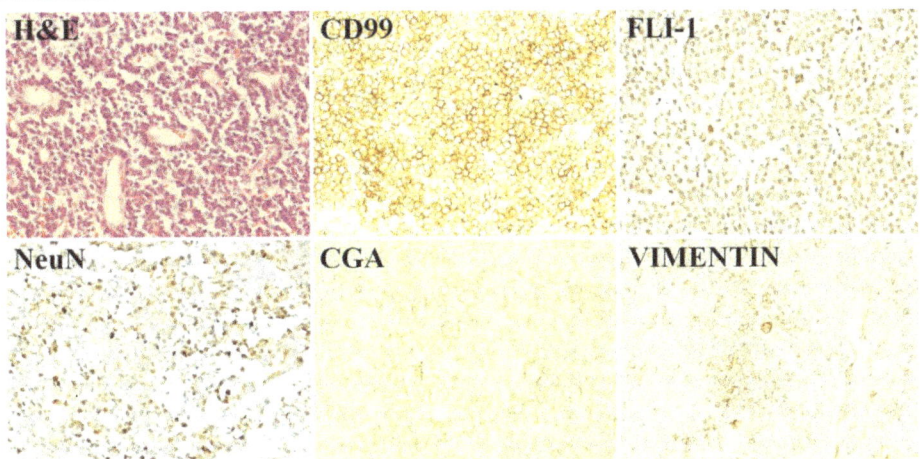

Fig. 2 Histopathologic examination showed small round blue cells forming Homer-Wright-type rosettes (H&E, ×400). Immunohistochemical staining revealed the tumor cells were positive for CD 99, FLI-1, NeuN, CGA and VIMENTIN (original magnification × 400)

Table 1 Summary of Reported Cases of ESFT Rising from the Adrenal Gland (F: female; M: male; IVC: inferior vena cava; Surg: surgery; Chemo: chemotherapy; RTx: radiotherapy; NR: not recorded)

Case Report (Reference Number)	Age	Gender	Chief Complaint	Position	Tumor Size (cm)	Initial Infiltration or Metastasis	Treatment	Outcome at Time of Report
9	17	F	NR	NR	NR	Liver, lung, lymph node	Chemo + RTx	Dead
	8	M	NR	NR	NR	Bone, lung	Surg + chemo + RTx	Dead
	4	M	NR	NR	NR	Lung	Surg + chemo + RTx	Dead
10	46	F	NR	NR	NR	NR	NR	NR
	20	F	NR	NR	NR	NR	NR	NR
	48	F	NR	NR	NR	NR	NR	NR
11	32	F	Abdominal pain	Left	10	Liver	Surg + adjuvant chemo	Dead
12	57	M	Lower extremity pain, edema	Right	15	None	Surg	NR
13	11	M	Abdominal tumor	Right	13	Peritoneum	Surg + chemo + RTx	Dead
14	28	F	Recurrent mass	Right	10	Lung	Surg + chemo	NR
15	25	F	Abdominal pain	Left	15.2	IVC, lung	NR	NR
	24	F	Flank pain	NR	8.4	Supraclavicular lymph node	NR	NR
16	53	F	Adrenal tumor	Right	3	None	Surg	Alive
17	30	M	NR	Right	12	IVC tumor embolus	Surg + RTx	Dead
	21	F	NR	Left	10	Liver	None	Dead
	24	F	NR	Left	9	Pelvic lymph node	Surg + chemo	Metastasis
	22	M	NR	Left	17	IVC tumor embolus	Surg + chemo	Local recurrence
18	20	F	Flank pain, anorexia, weight loss	Right	Large	Lung	Neo-adjuvant chemo	Unknow
5	17	F	Flank pain	Right	5	None	Surg + adjuvant chemo + RTx	Alive
19	26	F	Flank pain	Left	Large	IVC tumor thrombus	Surg + chemo + RTx	Alive
20	17	M	Swelling, abdominal pain	Right	21.3	Liver, lung	Systemic chemotherapy	Alive
21	17	F	Abdominal Pain, fever	Left	15	None	Surg + adjuvant chemo + RTx	Recurrence
22	26	F	Flank pain	Left	11.3	IVC tumor thrombus	Surg + adjuvant chemo + RTx	Alive
23	63	M	None	Left	3.2	None	Surg + adjuvant chemo	Alive
24	40	F	Abdominal pain, swelling, respiratory distress	Left	14.6	Retroperitoneal muscles	Surg + adjuvant chemo	Alive
25	37	F	Loin pain	Left	8	Kidney	Surg	Alive
26	26	M	None	Right	8	None	None	Dead
27	37	F	Flank pain, abdominal pain	Left	12	Crus of diaphragm, kidney	Surg + adjuvant chemo	Alive
28	17	F	Abdominal pain	Left	3.3	None	Surg + adjuvant chemo + RTx	Alive
29	23	M	Flank pain, weight loss	Right	15	Kidney, head of pancreas, liver	None	Unknow
	27	M	Pain	Right	NR	Kidney, liver, pancreas	Chemo	Dead
30	48	F	Abdominal pain, swelling	Left	12	None	Surg	Recurrence
Present case	57	M	Swelling	Right	10.6	None	Surg + adjuvant chemo	Dead

hemorrhage and necrosis. ESFT are mainly represented by the existence of typical Homer-Wright-type rosette or other types of rosettes [17, 31].

Immunohistochemical markers such as CD99, FLI-1, HNK-1 and CAV-1 are commonly expressed in ESFT and provide valuable support to the definitive diagnosis. CD99, a 32-kDa cell surface glycoprotein, is encoded by the MIC2 gene and extremely sensitive for ESFT [4, 14]. The sensitivity is as high as 95% although the specificity is low [14, 31]. Its expression is also observed in T-lymphoblastic lymphoma, rhabdomyosarcoma, synovial sarcoma, and small cell anaplastic osteosarcoma [32–35]. ESFT can be potentially misdiagnosed based merely on expression of CD99. Even so, CD99 is still the most reliable immunohistochemical marker for ESFT. FLI-1, as well as HNK-1, appears reliable but less sensitive for ESFT than CD99 [4, 31]. All authors agree that both markers are expressed in various other round cell tumors [36]. CD99 and FLI-1 are mainly used for the diagnosis of ESFT and an immunohistochemical panel consisting at least these two makers is recommended [37–39]. CAV1, a membrane protein, its high expression is associated with the anchorage-independent growth [40, 41]. Express CAV1 have been shown to be more aggressive and metastatic [41]. CAV1 appears as a diagnostic immunohistochemical marker of ESFT being positive in CD99-negative cases [31]. In addition, markers of NSE, VIMENTIN, cytokeratin and S-100 have been detected in a subset of ESFT by immunohistochemistry.

At present, cytogenetic analysis is the "gold standard" for diagnosis of ESFT. Conventional tests are valuable to make the definitive diagnosis such as Southern blot, Northern blot analyses, FISH and RT-PCR [14, 39, 42]. The diagnosis of our case, ESFT rising from the adrenal gland, was not based on the cytogenetic findings. However, it was supported by the histopathological findings of poorly differentiated, small round blue cells forming typical Homer-Wright rosettes and the immunohistochemical findings of strongly positive for CD99, FLI-1 and negative for differentiation markers such as epithelial sufficiently.

ESFT is an aggressive malignancy with very poor prognosis [6]. Multimodality regimens including surgical resection, adjuvant chemotherapy and radiation therapy are often required [43]. Current surgical approaches include open, laparoscopic and robotic resection. The latter two are more difficult to perform because the large tumor is often accompanied by liquefaction and/or necrosis. Jacob Stephenson et al. [5] reported a ESFT arising from adrenal gland, during operation with the robotic assistance, the tumor capsule was ruptured, which may lead to metastasis and increase the dose of chemotherapy and radiotherapy. Hence, the surgical approach should be selected in accordance with patient's condition.

Cooperative group studies have led to chemotherapy regimens using the same drugs (vincristine, doxorubicin, cyclophosphamide, ifosfamide, and etoposide), although the exact regimens differ in Europe and North America [2]. Only 16 cases of ESFT arising from the adrenal gland have been reported since 2011. Eleven of these sixteen patients received surgery. Nine received adjuvant chemotherapy and five received radiation treatment. Only two patients with small mass and no evidence of metastasis are alive and disease free. The two long-term survival of patients received multimodality regimens using a combination of complete surgery, as well as chemotherapy and radiotherapy (Table 1). We conclude that complete surgery is the treatment of choice for ESFT. Adjuvant chemotherapy and postoperative radiotherapy have shown significant improvements in survival. The tumor size and metastases are predictors for survival and effect prognosis obviously.

Conclusion

ESFT rising from the adrenal gland is a rare clinical entity. Histopathological evidence of Homer-Wright is crucial for ESFT diagnosis. The neural markers, such as CD99, FLI-1, HNK-1 and CAV-1, may play a valuable role in the immunohistochemical diagnosis of ESFT. The definitive diagnosis of ESFT requires a combination of immunohistochemical examination, as well as histopathologic evaluation, although the "gold standard" will obviously remain cytogenetic analysis. Complete surgery is the treatment of choice for ESFT. Adjuvant chemotherapy and postoperative radiotherapy have shown significant improvements in survival. The tumor size and metastases are predictors for survival and effect prognosis obviously.

Abbreviations
CAV-1: Caveolin-1; CD99: Cluster of differentiation 99; CGA: Chromogranin A; CT: Computed tomography; ES: Ewing's sarcoma; ESFT: Ewing's sarcoma family of tumor; LCA: Leukocyte common antigen; NSE: Neuron-specific enolase; PNET: Primitive neuroectodermal tumor; SYN: Synaptophysin

Acknowledgments
The authors thank the patient and his families for allowing us to publish this case report. We also thank Professor Meishan Jin (Department of Pathology, First Hospital of Jilin University, Changchun 130021, China) as the pathologist for reviewing and confirming the histological diagnosis for our patient.

Authors' contributions
HG and SQC wrote the manuscript and made the revisions. SKL, KXW, EPL and FPL participated in data collection. YCH collected cases and do the check. All authors read and approved the final manuscript.

Competing interests
The authors declare that they have no competing interests.

Consent for publication

Written informed consent was obtained from the patient for publication of this case report and any accompanying images. The data do not contain any information that could identify the patient. A copy of the written consent is available for review by the editor of this journal.

Author details

[1]Department of Urology, First Hospital of Jilin University, Changchun, Jilin 130021, China. [2]Department of Urology, The First Affiliated Hospital of Xinxiang Medical University, Xinxiang, Henan 453100, China.

References

1. Gupta AA, Pappo A, Saunders N, Hopyan S, Ferguson P, Wunder J, O'Sullivan B, Catton C, Greenberg M, Blackstein M. Clinical Outcome of Children and Adults With Localized Ewing Sarcoma Impact of Chemotherapy Dose and Timing of Local Therapy. Cancer. 2010;116(13):3189–94.

2. Balamuth NJ, Womer RB. Ewing's sarcoma. Lancet Oncology. 2010;11(2):184–92.

3. Fagone P, Nicoletti F, Salvatorelli L, Musumeci G, Magro G. Cyclin D1 and Ewing's sarcoma/PNET: A microarray analysis. Acta Histochem. 2015;117(8):824–8.

4. Hung YP, Fletcher CDM, Hornick JL. Evaluation of NKX2-2 expression in round cell sarcomas and other tumors with EWSR1 rearrangement: imperfect specificity for Ewing sarcoma. Mod Pathol. 2016;29(4):370–80.

5. Stephenson J, Gow KW, Meehan J, Hawkins DS, Avansino J. Ewing sarcoma/primitive neuroectodermal tumor arising from the adrenal gland in an adolescent. Pediatr Blood Cancer. 2011;57(4):691–2.

6. Tilan JU, Krailo M, Barkauskas DA, Galli S, Mtaweh H, Long J, Wang H, Hawkins K, Lu C, Jeha D, et al. Systemic Levels of Neuropeptide Y and Dipeptidyl Peptidase Activity in Patients With Ewing Sarcoma-Associations With Tumor Phenotype and Survival. Cancer. 2015;121(5):697–707.

7. Hameiri-Grossman M, Porat-Klein A, Yaniv I, Ash S, Cohen IJ, Kodman Y, Haklai R, Elad-Sfadia G, Kloog Y, Chepurko E, et al. The association between let-7, RAS and HIF-1 alpha in Ewing Sarcoma tumor growth. Oncotarget. 2015;6(32):33834–48.

8. Lee J, Hoang BH, Ziogas A, Zell JA. Analysis of Prognostic Factors in Ewing Sarcoma Using a Population-Based Cancer Registry. Cancer. 2010;116(8):1964–73.

9. Marina NM, Etcubanas E, Parham DM, Bowman LC, Green A. Peripheral Primitive Neuroectodermal Tumor (Peripheral Neuroepithelioma) In Children - A Review Of The St Jude Experience And Controversies In Diagnosis And Management. Cancer. 1989;64(9):1952–60.

10. Renshaw AA, PerezAtayde AR, Fletcher JA, Granter SR. Cytology of typical and atypical Ewing's sarcoma PNET. Am J Clin Pathol. 1996;106(5):620–4.

11. Matsuoka Y, Fujii Y, Akashi T, Gosehi N, Kihara K. Primitive neuroectodermal tumour of the adrenal gland. BJU Int. 1999;83(4):515–6.

12. Pirani JF, Woolums CS, Dishop MK, Herman JR. Primitive neuroectodermal tumor of the adrenal gland. Journal of Urology. 2000;163(6):1855–6.

13. Kato K, Kato Y, Ijiri R, Misugi K, Nanba I, Nagai J-I, Nagahara N, Kigasawa H, Toyoda Y, Nishi T, et al. Ewing's sarcoma family of tumor arising in the adrenal gland—Possible diagnostic pitfall in pediatric pathology: Histologic, immunohistochemical, ultrastructural, and molecular study. Hum Pathol. 2001;32(9):1012–6.

14. Ahmed AA, Nava VE, Pham T, Taubenberger JK, Lichy JH, Sorbara L, Raffeld M, Mackall CL, Tsokos M. Ewing sarcoma family of tumors in unusual sites: Confirmation by RT-PCR. Pediatr Dev Pathol. 2006;9(6):488–95.

15. Kim MS, Kim B, Park CS, Song SY, Lee EJ, Park NH, Kim HS, Kim SH, Cho KS. Radiologic findings of peripheral primitive neuroectodermal tumor arising in the retroperitoneum. Am J Roentgenol. 2006;186(4):1125–32.

16. Komatsu S, Watanabe R, Naito M, Mizusawa T, Obara K, Nishiyama T, Takahashi K. Primitive neuroectodermal tumor of the adrenal gland. Int J Urol. 2006;13(5):606–7.

17. Zhang Y, Li H. Primitive Neuroectodermal Tumors of Adrenal Gland. Jpn J Clin Oncol. 2010;40(8):800–4.

18. Mohsin R, Hashmi A, Mubarak M, Sultan G, Shehzad A, Qayum A, Naqvi SA, Rizvi SA. Primitive neuroectodermal tumor/Ewing's sarcoma in adult uro-oncology: A case series from a developing country. Urology annals. 2011;3(2):103–7.

19. Saboo SS, Krajewski KM, Jagannathan JP, Ramaiya N. IVC tumor thrombus: an advanced case of rare extraosseous Ewing sarcoma of the adrenal gland. Urology. 2012;79(6):e77–78.

20. Zahir MN, Ansari TZ, Moatter T, Memon W, Pervez S. Ewing's sarcoma arising from the adrenal gland in a young male: a case report. BMC Res Notes. 2013;6:533. doi:10.1186/1756-0500-1186-1533.

21. Sasaki T, Onishi T, Yabana T, Hoshina A. Ewing's sarcoma/primitive neuroectodermal tumor arising from the adrenal gland: a case report and literature review. Tumori. 2013;99(3):e104–106. doi:10.1700/1334.14815.

22. Abi-Raad R, Manetti GJ, Colberg JW, Hornick JL, Shah JG, Prasad ML. Ewing sarcoma/primitive neuroectodermal tumor arising in the adrenal gland. Pathol Int. 2013;63(5):283–6.

23. Blas JV, Smith ML, Wasif N, Cook CB. Schlinkert RT. Ewing sarcoma of the adrenal gland: a rare entity. BMJ Case Rep. 2013;2013:bcr2012007753. doi:10.1136/bcr-2012-007753.

24. Dutta D, Shivaprasad KS, Das RN, Ghosh S, Chowdhury S. Primitive neuroectodermal tumor of adrenal: Clinical presentation and outcomes. J Cancer Res Ther. 2013;9(4):709–11.

25. Phukan C, Nirmal TJ, Kumar RM, Kekre NS. Peripheral primitive neuroectodermal tumor of the adrenal gland: A rare entity. Indian J Urol. 2013;29(4):357–9.

26. Yamamoto T, Takasu K, Emoto Y, Umehara T, Ikematsu K, Shikata N, Iino M, Matoba R. Latent adrenal Ewing sarcoma family of tumors: A case report. Leg Med. 2013;15(2):96–8.

27. Tsang YP, Lang BH, Tam SC, Wong KP. Primitive neuroectodermal adrenal gland tumour. Hong Kong Med J. 2014;20(5):444–6.

28. Yoon JH, Kim H, Lee JW, Kang HJ, Park HJ, Park KD, Park B-K, Shin HY, Park JD, Park S-H, et al. Ewing Sarcoma/Peripheral Primitive Neuroectodermal Tumor in the Adrenal Gland of an Adolescent: A Case Report and Review of the Literature. J Pediatr Hematol Oncol. 2014;36(7):E456–9.

29. Bhatt Krutika R, Trivedi Priti P, Shah Manoj J. Adult Neuroblastoma of Adrenal gland: Two case report. The Southeast Asian Journal of Case Report and Review. 2015;4(3):1742–8.

30. Zhang L, Yao M, Hisaoka M, Sasano H, Gao H. Primary Ewing sarcoma/primitive neuroectodermal tumor in the adrenal gland. APMIS. 2016;124(7):624-9.

31. Llombart-Bosch A, Machado I, Navarro S, Bertoni F, Bacchini P, Alberghini M, Karzeladze A, Savelov N, Petrov S, Alvarado-Cabrero I, et al. Histological heterogeneity of Ewing's sarcoma/PNET: an immunohistochemical analysis of 415 genetically confirmed cases with clinical support. Virchows Arch. 2009;455(5):397–411.

32. Ambros IM, Ambros PF, Strehl S, Kovar H, Gadner H, Salzerkuntschik M. MIC2 is a specific marker for ewings-sarcoma and peripheral primitive neuroectodermal tumors - evidence for a common histogenesis of ewings-sarcoma and peripheral primitive neuroectodermal tumors from MIC2 expression and specific chromosome aberration. Cancer. 1991;67(7):1886–93.

33. Gerald WL, Ladanyi M, de Alava E, Cuatrecasas M, Kushner BH, LaQuaglia MP, Rosai J. Clinical, pathologic, and molecular spectrum of tumors associated with t(11;22)(p13;q12): Desmoplastic small round-cell tumor and its variants. J Clin Oncol. 1998;16(9):3028–36.

34. Devaney K, Vinh TN, Sweet DE. Small-cell osteosarcoma of bone - an immunohistochemical study with differential diagnostic considerations. Hum Pathol. 1993;24(11):1211–25.

35. Riopel M, Dickman PS, Link MP, Perlman EJ. MIC2 Analysis In Pediatric Lymphomas And Leukemias. Hum Pathol. 1994;25(4):396–9.

36. Mhawech-Fauceglia P, Herrmann FR, Bshara W, Odunsi K, Terracciano L, Sauter G, Cheney RT, Groth J, Penetrante R. Friend leukaemia integration-1 expression in malignant and benign tumours: a multiple tumour tissue microarray analysis using polyclonal antibody. J Clin Pathol. 2007;60(6):694–700.

37. Saxena R, Sait S, Mhawech-Fauceglia P. Ewing sarcoma/primitive neuroectodermal tumor of the kidney: a case report. Diagnosed by immunohistochemistry and molecular analysis. Ann Diagn Pathol. 2006;10(6):363–6.

38. Zhong J, Chen N, Chen X, Gong J, Nie L, Xu M, Zhou Q. Peripheral primitive neuroectodermal tumor of the kidney in a 51-year-old female following breast cancer: A case report and review of the literature. Oncol Lett. 2015;9(1):108–12.

39. Pinto A, Dickman P, Parham D. Pathobiologic markers of the ewing sarcoma family of tumors: state of the art and prediction of behaviour. Sarcoma. 2011;2011:856190.

40. Drab M, Verkade P, Elger M, Kasper M, Lohn M, Lauterbach B, Menne J, Lindschau C, Mende F, Luft FC, et al. Loss of caveolae, vascular dysfunction, and pulmonary defects in caveolin-1 gene-disrupted mice. Science. 2001; 293(5539):2449–52.

41. Williams TM, Lisanti MP. Caveolin-1 in oncogenic transformation, cancer, and metastasis. Am J Physiol Cell Physiol. 2005;288(3):C494–506.

42. Vural C, Uluoglu O, Akyurek N, Oguz A, Karadeniz C. The evaluation of CD99 immunoreactivity and EWS/FLI1 translocation by fluorescence in situ hybridization in central PNETs and Ewing's sarcoma family of tumors. Pathol Oncol Res. 2011;17(3):619–25.

43. DuBois SG, Krailo MD, Gebhardt MC, Donaldson SS, Marcus KJ, Dormans J, Shamberger RC, Sailer S, Nicholas RW, Healey JH, et al. Comparative Evaluation of Local Control Strategies in Localized Ewing Sarcoma of Bone A Report From the Children's Oncology Group. Cancer. 2015;121(3):467–75.

26

An ectopic adreocortical adenoma of the renal sinus

Jiexiu Zhang[†], Bianjiang Liu[†], Ninghong Song, Qiang Lv[*], Zenjun Wang and Ming Gu

Abstract

Background: Ectopic adrenal tumors are very rare, especially in the renal sinus in adults. An unusual case of ectopic adrenal cortical adenoma in the right renal sinus is reported here.

Case presentation: This patient was a 37-year-old woman. She was admitted to our hospital for hypertension and bilateral limb weakness. Computed tomography (CT) revealed a mass in right renal sinus. It was initially considered a tumor of the renal pelvis. Further computed tomographic angiography (CTA) showed the mass to be located outside the renal pelvis. After adequate preoperative preparation (blood pressure control and serum potassium supplement), the patient underwent laparoscopic resection of retroperitoneal tumor. During the procedure, a soft tissue tumor 3.4*3.0 cm^2 in size with a golden color was found in the right renal sinus. The final immunohistochemistry examination showed an ectopic adreocortical adenoma.

Conclusion: Ectopic adrenal tumors are rare in the renal sinus and difficult to diagnose and treat. Large and functional tumors should be treated with complete resection. The procedure is sometimes difficult for tumors located deep in the renal sinus. The decision to perform an open or minimally invasive surgery should be made according to the surgeon's experience.

Keywords: Ectopic, Adrenal tumor, CTA, Laparoscopy

Background

The adrenals are derived from primordial mesenchyme in the wall of the dorsal coelom adjacent to the dorsal mesentery and urogenital structures [1]. Most ectopic adrenocortical tissues exist along the path of embryonic migration within the urogenital tract [1]. The most common sites of ectopic adrenocortical neoplasm include the celiac axis (32 %), broad ligament (23 %), adenexa of the testis (7.5 %), and spermatic cord (3–8 %) [2]. Adrenal neoplasm adjacent to the renal sinus is very rare. The present work reports an unusual case of ectopic adrenocortical adenoma in the right renal sinus.

Case presentation

The patient was a 37-year-old woman. She was admitted to our hospital for hypertension and bilateral limb weakness on December 10, 2014. She had begun to take oral antihypertensive drugs 2 years earlier. The blood pressure was well controlled initially. Since October, 2014, she had felt bilateral limb weakness. Biochemical tests in a local hospital showed a significant decrease in serum potassium levels. She came to our hospital's endocrinology department for further diagnosis and treatment. During hospitalization, her fasting blood glucose, cortisol, and aldosterone were found to be higher than normal levels. Catecholamine levels were normal. Serum potassium levels were significantly lower than normal level. Physical examination was normal. No symptoms of virilization were observed. Computed tomography (CT) of the adrenal area showed a right retroperitoneal mass (about 3.4*3.0 cm^2) compressing the renal pelvis. The native adrenals appeared normal on the imaging. Then she was transferred to our department.

* Correspondence: drq_lv@163.com

[†]Equal contributors

Department of Urology, The First Affiliated Hospital of Nanjing Medical University, Nanjing 210029, China

Computed tomographic angiography (CTA) showed the mass to be located in the right renal sinus. It had clear margins and obvious enhancement. The mass was about 2.99*2.88*2.23 cm^3 in size. The right renal vessel, renal pelvis and ureter were compressed by the mass (Fig. 1). A preliminary diagnosis of ectopic adrenal cortical adenoma was considered.

After adequate blood pressure control and serum potassium supplement, the patient underwent the laparoscopic resection of retroperitoneal tumor. During the operation, a mass 3.4*3.0 cm^2 in size of medium density was found in the right renal sinus. It was tightly surrounded by the renal artery, renal vein, renal pelvis, and ureter (Fig. 2). The tumor was completely resected without conversion to open surgery. No complications were observed. The operation took about 100 min. Blood loss was about 90 ml. The blood pressure and heart rate remained stable during operation. Peri-operative vital signs and related biochemical indicators were closely monitored and remained normal. The Foley catheter was removed 1 day after the operation and the drainage tube was removed 3 days after the operation. The postoperative hospital stay lasted 4 days. Pathologic examination showed ectopic adrenal tissue with adrenocortical adenoma. Further immunohistochemistry showed the tissue to be positive for synaptophysin (Fig. 3a), CD56 (Fig. 3b), vimentin (Fig. 3c), Ki-67(2 %) (Fig. 3d), calretinin, and inhibin-α and negative for chromogranin A, CD117, CD10, CK7, EMA, CK-pan, and melan-A. However, the concentration of pax-8 was ± (Fig. 4). Using the

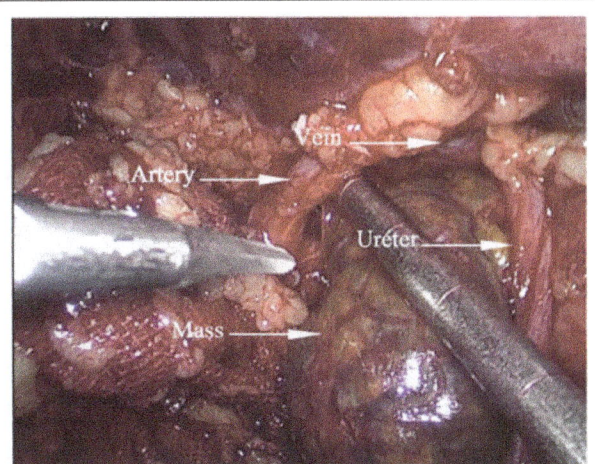

Fig. 2 The real time image of the ectopic adrenal tumor during the operation

results and HE staining, the tumor was diagnosed as an ectopic adreocortical adenoma of the right renal sinus. The patient was followed up for 1 month after the operation. Her blood pressure was normal. The bilateral limb weakness was significantly reduced. Abdominal CT showed native adrenals and no obvious mass in the renal sinus.

Conclusions

Ectopic adrenal tissue is estimated to occur in about 1 % of the adult population and up to 50 % of neonates [3]. It regresses usually in early infancy. The adrenal cortex is derived from the coelomic mesoderm of the urogenital ridge at the 5th week of gestational age and is separated at the 8th week. Ectopic adrenal tissue occurs when a fragment of the primitive adrenal gland sheds off during development. It may come to rest in any visceral organs, especially the kidneys, liver, and gonads. Rarer sites include the lung, spinal region, stomach, and brain [1, 4]. Ectopic adrenal tissue contains cortex and medulla if the breaking event occurs after the migration of neural crest tissue into the cortex. Otherwise, only cortex exists in ectopic adrenal tissue.

Most ectopic adrenal tissue has no obvious physiological function and causes no clinical symptoms. Few ectopic adrenal tumors can produce hormones. However, this can lead to physical changes such as hypertension, feebleness, crinosity, and palpitations. The reported case involved abnormal blood glucose, cortisol, and aldosterone levels, and obvious clinical symptoms. It should be considered a functional ectopic adrenal tumor. CT is sensitive enough to indicate the locations of ectopic adrenal masses. However, it can be difficult to determine whether a mass is inside or outside of the renal pelvis if it is adjacent to renal sinus. In these cases, CTA can help

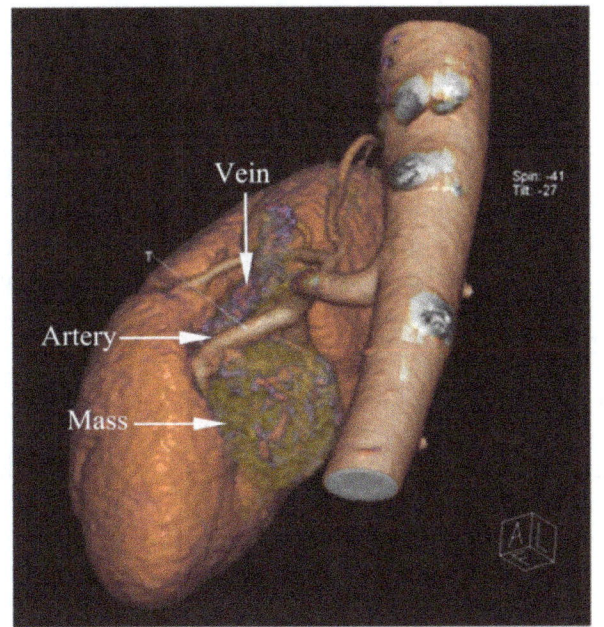

Fig. 1 The preoperative computed tomographic angiography (CTA) image of the ectopic adrenal tumor

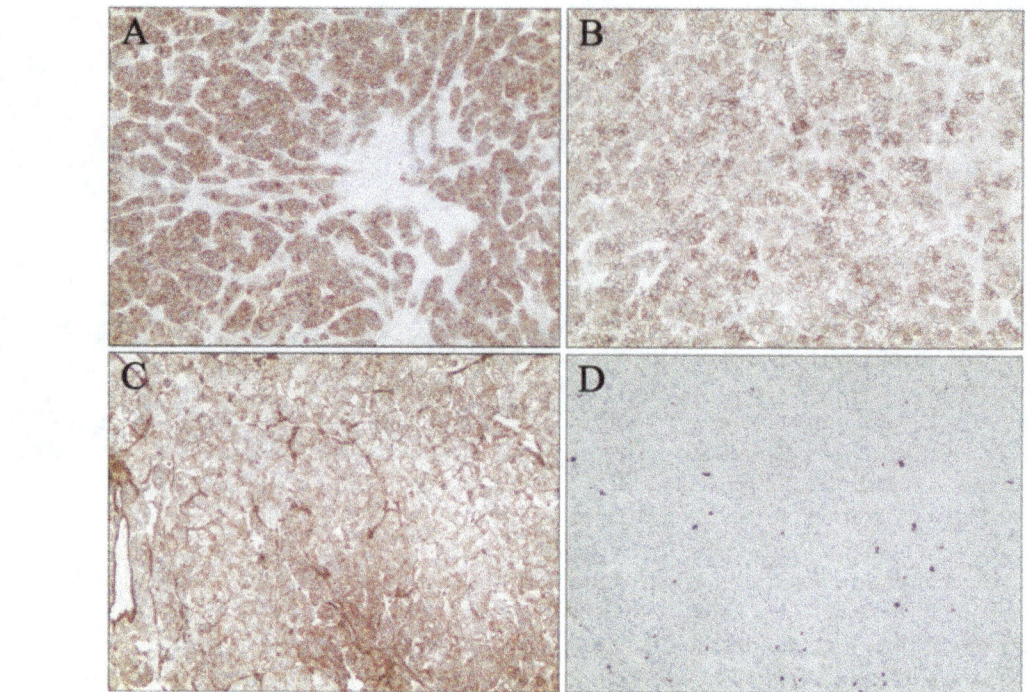

Fig. 3 Immunohistochemistry showed positive staining for synaptophysin (**a**), CD56 (**b**), vimentin (**c**), and Ki-67(2 %) (**d**). Magnification was × 100

determine the exact location. It is especially effective in the description of the relationship between mass and surrounding vessels, which is very important for this type of surgery.

Differentiating between benign and malignant ectopic adrenal tumor is a challenge. Routine pathological examinations are sometimes not always enough. Tumor weight and size, hormone levels, signs of vascular invasion, and high mitotic index are useful morphologic indicators to evaluate the carcinogenic potential. Large tumors (more than 100 g in weight or 5.0 cm in diameter), invasion of

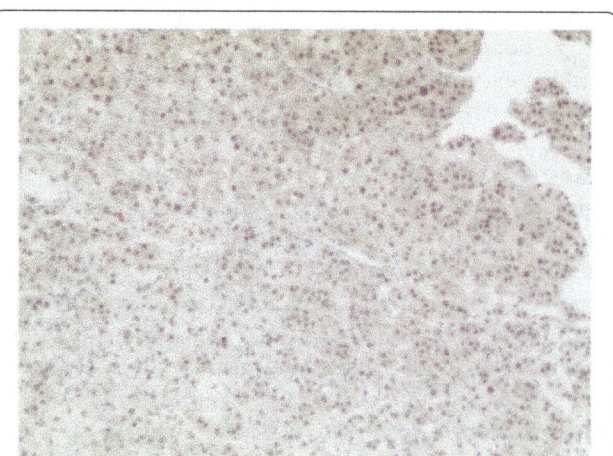

Fig. 4 Immunohistochemistry showed ± staining for pax-8. Magnification was × 100

surrounding tissues, and presence of metastasis, are indicators of malignancy [5, 6]. In addition, malignant tumor presents more commonly a mixed Cushing-virilization syndrome. The tumor in this report was much smaller than 100 g in weight and 3.4 cm in diameter. Only abnormal cortisol and aldsterone levels were detected. The tumor was completely resected from the renal sinus with an intact capsule. No invasion of surrounding tissues was detected. All signs indicated the benign tendency of this mass. Recently, some molecular markers have been used to differentiate adrenal carcinoma from benign tumors [7]. These new markers may help to distinguish the nature of tumor in the future.

The treatment of ectopic adrenal tumors includes conservative therapy and radical resection (open or minimally invasive surgery). If the tumor is small or nonfunctioning, watchful waiting is enough. Otherwise, the tumor should be resected although evincing no malignant tendency. In our study, the large tumor size (3.4 cm in diameter) and obvious clinical symptoms can serve at surgical indications. However, the procedure is complicated and difficult because tumors in the renal sinus are surrounded by the renal artery, renal vein, and ureter. Common complications include uncontrolled bleeding and side injury of renal pelvis or ureter. The choice of a surgical approach should depend on the surgeon's experience.

In summary, ectopic adrenal tumors of the renal sinus are rare and difficult to diagnose and treat. For large or functional tumors, complete resection should be performed. The procedure can be difficult if the tumor is located deep in the renal sinus. The decision to perform an open or minimally invasive surgery should be made according to the surgeon's experience.

Consent

Written informed consent was obtained from the patient for publication of this Case report and any accompanying images. A copy of the written consent is available for review by the Editor of this journal.

Abbreviations

CT: Computed tomography; CTA: Computed tomographic angiography.

Competing interests

The authors declare that they have no competing interests.

Authors' contributions

All authors participated in the study conception, design and coordination. ZJ, LB, and LQ performed the surgery and wrote the paper. SN and WZ collected the data. GM helped to revise the manuscript. All authors read and approved the final manuscript.

Acknowledgments

This work is supported by the grants from National Natural Science Foundation of China (81272832; 81200467) and by A Project Funded by the Priority Academic Program Development of Jiangsu Higher Education Institutions (JX10231802).

References

1. Ren PT, Fu H, He XW. Ectopic adrenal cortical adenoma in the gastric wall: case report. World J Gastroenterol. 2013;19:778–80.
2. Makino K, Kojima R, Nakamura H, Morioka M, Iyama K, Shigematsu K, et al. Ectopic adrenal cortical adenoma in the spinal region: case report and review of the literature. Brain Tumor Pathol. 2010;27:121–5.
3. Souverijns G, Peene P, Keuleers H, Vanbockrijck M. Ectopic localisation of adrenal cortex. Eur Radiol. 2000;10:1165–8.
4. Ye H, Yoon GS, Epstein JI. Intrarenal ectopic adrenal tissue and renal-adrenal fusion: a report of nine cases. Mod Pathol. 2009;22:175–81.
5. Lee PDK, Winter RJ, Green OC. Virilizing adrenocortical tumors in childhood: eight cases and review of the literature. Pediatrics. 1985;76:437–43.
6. Wolthers OD, Cameron FJ, Scheimberg I, Honour JW, Hindmarsh PC, Savage MO, et al. Androgen secreting adrenocortical tumors. Arch Dis Child. 1999; 80:46–50.
7. Choukair D, Beuschlein F, Zwermann O, Wudy SA, Haufe S, Holland-Cunz S, et al. Virilization of a young girl caused by concomitant ectopic and intra-adrenal adenomas of the adrenal cortex. Horm Res Paediatr. 2013;79:318–22.

27

The beneficial effect of alpha-blockers for ureteral stent-related discomfort: systematic review and network meta-analysis for alfuzosin versus tamsulosin versus placebo

Jong Kyou Kwon[1], Kang Su Cho[2], Cheol Kyu Oh[1], Dong Hyuk Kang[3], Hyungmin Lee[4], Won Sik Ham[5], Young Deuk Choi[5] and Joo Yong Lee[5*]

Abstract

Background: This study was carried out a network meta-analysis of evidence from randomized controlled trials (RCTs) to evaluate stent-related discomfort in patients with alfuzosin or tamsulosin versus placebo.

Methods: Relevant RCTs were identified from electronic databases. The proceedings of appropriate meetings were also searched. Seven articles on the basis of RCTs were included in our meta-analysis. Using pairwise and network meta-analyses, comparisons were made by qualitative and quantitative syntheses. Evaluation was performed with the Ureteric Stent Symptoms Questionnaire to assess the urinary symptom score (USS) and body pain score (BPS).

Results: One of the seven RCTs was at moderate risk of bias for all quality criteria; two studies had a high risk of bias. In the network meta-analysis, both alfuzosin (mean difference [MD];−4.85, 95 % confidence interval [CI];−8.53−−1.33) and tamsulosin (MD;−8.84, 95 % CI;−13.08−−4.31) showed lower scores compared with placebo; however, the difference in USS for alfuzosin versus tamsulosin was not significant (MD; 3.99, 95 % CI;−1.23−9.04). Alfuzosin (MD;−5.71, 95 % CI;−11.32−−0.52) and tamsulosin (MD;−7.77, 95 % CI;−13.68−−2.14) showed lower scores for BPS compared with placebo; however, the MD between alfuzosin and tamsulosin was not significant (MD; 2.12, 95 % CI;−4.62−8.72). In the rank-probability test, tamsulosin ranked highest for USS and BPS, and alfuzosin was second.

Conclusion: The alpha-blockers significantly decreased USS and BPS in comparison with placebo. Tamsulosin might be more effective than alfuzosin.

Keywords: Ureter, Stents, Adrenergic alpha-antagonists, Meta-analysis, Bayes theorem

Background

In 1978, the ureteral double-J stent was first described by Finney et al. [1, 2]. Ureteral double-J stent insertion has been one of the most common urologic procedures; however, indwelling stents are often accompanied by significant morbidity including voiding and storage symptoms, flank pain, hematuria, and infection [3]. Symptoms of stent discomfort, including bladder irritation symptoms and flank pain or discomfort, are generally treated with

oral analgesics, such as narcotics and antiinflammatory medications; however these medications are only moderately effective. Alpha-blockers alleviate bladder irritation due to stents, resulting in reduced incidence of dysuria, frequency, and pain compared to placebo [4]. Ureteral stent discomfort may be due to spasms of the ureteral smooth muscle that surrounds the indwelling foreign object and may run the length of the ureter. Further, irritation of the trigone, which also has alpha-1d receptors, may be caused by the intravesical lower coil of the stent. Alternatively, voiding may increase pressure on the renal pelvis and cause discomfort [5]. Several studies have investigated if alpha-blockers can alleviate symptoms related to stent placement [6]. In 2011, Lamb et al. reported a pair-

* Correspondence: joouro@yuhs.ac
[5]Department of Urology, Severance Hospital, Urological Science Institute, Yonsei University College of Medicine, 50-1 Yonsei-roSeodaemun-gu, Seoul 120-752, South Korea
Full list of author information is available at the end of the article

wise meta-analysis of randomized controlled trials (RCTs) indicating that orally administered alpha-blockers reduce stent-related discomfort and storage symptoms as evaluated by the Ureteric Stent Symptoms Questionnaire (USSQ) [7].

Newly introduced network meta-analysis is a meta-analysis in which multiple treatments are compared using direct comparisons of interventions within RCTs and indirect comparisons across trials based on a common comparator [8–10]. The present systematic review and network meta-analysis examined available RCTs to study the effects of alpha-blockers on stent-related symptoms.

Methods

Inclusion criteria

Published RCTs that accorded with the following criteria were included. (i) The design of study had an assessment for alpha-blockers to treat ureteral stent discomfort. (ii) A match was performed between the baseline characteristics of patients from two groups, including the total number of subjects and the values of each index. (iii) Alpha-blockers were analyzed with standard therapy or a placebo group. (iv) Standard indications for ureteral stenting, such as stone treatment, ureteroscopic procedures, and ureteral surgery including pyeloplasty, were accepted. (v) Endpoint outcome parameters were described using USSQ, including urinary symptom score (USS) and body pain score (BPS). (vi) The full text of the study was available in English. This report was prepared in compliance with the Preferred Reporting Items for Systematic Reviews and Meta-Analyses (PRISMA) statement (accessible at http://www.prisma-statement.org/).

Search strategy

A literature search of all publications before 31 January 2014 was performed in EMBASE and PubMed. Additionally, a cross-reference search of eligible articles was performed to check studies that were not found during the computerized search. Combinations of the following MeSH terms and keywords were used: tamsulosin, alfuzosin, doxazosin, terazosin, silodosin, prazosin, alpha, stent, discomfort, pain, complication, ureter, ureteral, ureteric, and randomized controlled trial.

Extraction of data

A researcher (JKK) screened all titles and abstracts identified by the search strategy. Other two researchers (JYL and DHK) independently evaluated the full text of each paper to determine whether a paper met the inclusion criteria. Disagreements were resolved by discussion until a consensus was reached or by arbitration mediated by another researcher (KSC).

Quality assessment for each study

After the final group of papers was agreed on, two researchers (JYL and JKK) independently evaluated the quality of each article. The Cochrane's risk of bias as a quality assessment tool for RCTs were used. The assessment included assigning a judgment of "yes," "no," or "unclear" for each domain to designate a low, high, or unclear risk of bias, respectively. If one or no domain was deemed "unclear" or "no," the study was classified as having a low risk of bias. If four or more domains were deemed "unclear" or "no," the study was classified as having a high risk of bias. If two or three domains were deemed "unclear" or "no," the study was classified as having a moderate risk of bias [11]. Quality assessment was performed with Review Manager 5 (RevMan 5.2.11, Cochrane Collaboration, Oxford, UK).

Heterogeneity tests

Heterogeneity on included studies was examined using the Q statistic and Higgins' I^2 statistic [12]. Higgins' I^2 measures the percentage of total variation due to heterogeneity rather than chance across studies. Higgins' I^2 was calculated as follows:

$$I^2 = \frac{Q\text{-df}}{Q} \times 100\%,$$

in which "Q" was Cochran's heterogeneity statistic, and "df" was the degrees of freedom.

An $I^2 \geq 50\%$ was considered to represent substantial heterogeneity. For the Q statistic, heterogeneity was deemed to be significant for p less than 0.10 [13]. If there was evidence of heterogeneity, the data were analyzed using a random-effects model. A summary estimate of the test sensitivity was obtained with 95 % confidence intervals (CIs) after secondary examination of heterogeneity in the random-effects model using radial plots [14]. Studies in which positive results were confirmed were assessed with a pooled specificity with 95 % CIs.

Statistical analysis

Outcome variables measured at specific time points were compared in terms of mean differences with 95 % CIs using a network meta-analysis. Analyses were based on non-informative priors for effect sizes and precision. Convergence and lack of auto-correlation were confirmed after four chains and a 50,000-simulation burn-in phase; finally, direct probability statements were derived from an additional 100,000-simulation phase. The probability that each group had the lowest rate of clinical events was assessed by Bayesian Markov Chain Monte Carlo modeling. Sensitivity analyses were performed by repeating the main computations with a fixed-effect method. Model fit was appraised by computing and comparing estimates for deviance and deviance information criterion. All statistical analyses were performed with Review Manager 5 and R (R version 3.0.3, R Foundation for Statistical Computing, Vienna, Austria; http://www.r-project.org) and the metafor and gemtc packages for pair-wise and network meta-analyses.

Results

Eligible studies

The database search retrieved 21 articles covering 88 studies for potential inclusion in the meta-analysis. Fourteen articles were excluded based on the inclusion/exclusion criteria; eight of the fourteen articles were retrospective models, and three articles were reported with different tools and variables. The other three articles were excluded, because they did not report final results. Using using pairwise and network meta-analyses, the remaining seven articles were included in the qualitative and quantitative syntheses (Fig. 1).

Data corresponding to confounding factors in each study are summarized in Table 1. Four studies included

outcome comparisons between alfuzosin versus placebo [15–18]. Two trials reported on therapeutic outcomes of tamsulosin versus placebo [19, 20], and a three-arm trial compared outcomes of alfuzosin, tamsulosin, and placebo [21].

Quality assessment

Figures 2 and 3 present the details of quality assessment, as measured by the Cochrane Collaboration risk-of-bias tool. Four trials exhibited a low risk of bias for all quality criteria, and two studies were classified as having a high risk of bias (Table 1). The most common risk factor for quality assessment was the risk of blinding of outcome assessment; the second most common concerns were allocation concealment and blinding participants and personnel.

Heterogeneity assessment

Forest plots of pairwise meta-analyses are demonstrated in Fig. 4. A heterogeneity test for USS showed the following: $\chi^2 = 96.43$ with 7 df ($P < 0.001$) and $I^2 = 93$ % in

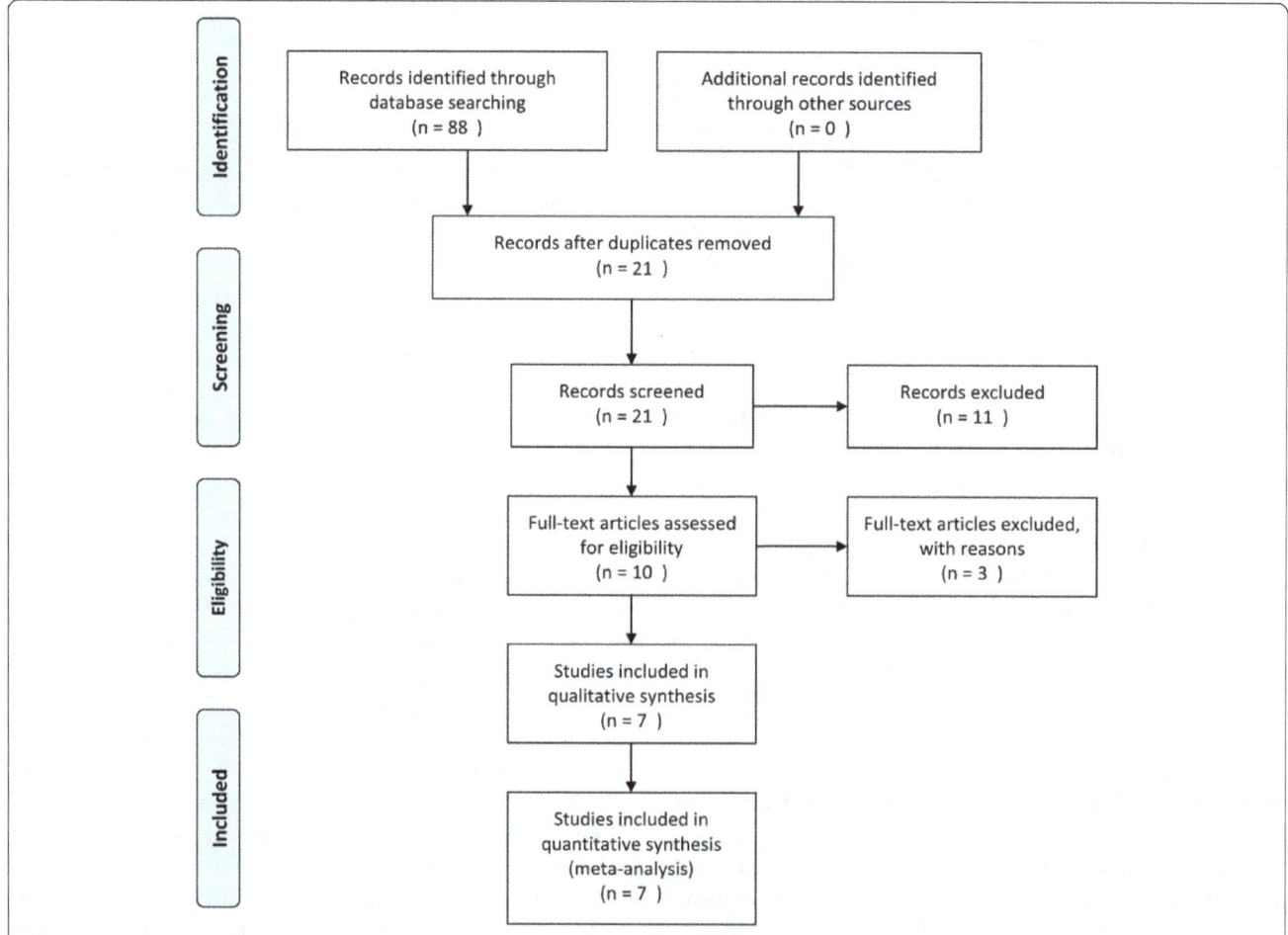

Fig. 1 Flow diagram of evidence acquisition. Seven studies were ultimately included in the qualitative and quantitative syntheses using pairwise and network meta-analyses

Table 1 Enrolled studies for this meta-analysis

Study	Study design	N	Tx	P	Alpha-blocker	Analgesic	Duration (day)	Stent Type	Stent Size	Length	Indication	Stone Size (mm) Tx	Stone Size (mm) P	Location	Measure	Quality assessment-risk bias
Beddingfield et al.[15]	RCT	55	26	29	Alfuzosin 10 mg	On demand	10	NA	NA	Adjusted	Post URS	6.35	7.2	55 % renal / 25 % renal/ureteric / 20 % ureteric	USSQ - urinary symptom score - body pain score - general health score - work performance score - sexual health score	Low
Damiano et al.[20]	RCT	75	38	37	Tamsulosin 0.4 mg	On demand	14	PU	7 Fr	Adjusted	Post URS	NA	NA	NA	USSQ - urinary symptom score - body pain score	Intermediate
Deliveliotis et al.[16]	RCT	100	50	50	Alfuzosin 10 mg	On demand	28	PU	5 Fr	Adjusted	Conservative treatment for stone, <10 mm, hydronephrosis	7.6	7.1	19 upper / 23 mid / 48 lower	USSQ - urinary symptom score - body pain score - general health score - sexual health score	Low
Dellis et al.[21]	RCT	150	100	50*	Alfuzosin 10 mg Tamsulosin 0.4 mg	On demand	28	NA	6 Fr	Adjusted	Post ESWL, URS	NA	NA	NA	USSQ - urinary symptom score - body pain score - general health score	Low

Table 1 Enrolled studies for this meta-analysis *(Continued)*

Study	Design	Total	Tx	P	Drug	Dosing		Material	Size		Procedure				Stone location	Outcome	Outcomes	Quality
Nazim et al.[17]	RCT	130	65	65	Alfuzosin 10 mg	On demand	7	PU	4.7 Fr / 6 Fr	NA	Post URS	NA	NA	NA	40 upper / 28 mid / 62 lower	VAS USSQ	- urinary symptom score - body pain score - work performance score - sexual health score	High
Park et al.[18]	RCT	32	20	12	Alfuzosin 10 mg	NA	42	PU	6 Fr	Adjusted	Post URS, PCNL, Lap Pyelo, endo-ureterotomy	NA	NA	NA		USSQ	- urinary symptom score - body pain score - general health score - work performance score - sexual health score	High
Wang et al.[19]	RCT	154	79	75	Tamsulosin 0.4 mg	On demand	7	Sil	7 Fr	Adjusted	Post URS	9	9.4		16 upper / 49 mid / 89 lower	USSQ	- urinary symptom score - body pain score - general health score - work performance score - sexual health score	Low

Adjusted, stent length is height adjusted; NA, not available; Tx, Treatment group, P, placebo; PU, Polyurethane; Sil, Silicone;USSQ, Ureteric Stent Symptom Questionnaire; VAS, visual analogue scale; URS, ureteroscopy; PCNL, percutaneous nephrolithotomy; Lap Pyelo, laparoscopic pyeloplasty

*50 patients received alfuzosin 10 mg, and another 50 patients received tamsulosin 0.4 mg

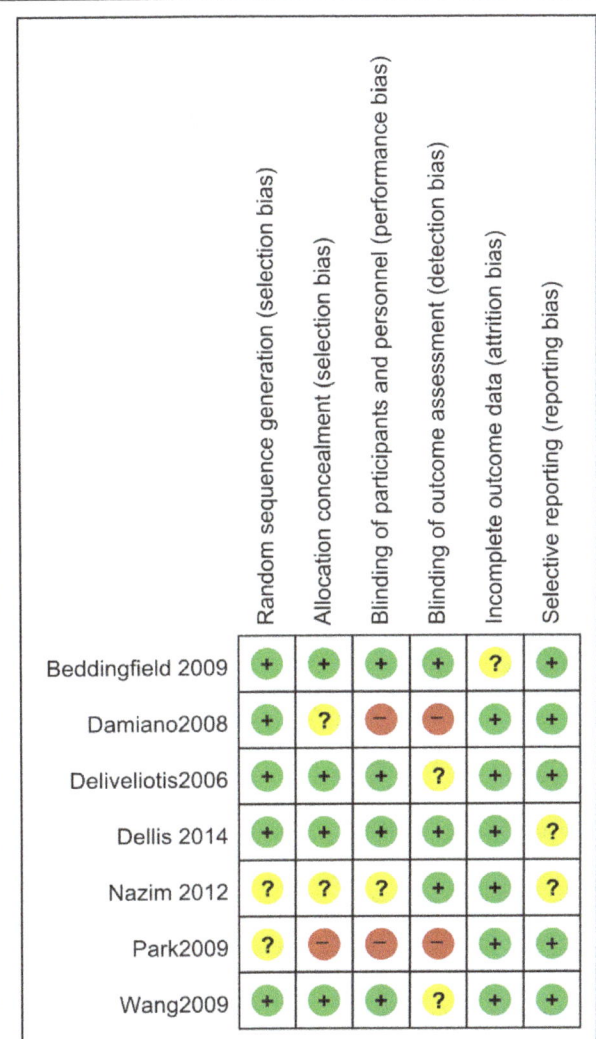

Fig. 2 Risk of bias graph. We reviewed the risk of bias in each study included in this meta-analysis and presented the results as percentages. Four trials exhibited a low risk of bias for all quality criteria, and two studies were classified as having a high risk of bias

the analysis of alpha-blockers, including alfuzosin and tamsulosin versus placebo. Notable heterogeneities were detected in the analyses of all studies; thus, random-effects models were used to further assess these variables. In the analysis of BPS, a heterogeneity test demonstrated homogeneity with $\chi^2 = 44.66$ with 8 df ($P < 0.001$) and $I^2 = 82$ %. Pairwise meta-analyses with random-effects models were also performed. None of the variables demonstrated heterogeneity in radial plots after selecting effect models for USS and BPS (Fig. 5).

Publication bias
Funnel plots from pairwise meta-analyses are demonstrated in Fig. 6; however, with few studies, it was difficult to assess publication bias, although some degree of bias is suspected.

Pairwise meta-analysis for urinary symptom and body pain scores
The forest plot using the random-effects model demomstrated an MD of −5.69 for USS (95 % CI [−8.84−−2.53], $P < 0.001$) between alpha-blockers and placebo (Fig. 4a). In subanalyses, both alfuzosin (MD; −4.12, 95 % CI [−5.51−−2.73], $P < 0.001$) and tamsulosin (MD; −7.83, 95 % CI [−14.35−−1.31], $P = 0.02$) had low MDs versus placebo. According to the forest plot for BPS, alpha-blockers were superior to placebo, with an MD of −6.20 (95 % CI [−8.74−−2.13], $P < 0.001$) (Fig. 4b). In the subanalysis of alfuzosin versus placebo, alfuzosin showed an MD of −4.21 (95 % CI [−5.56−−2.85], $P < 0.001$). Between tamsulosin and placebo, the random-effects model demonstrated an MD of −7.71 (95 % CI [−13.28−−2.13], $P = 0.007$) for BSP.

Network meta-analysis for urinary symptom and body pain scores
Alfuzosin had a lower In USS than that of placebo (MD; −4.85, 95 % CI [−8.53−−1.33]). Tamsulosin also had a lower score than that of placebo (MD; −8.84, 95 % CI [−13.08−−4.31]. However, there was not a significant difference in MD between alfuzosin and tamsulosin

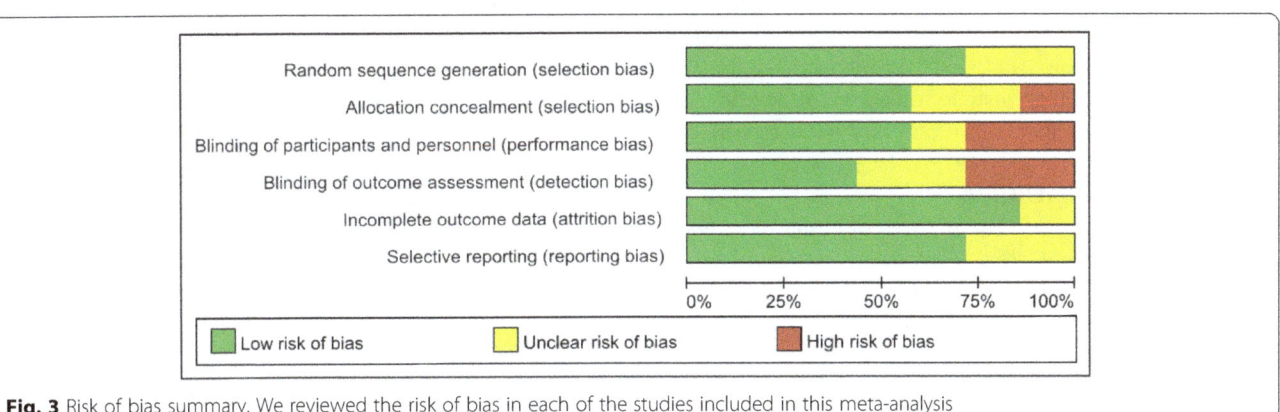

Fig. 3 Risk of bias summary. We reviewed the risk of bias in each of the studies included in this meta-analysis

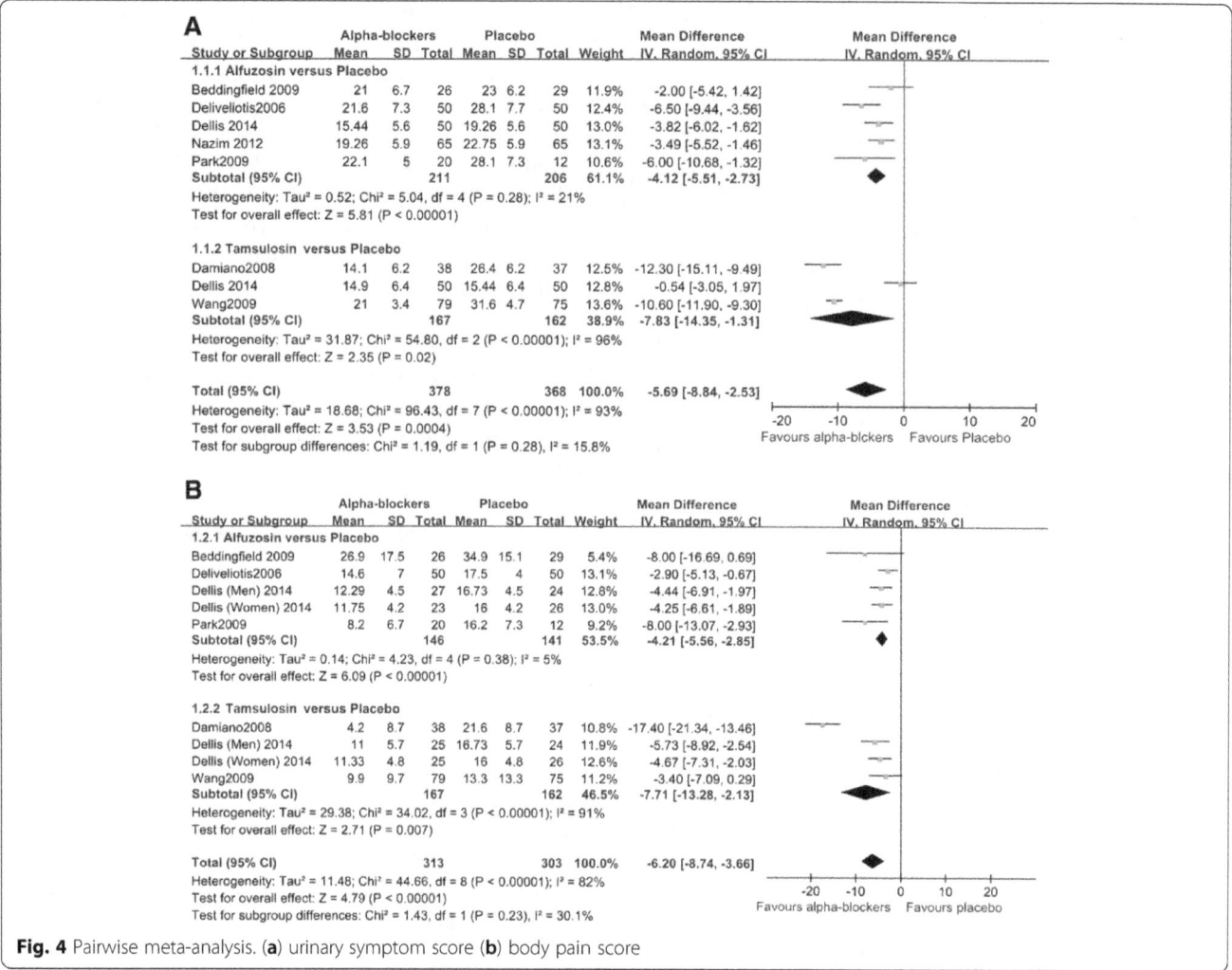

Fig. 4 Pairwise meta-analysis. (**a**) urinary symptom score (**b**) body pain score

according to network meta-analysis (MD; 3.99, 95 % CI [−1.23–9.04]). There were significant differences in the BPS achieved with alfuzosin versus placebo (MD; −5.71, 95 % CI [−11.32−−0.52]) and in tamsulosin versus placebo (MD; −7.77, 95 % CI [−13.68−−2.14]). Comparison of the BPS achieved with tamsulosin versus alfuzosin showed an MD of 2.12 (95 % CI [−4.62–8.72]), which was not significant (Fig. 7). In the rank-probability test, tamsulosin had the highest rank for USS, followed by alfuzosin. Tamsulosin was also ranked highest for BPS in the rank-probability test, followed by alfuzosin. The placebo was ranked lowest for USS and BPS (Fig. 8).

Discussion and conclusion

Recently, two pair-wise meta-analyses of alpha-blockers in patients with ureteral stent discomfort were published. Yakoubi et al. conducted a meta-analysis of four RCTs [22]. However, they did not distinguish the types of alpha-blockers analyzed by each domain. Alpha-blockers reduced the scores for urinary symptoms, body pain, and general health index score but did not achieve significant

changes in quality of work, sexual matters, or scores for additional problems. However, there were limits, as few studies were analyzed; in particular, only three studies were analyzed for quality of work and two for additional problems. Lamb et al. conducted a meta-analysis of five RCTs by distinguishing between alfuzosin and tamsulosin [7]; however, there was possible error in the effects-model with regards to heterogeneity. However, these meta-analyses showed decreased scores for both urinary symptoms and body pain after use of alpha-blockers.

More recently, Dellis et al. evaluated the effects of two different alpha-blockers for improving symptoms and quality of life in patients with indwelling ureteral stents in an RCT [21]. They prescribed alfuzosin, tamsulosin, or placebo to 50 patients and examined USSQ accordingly. Patients who received alpha-blockers had significantly decreased urinary symptoms, body pain, general health index, and sexual life scores compared to those of the control group. However, there was no difference in the quality of work score. Further, there was no difference between the alpha-blocker groups.

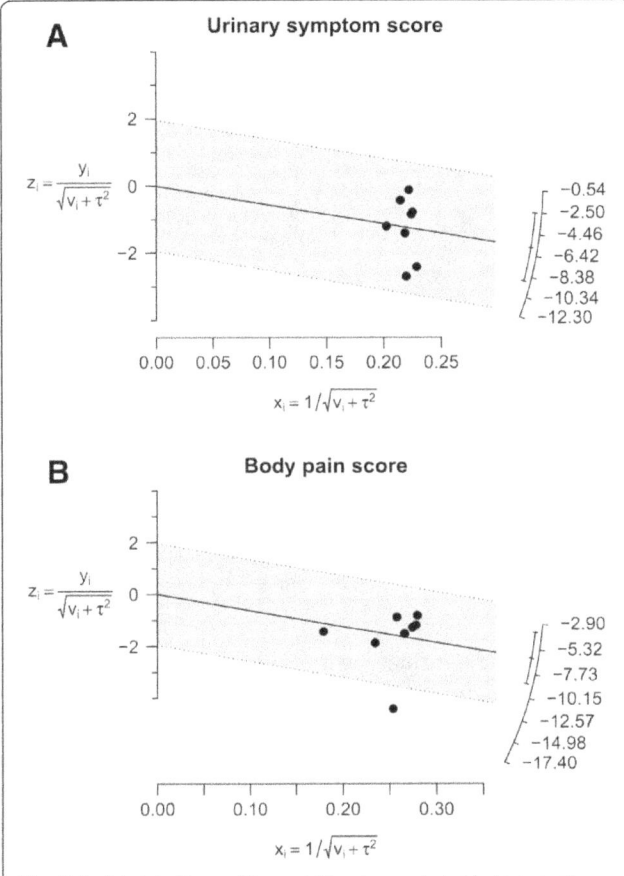

Fig. 5 Radial plots. None of the variables demonstrated heterogeneity after selecting effect models for each variable in the radial plots. (**a**) urinary symptom score (**b**) body pain score

The goal of this study was to ascertain the difference between tamsulosin and alfuzosin in alleviating stent discomfort by comparing the effectiveness of alpha-blockers to placebo in seven RCTs based on urinary symptoms and body pain scores. In most studies, continuous treatment had been carried out before the removal of ureter stents. We divided alpha-blockers into alfuzosin and tamsulosin to conduct subgroup and network meta-analyses. In the subgroup analysis, two alpha-blockers appeared to significantly decrease urinary symptoms and body pain scores compared to those of the placebo. There was no statistical significance between alfuzosin and tamsulosin in network meta-analysis both in urinary symptoms and body pain scores, which was consistent with the results of previous studies. However, after conducting network meta-analysis using a rank-probability test, the effectiveness of tamsulosin appeared to be better than that of alfuzosin in both urinary symptoms and body pain scores (Fig. 8).

We suggested that the difference in efficacy between the two alpha-blockers arises from the physiologic characteristics of ureteral receptor distribution. The ureter contains two continuous thin muscle layers with a loosely spiraled internal layer and a more tightly spiraled external layer. A third outer longitudinal layer is located in the lower third of the ureter. The lower ureter is consisted of transitional epithelium, a connective tissue layer, and three layers of smooth muscle [23]. Peristalsis of ureter is initiated by spontaneous activity of the renal pelvis pacemaker cell and is essentially regulated by the myogenic mechanism and neurogenic factors; electrical and mechanical activities are conducted to inactive distal regions [24]. The histologic characteristics of the three smooth muscle layers in the lower portion of ureter and the denser innervation of the lower portion of ureter have become subjects of research interest. The alpha-1d receptor has the highest

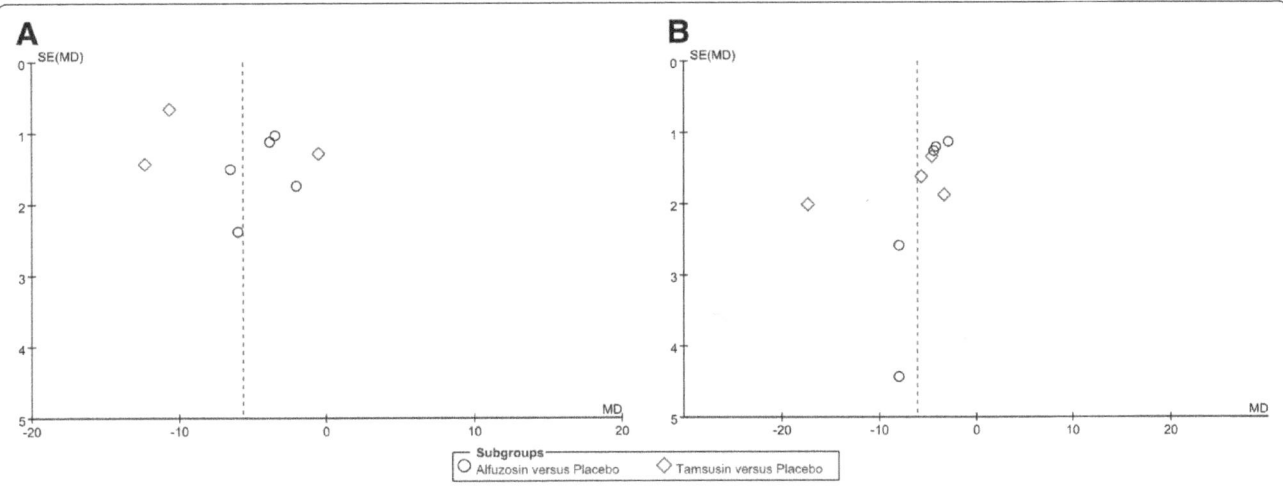

Fig. 6 Funnel plots. (**a**) urinary symptom score (**b**) body pain score. It was difficult to assess publication bias with few studies, although some degree of bias is suspected

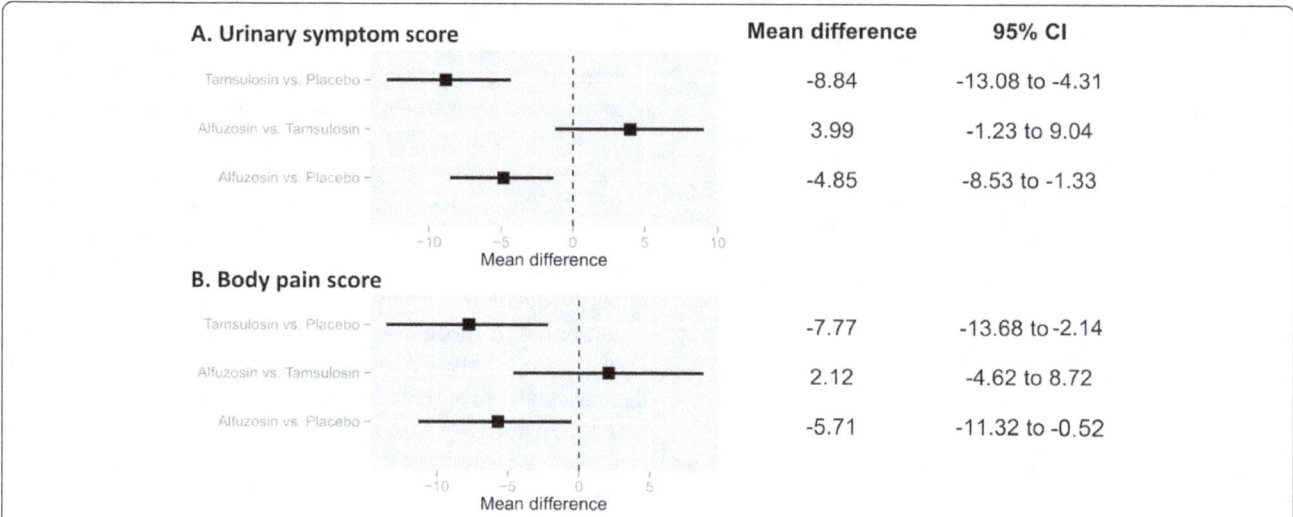

Fig. 7 Network meta-analysis. (**a**) urinary symptom score (**b**) body pain score. Alfuzosin and tamsulosin had a lower score both in USS and BPS than in the placebo. However, there was not a significant difference in MD between alfuzosin and tamsulosin according to network meta-analysis

density in the lower portion of ureter. Tamsulosin is a subtype selective alpha-1a and alpha-1d blocker, whereas alfuzosin is a subtype non-selective alpha-1 blocker [25]. The two alpha-blockers may elicit different levels of efficacy due to differences in selectivity and the distribution of the alpha-1d receptor in the lower ureter. However, it remains unclear if subtype selectivity makes a significant contribution to the differences in efficacy of alpha-blockers. In the near future, prospective trials should compare several alpha-blockers, including silodosin and naftopidil, to confirm our results.

A limitation of our study was that only two subdomains were included, urinary symptoms and body pain scores, as not all the RCTs involved in this study had available USSQ domains besides urinary symptoms and body pain scores (Table 1). These may cause a bias in the efficacy of the two alpha-blockers, which can be influenced by other symptoms and quality of life. All RCTs included in the present study used USSQ, which comprehensively assesses not only urinary symptoms and pain, but also sexual symptoms and quality of life. Although urinary symptoms and pain are the most problematic among stent-related symptoms of discomfort, low abdominal pain or discomfort, infection, and hematuria are also bothersome to patients. Furthermore, alpha-blockers can cause side effects on the central nervous system, sexual function, ejaculatory function, and cardiovascular system [26]. Therefore, it is important to compare not only the efficacy between the

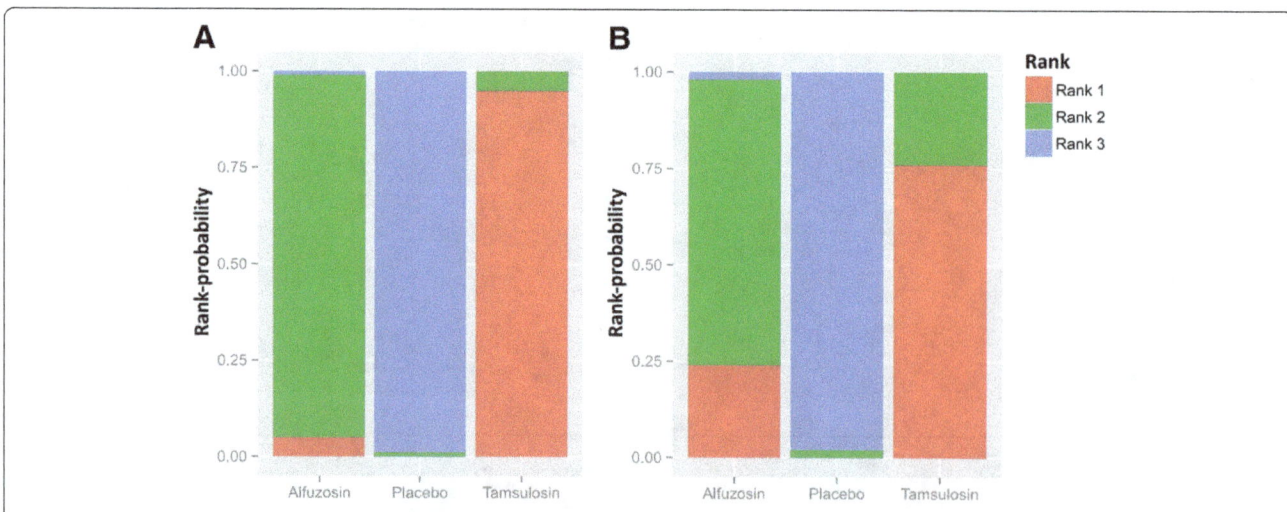

Fig. 8 Rank-probability test of network meta-analyses. (**a**) urinary symptom score (**b**) body pain score. Tamsulosin had the highest rank for USS, followed by alfuzosin. Tamsulosin was also ranked highest for BPS in the rank-probability test, followed by alfuzosin. The placebo was ranked lowest for USS and BPS

two medications but also the side effects. In addition, comparison of USSQ domains may also need to be considered. Some degree of publication bias was also a limitation of this study. However, Sutton et al. reviewed 48 articles from the Cochrane Database of Systematic Reviews and showed publication or related biases were common within the sample of meta-analyses assessed [27]. Moreover, they found that these biases did not affect the conclusions in most cases. Another limitation was that we did not take into consideration the possible effects of stent factors on stent discomfort. Although six out of seven RCTs reported that stent insertion was performed with height adjustment and the differences of stent materials were also considered, there was no consideration as to whether the stent was placed correctly or not. Lee et al. [28]. reported that only storage symptoms of the tamsulosin group were significantly lower than those of the analgesic group in the appropriate stent position. However, this medication effect was not observed in the inappropriate stent position group, and total IPSS and storage symptom scores were significantly higher than in the appropriate stent position group. The appropriate stent position might be one of the points to be considered when conducting the research on stent discomfort.

Conclusions

Ureteral stent-related symptoms are effectively alleviated with alpha-blockers. Tamsulosin might be more effective than alfuzosin. However, additional randomized controlled trials with alfuzosin and tamsulosin need to be performed for patients with ureteral stents.

Abbreviations
RCTs: Randomized controlled trials; USSQ: Ureteric Stent Symptoms Questionnaire; USS: Urinary symptom score; BPS: Body pain score.

Competing interests
All the authors declare that they have no competing interests.

Authors' contributions
Systematic review and meta-analysis JYL, KJK, KSC, DHK, HL, WSH, YDC. Identification of studies, critical evaluation and discussion. JYL, KJK, KSC, CKO, DHK, HL. All authors read and approved the final manuscript.

Acknowledgements
None

Author details
[1]Department of Urology, Haeundae Paik Hospital, Inje University College of Medicine, Busan, South Korea. [2]Department of Urology, Gangnam Severance Hospital, Urological Science Institute, Yonsei University College of Medicine, Seoul, South Korea. [3]Department of Urology, Yangpyeong Health Center, Yangpyeong, South Korea. [4]Division of Epidemic Intelligence Service, Korea Centers for Disease Control and Prevention, Osong, South Korea. [5]Department of Urology, Severance Hospital, Urological Science Institute, Yonsei University College of Medicine, 50-1 Yonsei-roSeodaemun-gu, Seoul 120-752, South Korea.

References
1. Finney RP. Experience with new double J ureteral catheter stent. J Urol. 1978;120(6):678–81.
2. Hepperlen TW, Mardis HK, Kammandel H. Self-retained internal ureteral stents: a new approach. J Urol. 1978;119(6):731–4.
3. Mendez-Probst CE, Fernandez A, Denstedt JD. Current status of ureteral stent technologies: comfort and antimicrobial resistance. Curr Urol Rep. 2010;11(2):67–73.
4. Chew BH, Lange D. Ureteral stent symptoms and associated infections: a biomaterials perspective. Nat Rev Urol. 2009;6(8):440–8.
5. Thomas R. Indwelling ureteral stents: impact of material and shape on patient comfort. J Endourol. 1993;7(2):137–40.
6. Lim KT, Kim YT, Lee TY, Park SY. Effects of tamsulosin, solifenacin, and combination therapy for the treatment of ureteral stent related discomforts. Korean J Urol. 2011;52(7):485–8.
7. Lamb AD, Vowler SL, Johnston R, Dunn N, Wiseman OJ. Meta-analysis showing the beneficial effect of alpha-blockers on ureteric stent discomfort. BJU Int. 2011;108(11):1894–902.
8. Caldwell DM, Ades AE, Higgins JP. Simultaneous comparison of multiple treatments: combining direct and indirect evidence. BMJ. 2005;331(7521):897–900.
9. Mills EJ, Thorlund K, Ioannidis JP. Demystifying trial networks and network meta-analysis. BMJ. 2013;346:f2914.
10. Yuan J, Zhang R, Yang Z, Lee J, Liu Y, Tian J, et al. Comparative effectiveness and safety of oral phosphodiesterase type 5 inhibitors for erectile dysfunction: a systematic review and network meta-analysis. Eur Urol. 2013;63(5):902–12.
11. Chung JH, Lee SW. Assessing the quality of randomized controlled urological trials conducted by korean medical institutions. Korean J Urol. 2013;54(5):289–96.
12. Higgins JP, Thompson SG, Deeks JJ, Altman DG. Measuring inconsistency in meta-analyses. BMJ. 2003;327(7414):557–60.
13. Fleiss JL. Analysis of data from multiclinic trials. Control Clin Trials. 1986;7(4):267–75.
14. Galbraith RF. A note on graphical presentation of estimated odds ratios from several clinical trials. Stat Med. 1988;7(8):889–94.
15. Beddingfield R, Pedro RN, Hinck B, Kreidberg C, Feia K, Monga M. Alfuzosin to relieve ureteral stent discomfort: a prospective, randomized, placebo controlled study. J Urol. 2009;181(1):170–6.
16. Deliveliotis C, Chrisofos M, Gougousis E, Papatsoris A, Dellis A, Varkarakis IM. Is there a role for alpha1-blockers in treating double-J stent-related symptoms? Urology. 2006;67(1):35–9.
17. Nazim SM, Ather MH. Alpha-blockers impact stent-related symptoms: a randomized, double-blind, placebo-controlled trial. J Endourol Endourol So. 2012;26(9):1237–41.
18. Park SC, Jung SW, Lee JW, Rim JS. The effects of tolterodine extended release and alfuzosin for the treatment of double-j stent-related symptoms. J Endourol. 2009;23(11):1913–7.
19. Wang CJ, Huang SW, Chang CH. Effects of specific alpha-1A/1D blocker on lower urinary tract symptoms due to double-J stent: a prospectively randomized study. Urol Res. 2009;37(3):147–52.
20. Damiano R, Autorino R, De Sio M, Giacobbe A, Palumbo IM, D'Armiento M. Effect of tamsulosin in preventing ureteral stent-related morbidity: a prospective study. J Endourol. 2008;22(4):651–6.
21. Dellis AE, Keeley Jr FX, Manolas V, Skolarikos AA. Role of alpha-blockers in the treatment of stent-related symptoms: a prospective randomized control study. Urology. 2014;83(1):56–61.
22. Yakoubi R, Lemdani M, Monga M, Villers A, Koenig P. Is there a role for alpha-blockers in ureteral stent related symptoms? A systematic review and meta-analysis. J Urol. 2011;186(3):928–34.
23. Cha WH, Choi JD, Kim KH, Seo YJ, Lee K. Comparison and efficacy of low-dose and standard-dose tamsulosin and alfuzosin in medical expulsive therapy for lower ureteral calculi: prospective, randomized, comparative study. Korean J Urol. 2012;53(5):349–54.
24. Lang RJ, Exintaris B, Teele ME, Harvey J, Klemm MF. Electrical basis of peristalsis in the mammalian upper urinary tract. Clin Experimental Pharmacol Physiol. 1998;25(5):310–21.
25. Yoo TK, Cho HJ. Benign prostatic hyperplasia: from bench to clinic. Korean J Urol. 2012;53(3):139–48.
26. Andersson KE, Gratzke C. Pharmacology of alpha1-adrenoceptor antagonists in the lower urinary tract and central nervous system. Nat Clin Pract Urol. 2007;4(7):368–78.
27. Sutton AJ, Duval SJ, Tweedie RL, Abrams KR, Jones DR. Empirical assessment of effect of publication bias on meta-analyses. BMJ. 2000;320(7249):1574–7.
28. Lee SJ, Yoo C, Oh CY, Lee YS, Cho ST, Lee SH, et al. Stent position is more important than alpha-blockers or Anticholinergics for stent-related lower urinary tract symptoms after ureteroscopic Ureterolithotomy: a prospective randomized study. Korean J Urol. 2010;51(9):636–41.

28

The susceptibility to fosfomycin of Gram-negative bacteria isolates from urinary tract infection in the Czech Republic: data from a unicentric study

Miroslav Fajfr[1,2*], Miroslav Louda[2,3], Pavla Paterová[1,2], Lenka Ryšková[1,2], Jaroslav Pacovský[2,3], Josef Košina[2,3], Helena Žemličková[1,2] and Miloš Broďák[2,3]

Abstract

Background: Against a background of rapid increase of β-lactamase-producing or multi-resistant pathogenic bacteria and the resulting lack of effective antibiotic treatment, some older antibiotics have been tested for new therapeutic uses. One of these is fosfomycin, to which according to studies these resistant bacteria are very sensitive. Our study was designed because there is no data on the fosfomycin susceptibility rate in the Czech Republic.

Method: In this study from January 2013 to June 2014 3295 unique isolates of Gram-negative bacteria which had caused urinary tract infections were examined. The antibiotic susceptibility was measured by disk diffusion test. Both EUCAST and CLSI guidelines criteria (for fosfomycin only) were used for the antibiotic susceptibility evaluation.

Results: The most frequently tested bacterial isolates were *Escherichia coli* (51.3%, $n = 1703$), *Klebsiella pneumoniae* (19.4%, $n = 643$) and *Proteus* spp. (11.8%, $n = 392$). Among all isolates 29.0% ($n = 963$) were resistant to fluoroquinolones, 11.3% ($n = 374$) produced extended spectrum β-lactamase and 4.2% ($n = 141$) produced AmpC β-lactamase. The overall in vitro susceptibility was significantly higher for fosfomycin compared to the other tested per-oral antibiotics (nitrofurantoin, ampicillin, co-trimoxazole, ciprofloxacin and cefuroxime) against all tested Gram-negative rod isolates (excluding *Morganella morgani* and *Acinetobacter* spp. isolates). Fosfomycin also remained highly active against those isolates with extended spectrum β-lactamase (ESBL) production (95.8% in *Escherichia coli* isolates and 85.3% in *Klebsiella pneumoniae* isolates), unlike other tested per-oral antibiotics, which showed significant ($p < 0.0001$) susceptibility decrease.

Conclusion: We have confirmed in the Czech Republic the very high susceptibility to fosfomycin trometamol of urinary tract infection pathogens, particularly Gram-negative rods including those producing β-lactamase.

Keywords: Fosfomycin, Urinary tract infection, Susceptibility

* Correspondence: miroslav.fajfr@fnhk.cz
[1]Institute of Clinical Microbiology, University Hospital Hradec Kralové,
Sokolska 581, Hradec Králové 50005, Czech Republic
[2]Charles University in Prague, Faculty of Medicine in Hradec Kralové, Simkova
870, Hradec Kralove 500 38, Czech Republic
Full list of author information is available at the end of the article

Background

Fosfomycin (Phosphomycin) as a new antimicrobial substance was first introduced in 1969. It is characterized as an anti-cell wall bactericidal antibiotic with a wide spectrum of antimicrobial activity, both to Gram-negative and Gram-positive bacteria [1]. It was used for many years as a highly effective antimicrobial drug especially for the treatment of urinary tract infections (UTIs), but with the advent of new antibiotics such as β-lactams or fluoroquinolones, it became somewhat obsolete. In the past decade there have been reports of a rapid increase in resistant pathogens, including extended spectrum β-lactamase (ESBL) producers or multi-drug resistant (MDR) pathogens (defined as non-susceptible to at least one agent in three or more antimicrobial categories) [2, 3]. Due to the lack of an effective antimicrobial drug for these cases, some older antibiotics were tested to evaluate their effectivity against multi-resistant bacteria. One such was fosfomycin, which according to the results of previously published studies had shown very good in vitro activity against resistant bacteria such as ESBL-producers, carbapenem-resistant *Klebsiella pneumoniae*, multi-resistant *Pseudomonas aeruginosa*, vancomycin-resistant enterococci (VRE) and methicillin-resistant *Staphylococcus aureus* (MRSA) [4–6]. All this evidence has generated higher interest in the use of fosfomycin in the last 5 years.

Fosfomycin for a long time has not been available in the Czech Republic, but since October 2014 has been available as the per-oral formulation, fosfomycin trometamol. Since there was no data on the susceptibility to fosfomycin of Czech bacterial isolates, we carried out this one-and-half year study with the aim of determining the fosfomycin susceptibility of isolates collected from UTIs among hospitalised and ambulatory patients in the University Hospital, Hradec Kralove.

Methods

The sampling selection criteria for inclusion in the study allowed only samples from the urinary tract (urine, urethral swabs and samples from nephrostomies) examined in the Department of Clinical Microbiology, University Hospital Hradec Kralove. All Gram-negative bacterial isolates of significant quantity according to the European Association of Urology Guidelines 2015 [7] were collected throughout the whole study period (from January 2013 to June 2014). All duplicate isolates (the same bacterial isolates in significant quantity with the same antibiotic susceptibility in the same patient) were excluded. In total 3295 unique bacterial isolates were included. The isolates were from both hospitalised patients (55.1%, $n = 1814$) and hospital ambulant patients with a previous history of hospitalization (especially patients with chronic renal failure and patients after kidney transplantation) (44.9%, $n = 1481$). Our patients group did not include patients from the community. All study participants provided informed consent. The samples included in our research were processed strictly anonymously and therefore the approval of our ethical committee was not required. Nevertheless all sample processing and data evaluation were in compliance with the Helsinki Declaration.

Bacterial culture and identification

Bacteria were cultured in 5% sheep blood agar and MacConkey agar and then tested for antibiotic susceptibility. Bacterial identifications were made by short biochemical line test (TRIOS®) or by a Biotyper Brucker® Matrix-Assisted Laser Desorption Ionization Time-of-Flight Mass Spectrometry (MALDI-TOF-MS) device according to standard operational procedures.

Susceptibility testing

The susceptibility to fosfomycin, nitrofurantoin (in *E. coli* and *K. pneumoniae* isolates only), ampicillin, ampicillin/sulbactam (as a representative of aminopenicillins with β-lactamase inhibitors), trimethoprim-sulfamethoxazole (co-trimoxazole), ciprofloxacin and cefuroxime was determined by the disk diffusion method according to EUCAST guidelines. With the exception of fosfomycin, the EUCAST clinical breakpoints were used for interpretation of results [8]. For *K. pneumoniae* and nitrofurantoin susceptibility, the epidemiological cut-off value (ECOFF) 8 mm was used to distinguish susceptible and resistant isolates. All pathogens naturally resistant to tested antimicrobial substances were classified as resistant. As the current EUCAST version (2016) has no breakpoint available for the disk diffusion method for fosfomycin, the CLSI guidelines were used for interpretation of fosfomycin results [9]. The ESBL, AmpC or K1 β-lactamase producers were identified using the modified double disk synergy method according to the national recommendation [10]. For the ESBL quality control testing the *Klebsiella pneumoniae* strain ATCC700603 was used according to EUCAST guidelines. For AmpC quality control testing no testing strain is recommended in the EUCAST guidelines.

Statistical methods

Chi-square (χ^2) test in software STATISTICA CZ 12 (StatSoft®, USA) was used for statistical analysis. *P*-value was used for comparison of antibiotic susceptibility and significance levels in all analyses were taken to be $p \leq 0.05$. For the determination of the probability of inadequate antimicrobial coverage a weighted average was calculated of non-susceptibility for all uropathogens combined together in each of the patient groups [11].

Results

The bacterial isolates distribution

The most frequently found bacteria were *E. coli* (n = 1703, 51.3%), followed by *K. pneumoniae* (n = 643, 19.4%), *Proteus* species (*P. mirabilis* and *P. vulgaris*) (n = 392, 11.8%), and *Enterobacter* species (*E. cloacae, kobei, asburiae* and *aerogenes*) (n = 261, 7.9%). The other isolated Gram-negative bacteria were *Citrobacter* species (n = 97), *Morganella morganii* (n = 68), *P. aeruginosa* (n = 22) and *Providencia* species (n = 34). Of all the examined isolates 29.0% (n = 963) were resistant to ciprofloxacin. Overall 11.4% (n = 374) of isolates produced ESBL (mostly *K. pneumoniae*, n = 216), and 4.3% (n = 141) of isolates produced AmpC β-lactamase. In 414 cases (12.5% of all isolates) coproduction of AmpC or ESBL with resistance to ciprofloxacin was detected.

Susceptibility testing results

Escherichia isolates showed very good susceptibility against fosfomycin (97.0%), nitrofurantoin (96.6%) and cefuroxime (90.5%), but poorer susceptibility against other common first line antibiotics – co-trimoxazole (67.8%) and ciprofloxacin (75.8%). *Klebsiella* strains showed good susceptibility only against fosfomycin (80.4%), and other tested first line antibiotics were poorly active (from 52.4% to 43.5%). Fosfomycin was also the most active antibiotic for *Enterobacter* isolates (82.8% against 77.2% - 0.0% susceptibility for the other tested first line antibiotics). Other Gram-negative bacterial isolates were also highly susceptible to fosfomycin with the exception of *Providencia* (susceptible 44.1%) and *Morganella* (susceptible only 16.2%). Other susceptibility results for the main groups of Gram-negative bacteria are presented in Table 1.

Antibiotic susceptibility in common susceptible isolates and isolates producing β-lactamase (ESBL or AmpC)

For *E. coli* isolates only two antibiotics remained highly active against both common susceptible and β-lactamase producing isolates (ESBL or AmpC) – fosfomycin (respectively 97.4% and 92.0%) and nitrofurantoin (respectively 97.1% and 89.6%). The susceptibility of β-lactamase producing isolates was significantly lower ($p < 0.0001$) for all other tested first line antibiotics. A very similar situation was found also for *Enterobacter* isolates, for which there is susceptibility of both groups only for fosfomycin (no statistically significant decrease in β-lactamase producing isolates, $p = 0.1081$). Fosfomycin remained the only highly effective antibiotic against β-lactamase producing *K. pneumoniae* isolates; for all other tested antibiotics, β-lactamase producing isolates showed statistically significantly lower susceptibility ($p < 0.0001$). Further comparisons of the commonly susceptible and β-lactamase producing isolates are presented in Table 2.

Comparison of the susceptibility of the four most frequent Gram-negative bacterial isolates to fosfomycin with that of the other first line antibiotics

Fosfomycin showed relatively good activity against *Proteus* isolates which are primarily resistant to nitrofurantoin (82.5% of isolates were susceptible to fosfomycin). Additionally, *E. coli, K. pneumoniae* and *Enterobacter* species isolates resistant to nitrofurantoin remained susceptible to fosfomycin, between 78.6% and 88.1%. There was high resistance in all tested strains against ampicillin and ciprofloxacin; however, between 77.9% and 97.5% of ampicillin- or ciprofloxacin-resistant bacterial isolates were susceptible to fosfomycin.

Comparison of overall susceptibility to first line antibiotics according to patient status

All samples were allocated to one of three groups – patients from intensive care units (ICUs), from standard

Table 1 Overall in-vitro susceptibility of the main Gram-negative rods to commonly used per-oral antibiotics (N/D - not defined susceptibility according to used EUCAST guidelines)

	Fosfomycin		Nitrofurantoin		Ampicillin		Ampicillin-sulbactam		Cefuroxime		Ciprofloxacin		Co-trimoxazole	
	S%	R%	S%	R%	S%	R%	S%	R%	S%	R%	S%	R%	S%	R%
E. coli (n = 1703)	97.0	2.2	96.6	3.4	46.3	53.7	76.3	23.7	90.5	9.5	75.8	24.0	67.8	31.8
K. pneumoniae (n = 643)	80.4	10.0	64.9	35.1	0.0	100.0	43.5	56.5	51.9	48.1	52.4	47.0	49.4	50.3
Proteus sp.(n = 392)	78.3	16.6	N/D	N/D	38.8	61.2	84.5	15.5	81.6	18.4	68.9	28.8	51.3	47.7
Enterobacter sp.(n = 261)	82.8	11.1	N/D	N/D	0.0	100.0	0.0	100.0	N/D	N/D	77.2	19.7	71.4	27.8
Citrobacter sp. (n = 97)	100.0	0.0	N/D	N/D	0.0	100.0	40.2	59.8	N/D	N/D	90.7	9.3	76.3	23.7
M. morganii (n = 68)	16.2	75.0	N/D	N/D	0.0	100.0	0.0	100.0	N/D	N/D	72.1	22.0	61.8	33.8
Providencia sp. (n = 34)	44.1	50.0	N/D	N/D	0.0	100.0	0.0	100.0	N/D	N/D	61.8	38.2	73.5	26.5

E. coli Escherichia coli, K. pneumoniae Klebsiella pneumoniae, Proteus sp. Proteus species, Enterobacter sp. Enterobacter species, Citrobacter sp. Citrobacter species, M. morganii Morganella morganii, Providencia sp. Providencia species

Table 2 - Comparison of the susceptibility to commonly used first-line antibiotics and chemotherapeutics of the common susceptible isolates with that of isolates producing β-lactamase (ESBL or AmpC)

Antibiotic	Escherichia coli (n = 1578)			Escherichia coli beta lactamase positive[a] (n = 125)			Klebsiella pneumoniae (n = 359)			Klebsiella pneumoniae beta lactamase positive[a] (n = 284)			Enterobacter species (n = 186)			Enterobacter species beta lactamase positive[a] (n = 75)		
	S%	I%	R%	S%	I%	R%	S%	I%	R%	S%	I%	R%	S%	I%	R%	S%	I%	R%
Fosfomycin	97.4	0.8	1.8	92.0	1.6	6.4	85.8	5.6	8.6	73.6	14.8	11.6	86.1	4.8	9.1	74.7	9.3	16.0
Ampicilin	50.0	0.0	50.0	0.0	0.0	100.0	0.0	0.0	100.0	0.0	0.0	100.0	0.0	0.0	100.0	0.0	0.0	100.0
Ampicilin-sulbactam	82.4	0.0	17.6	0.0	0.0	100.0	78.3	0.0	21.7	0.0	0.0	100.0	0.0	0.0	100.0	0.0	0.0	100.0
Cefuroxime	97.7	0.0	2.3	0.0	0.0	100.0	92.8	0.0	7.2	0.0	0.0	100.0	0.0	0.0	100.0	0.0	0.0	100.0
Ciprofloxacin	80.6	0.3	19.1	16.0	0.0	84.0	84.5	1.2	14.3	12.0	0.0	88.0	88.7	1.1	10.2	49.3	8.0	42.7
Co-trimoxazole	71.0	0.4	28.6	28.0	0.0	72.0	80.5	0.3	19.2	10.2	0.4	89.4	84.9	0.0	15.1	38.6	2.7	58.7
Nitrofurantoin	97.1	0.0	2.9	89.6	0.0	10.4	76.6	0.0	23.4	50.0	0.0	50.0	65.1	0.0	34.9	65.3	0.0	34.7

[a]beta lactamase positive means bacterial isolates producing ESBL or AmpC beta lactamase

hospital wards, and ambulatory. Resistance to all tested antibiotics was lowest in hospital ambulatory patients and highest in patients from ICUs. There was significantly higher resistance to all evaluated antibiotics in standard wards and ICUs compared with hospital out-patients ($p = 0.006$ to $p < 0.0001$), with one exception: there was lower resistance to fosfomycin in all groups ($p = 0.1173$ and $p = 0.2334$). Full data are presented in Table 3.

Discussion

The increasing incidence of urinary tract infection caused by Gram-negative bacteria with multiple drug resistance is well described worldwide and also by the European Antimicrobial Resistance Surveillance Network (EARS-Net), where this phenomenon has been reported in E. coli and K. pneumoniae isolates [12, 13]. The same data were obtained in our study: for example, more than 47% of K. pneumoniae isolates were resistant to fluoroquinolones, and 44% produce β-lactamase (ESBL or AmpC). These findings underlie the necessity for the increasing use of highly effective parenteral antibiotics such as aminoglycosides, 3rd generation cephalosporins or carbapenems in urinary tract infection treatment, and which also often requires hospitalisation. Per-oral treatment is mainly confined to mild infections such as uncomplicated cystitis.

Our study compared the susceptibility to commonly-used first line antibiotics (fosfomycin, nitrofurantoin, ampicillin, ampicillin-sulbactam, co-trimoxazole, ciprofloxacin, cefuroxime) of susceptible bacterial isolates and bacterial isolates evincing multiple resistance (ESBL or AmpC), with the aim of determining the feasibility of using per-oral antibiotics (especially fosfomycin trometamol) in the therapy of urinary tract infection caused by multiply-resistant pathogens.

Our study confirmed the leading role of E. coli in urinary tract infection, as nearly 51.0% of urinary samples contained this pathogen. The other most frequent isolates are also of Gram-negative rods, especially Klebsiella, Proteus or Enterobacter, which together comprised 40.0% of all tested isolates. The results were in congruence with studies from other countries [14, 15]. E. coli isolates were highly susceptible to fosfomycin and nitrofurantoin (97.0% and 96.6% respectively) and less susceptible to ciprofloxacin and trimethoprim-sulfamethoxazole (75.8% and 67.8%), which is in line with other studies from Europe and Asia [13, 15, 16]. A similar pattern was found in K. pneumoniae, where 80.4% of isolates were susceptible to fosfomycin, although other tested antibiotics showed susceptibility in the range 43.5% to 64.4%. In β-lactamase producing bacterial isolates (ESBL or AmpC), fosfomycin

Table 3 The comparison of overall antibiotic resistance according to patient status - patients from intensive care units (ICU), standard hospital wards (SHW) or from hospital ambulance (AMB)

		AMP-R (%)	AMS-R (%)	CRX-R (%)	CIP-R (%)	COT-R (%)	FUR-R (%)	FOS-R (%)
ICU	n = 639	79.3	47.7	40.1	35.4	45.4	33.0	11.3
SHW	n = 1175	75.6	44.0	33.2	37.9	44.1	30.6	7.8
AMB	n = 1481	63.8	32.3	25.7	17.7	26.8	25.7	9.1
Statistical evaluation (p-value)								
Ambulance versus intensive care units		<0.0001	< 0.0001	< 0.0001	< 0.0001	< 0.0001	0.0060	0.1173
Ambulance versus standard hospital wards		< 0.0001	< 0.0001	< 0.0001	< 0.0001	< 0.0001	0.,0052	0.2334

AMP-R ampicillin resistance, AMS-R ampicillin-sulbactam resistance, CRX-R cefuroxime resistance, CIP-R ciprofloxacin resistance, COT-R co-trimoxazole resistance, FUR-R nitrofurantoin resistance, FOS-R fosfomycin resistance showed the lowest proportion of resistant isolates. However, it is necessary to comment that comparison of antibiotics and chemotherapeutics is sometimes difficult due to the absence of EUCAST break points for many of them. A good example is nitrofurantoin, which according to EUCAST guidelines has a susceptibility range only for *E. coli*, but which according to CLSI guidelines has assessed break points for all *Enterobacteriacae*. The problematic assessment of susceptibility testing according to different guidelines is well known [17]. The good activity of fosfomycin against extended spectrum β-lactamase positive Gram-negative bacteria in comparison with other first line antibiotics has also been observed in other countries [15, 16, 18–20].

The evaluation of overall antibiotic susceptibility in relation to patient status revealed significantly lower resistance in bacterial isolates from ambulatory patients in comparison to those of hospitalized patients. With the exception of ICU isolates, and using resistance of 10% as the limit for use as a first line option for empirical therapy in non-life-threatening infections, only fosfomycin seems to have an adequate coverage amongst agents suitable for per oral therapy. In our study there were no samples from the community (from GPs), which is why our samples had higher resistance.

Our results showed fosfomycin trometamol as a promising antibiotic for urinary tract infection in our country. But according to some published studies, the increasing use of fosfomycin worldwide has led to increased levels of resistance in isolates. For example, in a Spanish study an increase of fosfomycin resistance was detected in *Escherichia coli* isolates from 0.0% in 2005 to 14.4% in 2011 [21]. A change in the guidelines for UTI therapy is required to prevent this side effect of mass use of fosfomycin trometamol for UTIs. We see the main future benefit of a per-oral fosfomycin formulation in our fosfomycin-naive population in the treatment of specific groups of patients with non-life-threatening urinary tract infections, such as in patients with long-term stents which were often colonised by multi-resistant Gram-negative bacteria. These patients are threatened frequently by chronic urinary tract infections, and after successful intra-venous antibiotic therapy during hospitalization they should be treated by continuous per-oral therapy at home. Of all the commonly available per-oral antibiotics only fosfomycin was shown in our study to be highly effective against multi resistant (ESBL or AmpC) Gram-negative bacteria.

Conclusion

We have confirmed in the Czech Republic the very high susceptibility to fosfomycin trometamol of urinary tract infection pathogens, particularly Gram-negative rods including those producing β-lactamase. Our results will be used to rationalise treatment of urinary tract infection by fosfomycin trometamol in our country.

Abbreviations
CLSI: The clinical and laboratory standards institute; EARS-Net: The European Antimicrobial Resistance Surveillance Network; ECOFF: The epidemiological cut-off value; ESBL: Extended spectrum β-lactamase; EUCAST: The European Committee on Antimicrobial Susceptibility Testing; ICU: Intensive care unit; MALDI-TOF-MS: Matrix-assisted laser desorption ionization time-of-flight mass spectrometry; MDR: Multi-drug resistance; MRSA: Methicillin-resistant *Staphylococcus aureus*; UTI: Urinary tract infection; VRE: Vancomycin-resistant enterococci

Acknowledgements
The authors are grateful to Ian McColl M.D., Ph.D. for assistance with the manuscript.

Funding
Supported by MH CZ – DRO (UHHK, 00179906) and by the programme PRVOUK P37/04.

Authors' contributions
MF and ML designed the research and defined the research aim; MF, ML, PP, LR, MB, JP, JK and HZ performed the research. MF and HZ analyzed the data and interpreted the results. All authors read and approved the final manuscript.

Competing interests
The authors declare that they have no competing interest.

Author details
[1]Institute of Clinical Microbiology, University Hospital Hradec Kralové, Sokolska 581, Hradec Králové 50005, Czech Republic. [2]Charles University in Prague, Faculty of Medicine in Hradec Kralové, Simkova 870, Hradec Kralove 500 38, Czech Republic. [3]Clinic of Urology, University Hospital Hradec Kralové, Sokolska 581, Hradec Králové 50005, Czech Republic.

References
1. Frimondt-Møller N. Chapter 73 – Fosfomycin, in Kucers' The Use of Antibiotics, 6th Edition. Lead Editor M. Lindsay Grayson. USA: CRC Press. 2010
2. Magiorakos AP, Srinivasan A, Carey RB, Carmeli Y, Falagas ME, Giske CG, Harbarth S, Hindler JF, Kahlmeter G, Olsson-Liljequist B, Paterson DL, Rice LB, Stelling J, Struelens MJ, Vatopoulos A, Weber JT, Monnet DL. Multidrug-resistant, extensively drug-resistant and pandrug-resistant bacteria: an international expert proposal for interim standard definitions for acquired resistance. Clin Microbiol Infect. 2012;18(3):268–81.
3. Kaase M, Szabados F, Anders A, Gatermann SG. Fosfomycin susceptibility in carbapenem-resistant Enterobacteriaceae from Germany. J Clin Microbiol. 2014;52(6):1893–7.
4. Falagas ME, Kastoris AC, Karageorgopoulos DE, Rafailidis PI. Fosfomycin for the treatment of infections caused by multidrug-resistant non-fermenting Gram-negative bacilli: a systematic review of microbiological, animal and clinical studies. Int J Antimicrob Agents. 2009;34(2):111–20.
5. Mihailescu R, Furustrand Tafin U, Corvec S, Oliva A, Betrisey B, Borens O, Trampuz A. High activity of Fosfomycin and Rifampin against methicillin-resistant staphylococcus aureus biofilm in vitro and in an experimental foreign-body infection model. Antimicrob Agents Chemother. 2014;58(5):2547–53.

6. Neuner EA, Sekeres J, Hall GS, van Duin D. Experience with fosfomycin for treatment of urinary tract infections due to multidrug-resistant organisms. Antimicrob Agents Chemother. 2012;56(11):5744–8.

7. The European Association of Urology. Guidelines on Urological Infection, version 2015. http://uroweb.org/guideline/urological-infections/?type= archive

8. The European Committee on Antimicrobial Susceptibility Testing. Breakpoint tables for interpretation of MICs and zone diameters. Version 5.0, 2015. http://www.eucast.org/ast_of_bacteria/previous_versions_of_ documents/.

9. The Clinical and Laboratory Standards Institute. Performance Standards for Antimicrobial Susceptibility Testing; Twenty – Third Informational Supplement. Pennsylvania 19087, USA, 2013.

10. Hrabák J, Bergerová T, Zemličková H, Urbášková P. Detection of extended-spectrum ß-lactamases, AmpC ß-lactamases, metallo-ß-lactamases and Klebsiella pneumoniae carbapenemases in Gram-negative rods. Zprávy EMI. 2009;18(3):100–6.

11. Koningstein M, van der Bij AK, de Kraker MEA, Monen JC, Muilwijk J, de Greeff SC, Geerlings SE, van Hall MA ISIS-AR Study Group. Recommendations for the empirical treatment of complicated urinary tract infections using surveillance data on antimicrobial resistance in the Netherlands. PLoS ONE. 2014;9(1):e86634. doi:10.1371/journal.pone.0086634.

12. Cassir N, Rolain JM, Brouqui P. A new strategy to fight antimicrobial resistance: the revival of old antibiotics. Front Microbiol. 2014;5:551. doi:10.3389/fmicb.2014.00551.

13. Gupta V, Rani H, Singla N, Kaisha N, Chander J. Determination of Extended-Spectrum- β-Lactamases and AmpC production in uropathogenic isolates of Escherichia coli and susceptibility to Fosfomycin. J Lab Physicians. 2013;5(2):90–3.

14. Miranda EJ, Oliveira GS, Roque FL, Santos SR, Olmos RD, Lotufo PA. Susceptibility to antibiotics in urinary tract infections in a secondary care setting from 2005-2006 and 2010-2011, in São Paulo, Brazil: data from 11,943 urine cultures. Rev Inst Med Trop Sao Paulo. 2014;56(4):313–24.

15. Qiao L-D, Chen S, Yang Y, Zhang K, Zheng B, Guo HF, Yang B, Niu YJ, Wang Y, Shi BK, Yang WM, Zhao XK, Gao XF, Chen M, Tian Y. Characteristics of urinary tract infection pathogens and their in vitro susceptibility to antimicrobial agents in China: data from a multicenter study. BMJ Open. 2013;3:e004152. doi:10.1136/bmjopen-2013-004152.

16. Sorlozano A, Jimenez-Pacheco A, de Dios Luna Del Castillo J, Sampedro A, Martinez-Brocal A, Miranda-Casas C, Navarro-Marí JM, Gutiérrez-Fernández J. Evolution of the resistance to antibiotics of bacteria involved in urinary tract infection: a 7-year surveillance study. Am J Infect Control. 2014;42(10):1033–8.

17. Perdigão-Neto LV, Oliveira MS, Rizek CF, Carrilho CM, Costa SF, Levin AS. Susceptibility of multiresistant gram-negative bacteria to fosfomycin and performance of different susceptibility testing methods. Antimicrob Agents Chemother. 2014;58(3):1763–7.

18. Liu HY, Lin HC, Lin YC, Yu SH, Wu WH, Lee YJ. Antimicrobial susceptibilities of urinary extended-spectrum beta-lactamase-producing Escherichia coli and Klebsiella pneumoniae to fosfomycin and nitrofurantoin in a teaching hospital in Taiwan. J Microbiol Immunol Infect. 2011;44(5):364–8.

19. Chislett RJ, White G, Hills T, Turner DP. Fosfomycin susceptibility among extended-spectrum beta-lactamase producing Escherichia coli in Nottingham, UK. J Antimicrob Chemother. 2010;65:1076–7.

20. Schmiemann G, Gágyor I, Hummers-Pradier E, Bleidorn. Resistance profiles of urinary tract infections in general practice - an observational study. BMC Urol. 2012;12:33. doi:10.1186/1471-2490-12-33.

21. Rodríguez-Avial C, Rodríguez-Avial I, Hernández E, Picazo JJ. Increasing prevalence of fosfomycin resistance in extended-spectrum-beta-lactamase-producing Escherichia coli urinary isolates (2005-2009-2011). Rev Esp Quimioter. 2013;26(1):43–6.

29

The efficacy and safety of silodosin for the treatment of ureteral stones

Diandong Yang, Jitao Wu, Hejia Yuan and Yuanshan Cui[*]

Abstract

Background: To evaluate the efficacy and safety of silodosin as a medical expulsive therapy for ureteral stones by means of a systematic review and meta-analysis.

Methods: We searched MEDLINE, EMBASE and the Cochrane Controlled Trials Register to identify randomized controlled trials (RCTs) of silodosin in the treatment of ureteral stones. The reference lists of retrieved studies were also investigated.

Results: Six RCTs, including 916 participants and comparing silodosin with controls, were used in the meta-analysis. Silodosin was superior to controls in terms of stone expulsion rate, the primary efficacy end point in all six RCTs (odds ratio [OR] for expulsion 2.16, 95 % confidence interval [CI] 1.62 to 2.86, p <0.00001). Silodosin was also more effective for secondary efficacy end points; the stone expulsion time (standardized mean difference [SMD] −3.66, 95 % CI −6.61 to −0.71; p =0.01) and analgesic requirements (SMD −0.89, 95 % CI −1.19 to −0.60; p < 0.00001) were significantly reduced compared with those of controls. Other than the incidence of abnormal ejaculation, which was higher in the silodosin groups (OR 2.84, 95 % CI 1.56 to 5.16, p =0.0006), few adverse effects were observed.

Conclusion: This meta-analysis indicates silodosin is an effective and safe treatment option for ureteral stones with a low occurrence of side effects.

Keywords: Silodosin, Ureteral stones, Meta-analysis, Randomized controlled trial

Abbreviations: RCT, Randomized controlled trial; OR, Odds ratio; CI, Confidence interval; SMD, Standardized mean difference; MET, Medical expulsive therapy; α1A-AR, α1A-adrenoceptor

Background

Urolithiasis is a multifactorial disease that is common in daily urological practice, and is also a substantial public health problem. After urinary tract infections and pathologic conditions of the prostate [1], urolithiasis is the third most common disease of the urinary tract, with an estimated prevalence of 2–3 % and a lifetime recurrence rate of approximately 50 % [2, 3]. To date, minimally invasive therapies, such as extracorporeal shock wave lithotripsy, ureterolithotripsy and percutaneous nephrolithotomy have proved to be effective treatments in many cases. Nevertheless, these procedures are expensive and are not without risk [4].

A conservative approach involving close monitoring can be used in most cases, and is becoming more popular as a result of advances in pharmacological therapy, which can reduce symptoms and facilitate stone expulsion [5, 6]. For example, medical expulsive therapy (MET) using α-adrenoceptor antagonists has emerged as an alternative strategy for the initial management of small distal ureteral stones [7].

Silodosin is a novel highly selective α1A-adrenoceptor (α1A-AR) blocker: *in vitro* its α1A-to-1B binding ratio is extremely high (162:1), suggesting that it has the potential to reduce dynamic neurally mediated smooth muscle relaxation in the ureter, while minimizing undesirable effects on blood pressure regulation [8].

The goal of this study was to perform a meta-analysis to evaluate the efficacy and safety of silodosin as a MET for ureteral stones to help address some of the current controversies over its use for this indication.

* Correspondence: doctorcuiys@163.com
Jitao Wu co-first author.
Department of Urology, Yantai Yuhuangding Hospital Affiliated to Medical College of Qingdao University, NO.20 East Yuhuangding Road, 264000 Yantai, China

Methods

Search strategy

MEDLINE (1966 to Jan 2015), EMBASE (1974 to Jan 2015) and the Cochrane Controlled Trials Register databases were searched to identify randomized controlled trials (RCTs) of silodosin in the treatment of ureteral stones; we also searched the reference lists of the retrieved studies. The following search terms were used: "silodosin"; "ureteral stones"; and "randomized controlled trial".

Inclusion criteria and trial selection

Randomized controlled trials that met the following criteria were included: (1) the study design included treatment with silodosin; (2) the study provided accurate data that could be analyzed, including the total number of subjects and the values of each outcome measured; and (3) the full text of the study could be accessed. When the same study was published in more than one journal or in different years, the most recent publication was used for the meta-analysis. If the same group of researchers studied a group of subjects with multiple experiments, then each study was included. A flow diagram of the study selection process is presented in Fig. 1.

Quality assessment

The quality of the retrieved RCTs was assessed using the Jadad scale [9]. All identified RCTs were included in the meta-analysis, regardless of the quality score. The methodological quality of each study was assessed according to the means of allocation of participants to the arms of the study, the concealment of allocation procedures, blinding and data loss due to attrition. The studies were then classified qualitatively according to the guidelines published in the *Cochrane Handbook for Systematic Reviews of Interventions* v.5.1.0 [10]. Each study was rated according to these quality assessment criteria, and assigned to one of the three following quality categories: A, if all quality criteria were adequately met the study was deemed to have a low risk of bias; B, if one or more of the quality criteria was only partially met or was unclear the study was deemed to have a moderate risk of bias; or C, if one or more of the criteria was not met or not included the study was deemed to have a high risk of bias. Differences were resolved by discussion among the authors.

Data extraction

The following information was collected for each study: (1) the name of the RCT; (2) the study design and sample size; (3) the therapy that the patients received; (4) the country in which the study was conducted; and (5) data including the stone expulsion rate, stone expulsion time, analgesics required and incidence of adverse events, including abnormal ejaculation in male participants.

Statistical analysis and meta-analysis

The meta-analysis of comparable data was carried out using RevMan v.5.1.0 (Cochrane Collaboration, Oxford, UK) [10]. We estimated the relative risk for dichotomous outcomes and the standardized mean difference (SMD) for continuous outcomes pooled across studies by using the DerSimonian and Laird random-effects model [11]. The corresponding 95 % confidence interval (CI) was calculated, if the result of analysis showed $p > 0.05$, we considered the studies homogeneous and so chose a fixed-effect model for meta-analysis; otherwise, a random-effect model was used. We quantified inconsistency using the I^2 statistic, which describes the proportion of heterogeneity across studies that is not due to chance, thus describing the extent of true inconsistency in results across trials [12]. $I^2 < 25$ % reflects a small amount of inconsistency and $I^2 > 50$ % reflects significant inconsistency.

Results

Characteristics of the individual studies

The database search produced 114 articles that could have been included in our meta-analysis. Based on the inclusion and exclusion criteria, 99 articles were excluded after reading the titles and abstracts of the articles; nine articles were not RCTs. In all, six articles [13–18], reporting data from three RCTs that compared silodosin with tamsulosin, two RCTs that compared silodosin with placebo and one RCT that compared silodosin with naftopidil were included in the analysis (Fig. 1). The baseline characteristics of the studies included in our meta-analysis are listed in Table 1.

Quality of the individual studies

Two of the six RCTs were double-blinded, and included descriptions of the randomization processes used. Three RCTs included a power calculation to determine the optimal sample size (Table 2). The quality of all identified studies was categorized as A or B, and the final Jadad score for each study ranged from 3 to 5 points (Table 2). A funnel plot suggested there was no bias (Fig. 2).

Efficacy

Stone expulsion rate

Six RCTs with 916 participants (457 in the silodosin groups and 459 in the control groups, Fig. 3) reported stone expulsion rate as the primary outcome measure. According to our analysis, no heterogeneity was found between the trials ($P = 0.39$) (Fig. 3), and a fixed-effects model was thus chosen for the analysis. Silodosin

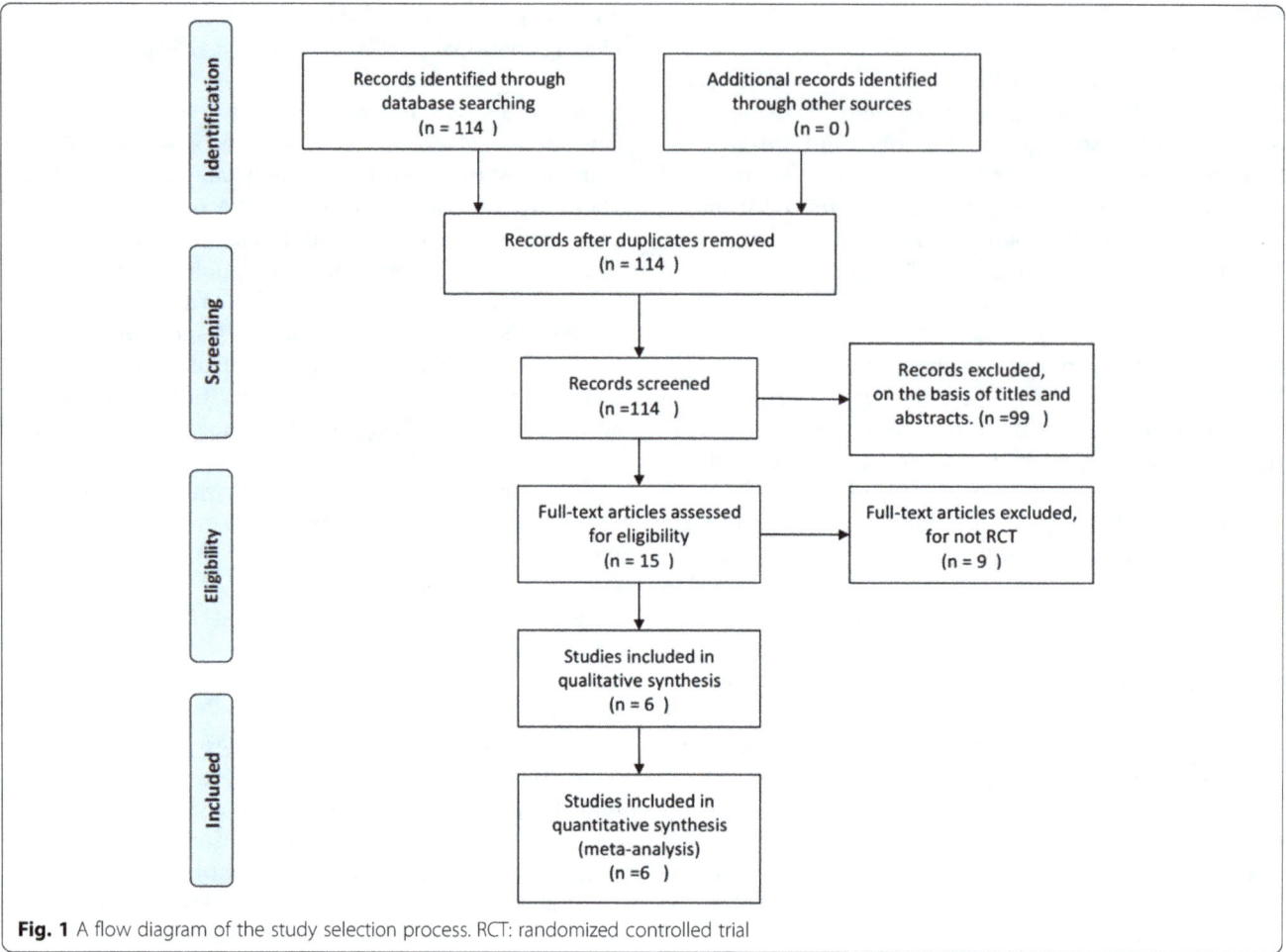

Fig. 1 A flow diagram of the study selection process. RCT: randomized controlled trial

showed a significantly superior stone expulsion rate compared with controls (OR 2.16, 95 % CI 1.62 to 2.86; p <0.00001).

Stone expulsion time

Four RCTs with 541 participants (270 in the silodosin groups and 271 in the control groups, Fig. 3) reported stone expulsion times as a secondary outcome. According to our analysis, heterogeneity was found between the trials (P = 0.0001). A random-effects model was chosen for the analysis. The stone expulsion time was significantly shorter in the silodosin groups than controls (SMD –3.66, 95 % CI –6.61 to –0.71; p =0.01).

Analgesia required

Two of the RCTs (consisting of 367 participants, with 185 in the silodosin groups and 182 in the control groups, Fig. 3) reported the analgesics required during stone expulsion. According to our analysis, no heterogeneity was found between the trials (P = 0.85). A fixed-effects model was chosen for the analysis. Expulsion using silodosin was associated with a significantly lower analgesic requirement than that in controls (SMD –0.89, 95 % CI –1.19 to –0.69; p <0.00001).

Side effects and safety
Abnormal ejaculation

Six RCTs with 916 participants (457 in the silodosin groups and 458 in the control groups, Fig. 3) reported the incidence of abnormal ejaculation (Fig. 4). The effect size for the purposes of meta-analysis was denoted as the OR. According to our analysis based on a fixed-effects model, no heterogeneity was found between the trials (P = 0.47). The pooled estimate of OR was 2.84 (95 % CI 1.56 to 5.16, p =0.0006). This suggests that abnormal ejaculation was more common among patients treated with silodosin than among control-treated patients.

Subgroup analysis

We divided the included studies into three groups on the basis of the treatment given to the control groups: tamsulosin, naftopidil or inactive placebo. According to

Table 1 Study and patient characteristics

Study	Therapy in experimental group	Therapy in control group	Country	Sample size		Administration method	Duration of treatment	Dosage	Stone location and size range
				experimental	Control				
Itoh Y 2011	silodosin	blank control	Japan	95	92	Oral	8 wk	8mg/d	symptomatic unilateral ureteral calculi of less than 10 mm
Tsuzaka Y 2011	silodosin	naftopidil	Japan	35	39	Oral	6 wk	8mg/d	symptomatic≤10 mm ureteral stones
Guptas S 2013	silodosin	tamsulosin	India	50	50	Oral	4 wk	8mg/d	unilateral, uncomplicated middle or lower ureteral stones ≤10 mm
Dell'Atti L 2014	silodosin	tamsulosin	Italy	68	68	Oral	3 wk	8mg/d	single, unilateral, radiopaque, proximal ureteral stone (range 4–10 mm in size)
Sur RL 2014	silodosin	placebo	USA	119	120	Oral	4 wk	8mg/d	unilateral ureteral calculus of 4–10 mm
Kumar S 2015	silodosin	tamsulosin	India	90	90	Oral	4 wk	8mg/d	distal ureteric stones of size 5–10 mm

our analysis, no heterogeneity was found between the trials ($P > 0.05$); therefore, we chose a fixed-effects model for the analysis. Stone expulsion rates were significantly higher in those treated with silodosin compared with tamsulosin (OR 1.65, 95 % CI 1.12 to 2.43; p =0.01), naftopidil (OR 2.83, 95 % CI 1.80 to 4.45; p <0.00001) or inactive placebo (OR 3.36, 95 % CI 1.13 to 9.96; p =0.03, Fig. 5).

We further divided the included studies into two groups according to stone location: proximal or distal. According to our analysis, no heterogeneity was found between the trials ($P > 0.05$); therefore, a fixed-effects model was chosen. Stone expulsion rates were significantly higher in those treated with silodosin compared with control in spite of the stone location. (proximal OR 2.1, 95 % CI 1.12 to 3.92; p =0.02 or distal OR 2.53, 95 % CI 1.61 to 3.99; p <0.00001, Fig. 6).

Discussion

The introduction of more effective drugs has seen significant improvements in the medical management of ureteral stones. The likelihood of a ureteral stone passing depends on several factors, which include the stone size and location, and the condition of the ureter [19]. The stimulation of the α1-AR in the ureter increases the force of ureteric contraction and the frequency of ureteric peristalsis. Blockade of the α1-AR inhibits basal tone, reduces peristaltic amplitude and frequency, and decreases intraluminal pressure while increasing the rate of fluid transport and the chances of stone expulsion. Expression of the α1A- and α1D-AR subtypes is greater in the distal ureter [20]. Silodosin is a highly selective α1A-AR blocker, and it has been demonstrated *in vitro* that silodosin's α1A-to-1B binding ratio is extremely high (162:1).

Our meta-analysis found that silodosin 8 mg/day for 3–8 weeks is superior to controls (tamsulosin 0.4 mg/day, naftopidil 50 mg/day or inactive placebo) in improving the stone expulsion rate, reducing the stone expulsion time and analgesic requirements. According to our analysis, no heterogeneity was found between the trials, allowing us to use a fixed-effects model for the analysis. We may therefore conclude that silodosin 8 mg/day treats stones more

Table 2 Quality assessment of individual study

Study	Allocation sequence generation	Allocation concealment	Blinding	Loss to follow-up	Calculation of sample size	Statistical analysis	Level of quality	Jadad Score(5-point)
Itoh Y 2011	B	B	A	6	NO	Student's t-test	B	3
Tsuzaka Y 2011	B	B	A	10	NO	Student's t-test	B	3
Guptas S 2013	A	B	A	0	NO	Student's t-test	A	4
Dell'Atti L 2014	B	A	A	3	YES	Student's t-test	A	4
Sur RL 2014	A	A	A	6	YES	Wilcoxon test	A	5
Kumar S 2015	A	A	A	6	YES	chi-square test	A	5

A - all quality criteria met (adequate): low risk of bias. B - one or more of the quality criteria only partly met (unclear): moderate risk of bias
C - one or more criteria not met (inadequate or not used): high risk of bias

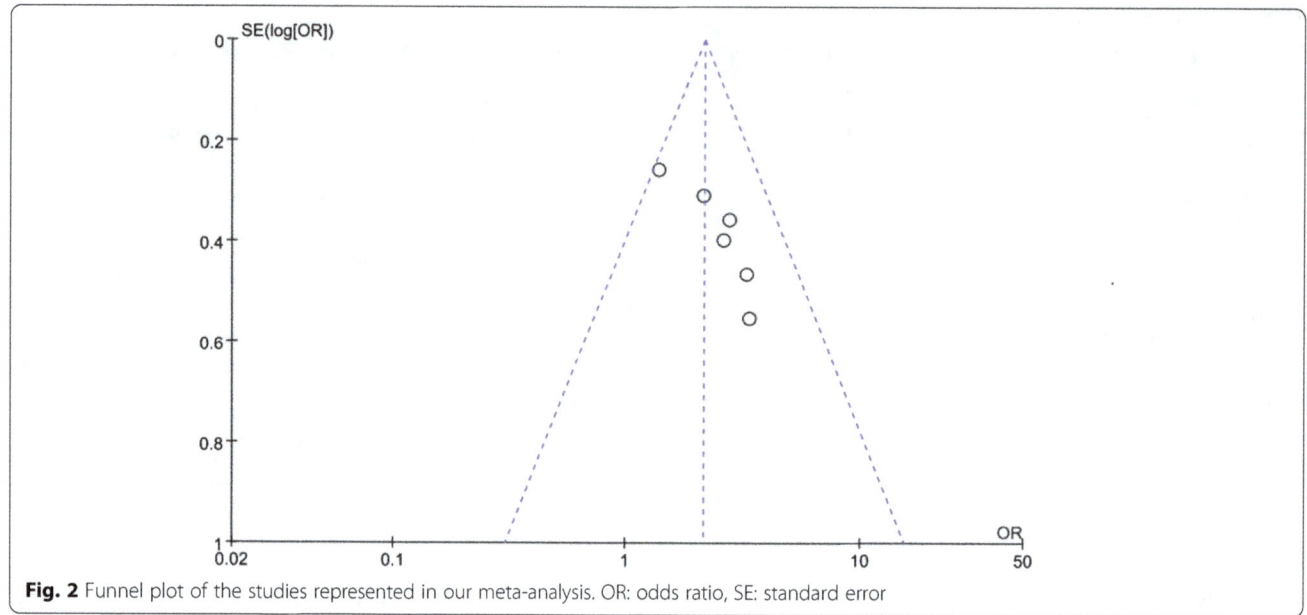

Fig. 2 Funnel plot of the studies represented in our meta-analysis. OR: odds ratio, SE: standard error

effectively than tamsulosin 0.4 mg/day, naftopidil 50 mg/day or placebo. Our subgroup analysis showed that stone expulsion rates were significantly higher in those treated with silodosin compared with those treated with a control, regardless of stone location. It is worth noting that stone expulsion rates ranged from 57.7 % to 80.9 % in cases involving proximal ureteral stones, and 69.8 % to 93.8 % in distal ureteral stones. Therefore, it seems that the stone expulsion rate for distal ureteral stones is higher than for proximal ureteral stones. Stone size has been identified as

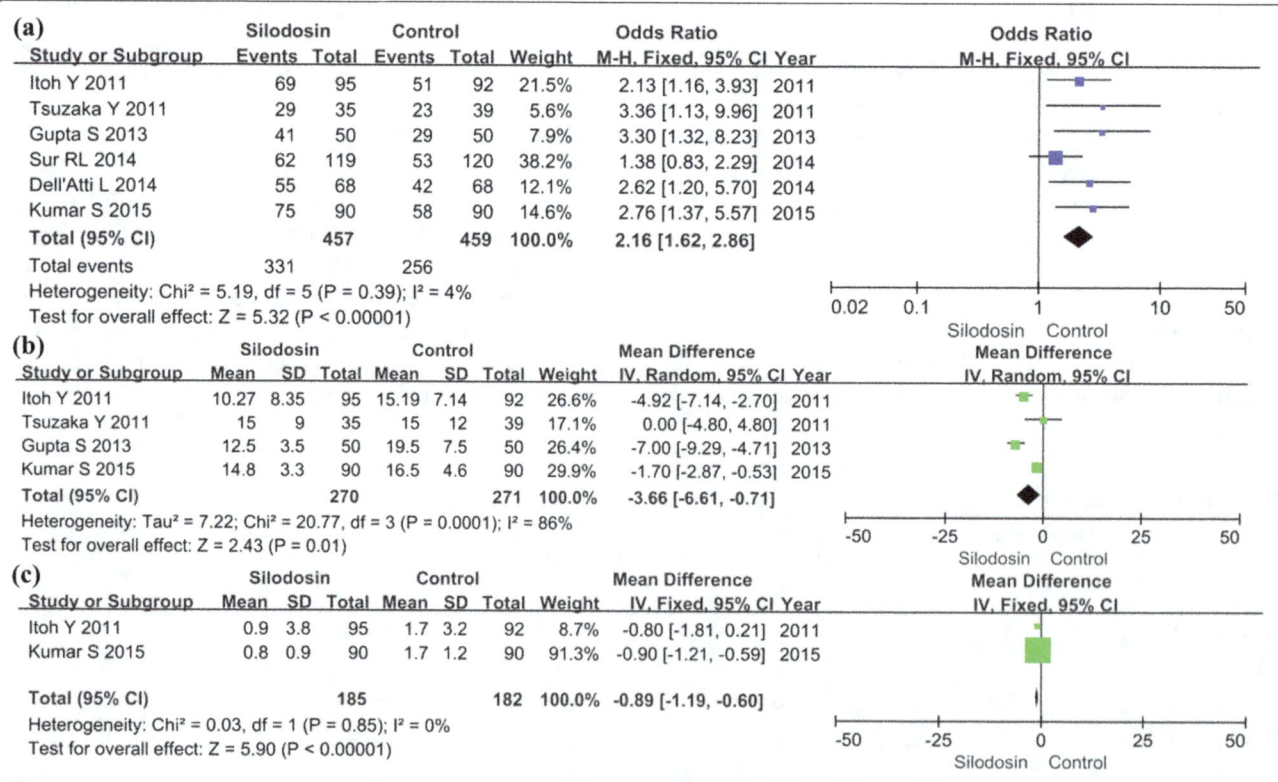

Fig. 3 Forest plots showing changes in (**a**) the stone expulsion rate, (**b**) stone expulsion time and (**c**) analgesics were required. MH: mantel haenszel, CI: confidence interval, SD: standard deviation, IV: inverse variance

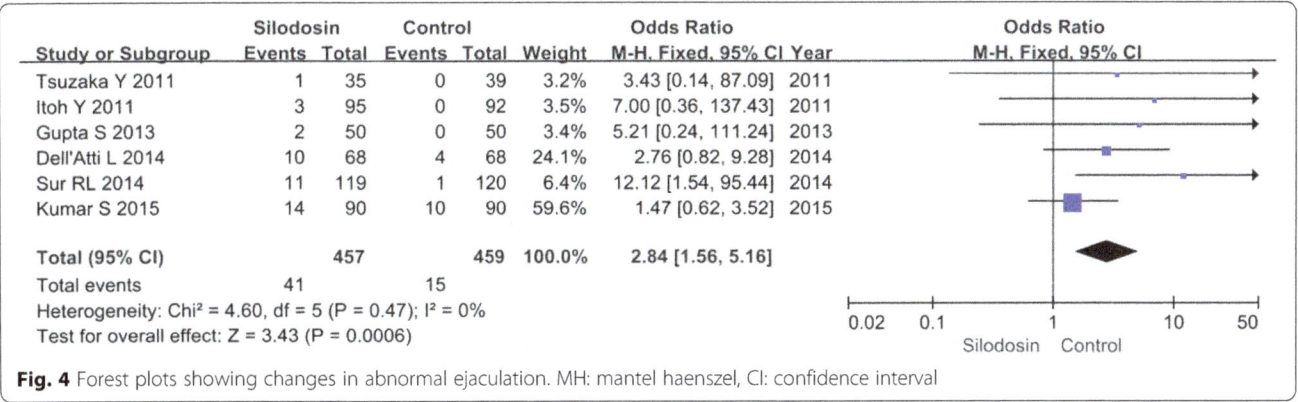

Fig. 4 Forest plots showing changes in abnormal ejaculation. MH: mantel haenszel, CI: confidence interval

an important predictive factor for expulsion: the trials we chose examined those ≤10 mm in diameter, so we cannot draw any conclusions about the role of silodosin in the treatment of larger ureteral calculi.

The α1A/D selective AR-blocker tamsulosin is recognized as a safe and effective drug that also enhances spontaneous passage of distal ureteral stones ≤10 mm in diameter [21]. Recent studies have demonstrated that the α1A subtype plays the most important role in mediating phenylephrine-induced contraction of the isolated human ureter [22]. Kobayashi et al. found that silodosin enhanced noradrenaline-induced contraction of the

human ureter more than the selective α1D-AR antagonist BMY-7378 [23]. The mechanism of action of silodosin presumably includes blockade of the α-adrenergic receptors, thereby relaxing the ureter and potentially providing a spasmolytic effect [24].

Our meta-analysis suggests that there is a higher incidence of retrograde ejaculation in patients treated with silodosin than active or inactive controls. The incidence of side effects was similar to that reported by other authors [25]. Nonetheless, retrograde ejaculation does not appear to be particularly troublesome, and only a small proportion of participants enrolled in clinical studies

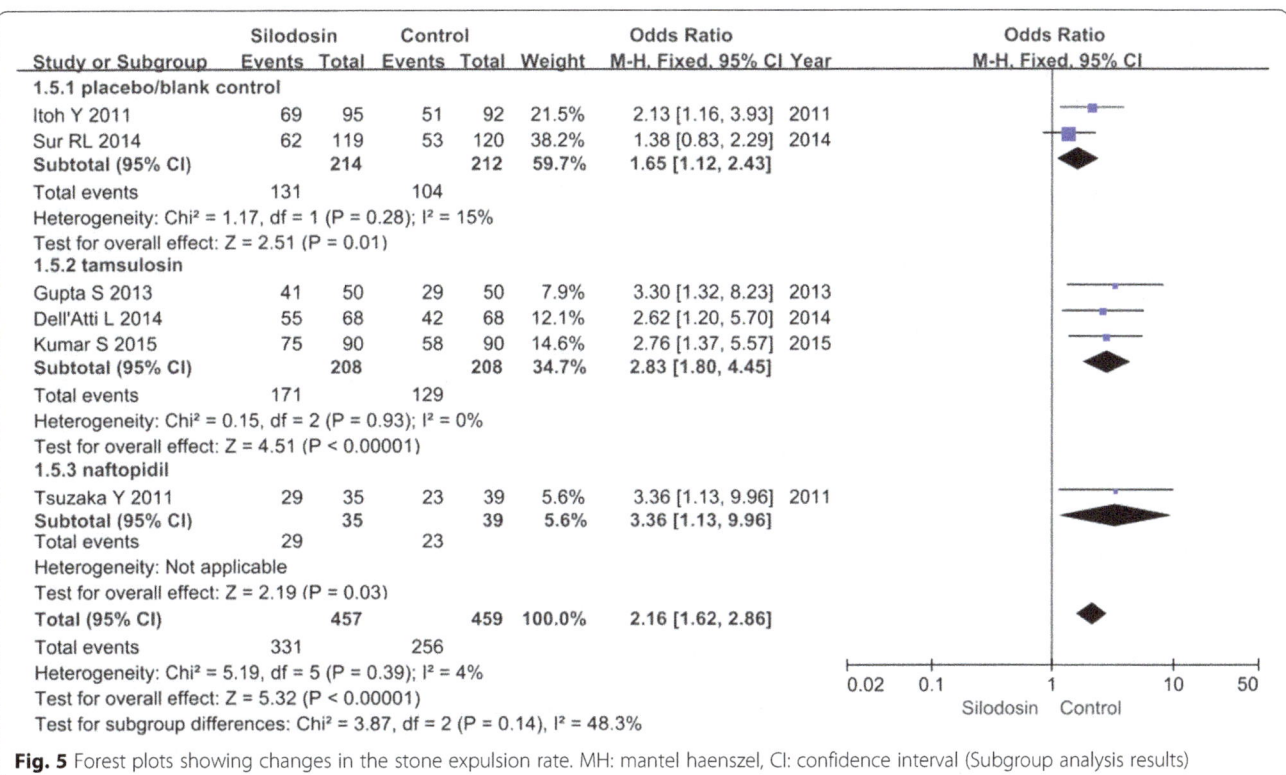

Fig. 5 Forest plots showing changes in the stone expulsion rate. MH: mantel haenszel, CI: confidence interval (Subgroup analysis results)

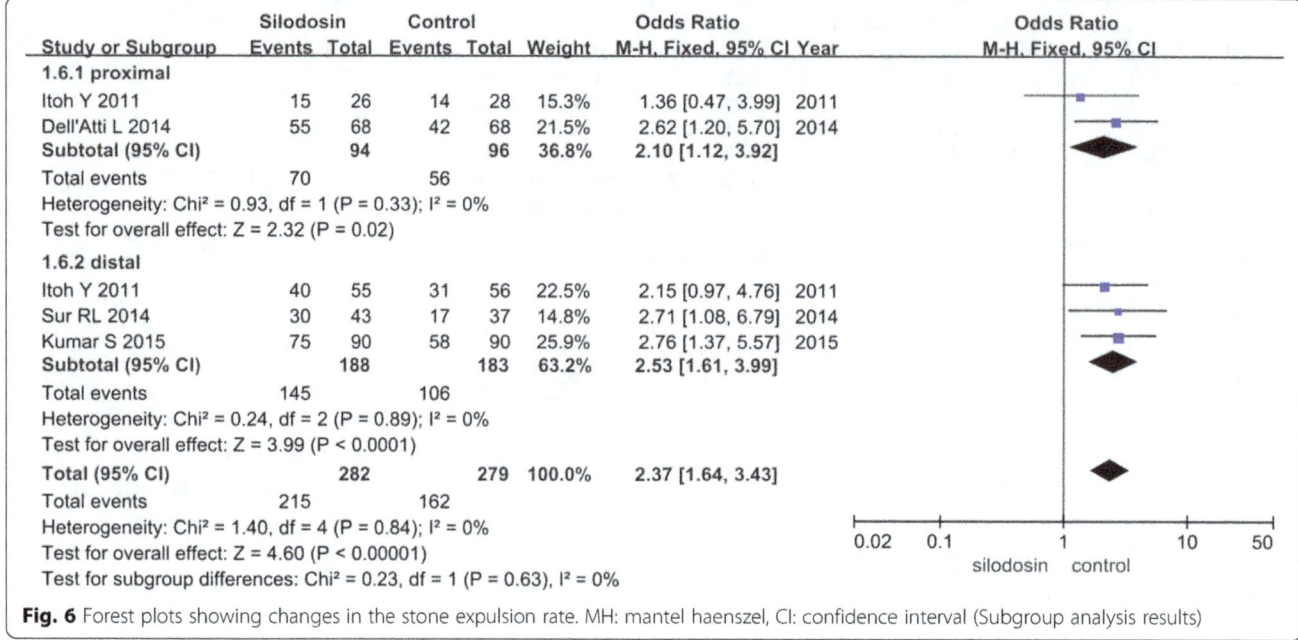

Fig. 6 Forest plots showing changes in the stone expulsion rate. MH: mantel haenszel, CI: confidence interval (Subgroup analysis results)

who report this adverse effect discontinued treatments because of it [26]. Furthermore, retrograde ejaculation resolves completely within a few days of discontinuing treatment [26]. Silodosin appears to relax the smooth muscles of the lower urinary tract and the genital tract enough to induce retrograde ejaculation, reflected in the finding that patients who had the greatest relief from lower urinary tract symptoms had a higher likelihood of retrograde ejaculation. This observation suggests that retrograde ejaculation is an indirect indicator of the extent of the smooth muscle relaxation that silodosin induces. Other than retrograde ejaculation, the type and incidence of adverse events reported by those taking silodosin were similar to those taking tamsulosin, naftopidil or an inactive control. Besides, Imperatore V et al. conducted a retrospectively controlled study demonstrated that MET with silodosin is associated with a lower incidence of side effects related to peripheral vasodilation but an higher incidence of retrograde ejaculation when compared to tamsulosin [27].

Our meta-analysis was based on data collected entirely from RCTs that we considered to be at low risk of bias. This suggests that our findings could be sufficiently sound to inform everyday clinical practice. Importantly, however, the number of included studies was small and there were a variety of control groups; therefore, a certain amount of clinical heterogeneity seems inevitable. Furthermore, we cannot account for the possible influence of unpublished studies, which could have introduced an unrecognized bias into our analysis. The longer-term efficacy and safety of silodosin cannot therefore be extrapolated from our findings. More high-quality trials with larger sample sizes

are needed to establish fully the role of silodosin in the treatment of distal ureteral stones.

Conclusions
This meta-analysis indicates silodosin is an effective and safe treatment option for ureteral stones with a low occurrence of side effects.

Acknowledgement
We thank *Edanz Group (liwenbianji)* for assisting in the preparation of this manuscript.

Authors' contributions
CYS designed the research, interpreted the data and revised the paper. YDD, WTT, and YHJ performed the data extraction, carried out the meta-analysis and drafted the paper. All of the authors approved the submitted and final versions.

Competing interests
The authors declare that they have no competing interests.

References
1. Stefanos PJ, Michael C. Trussa, Treatment strategies of ureteral stones. EAU-EBU Up-date Series. 2006;4:184–90.
2. Sakhaee K, Maalouf NM, Sinnott B. Clinical review. Kidney stones 2012: pathogenesis, diagnosis, and management. J Clin Endocrinol Metab. 2012; 97:1847–60.
3. Bihl G, Meyers A. Recurrent renal stone disease-advances in pathogenesis and clinical management. Lancet. 2011;358:651–6.
4. Dellabella M, Milanese G, Muzzonigro G. Randomized trial of the efficacy of tamsulosin, nifedipine and phloroglucinol in medicalexpulsive therapy for distal ureteral calculi. J Urol. 2005;174:167–72.
5. Borghi L, Meschi T, Amato F, Novarini A, Giannini A, Quarantelli C, et al. Nifedipine and methylprednisolone in facilitating ureteral stone passage: a randomized, double-blind, placebo-controlled study. J Urol. 1994;152:1095–8.

6. Porpiglia F, Destefanis P, Fiori C, Fontana D. Effectiveness of nifedipine and deflazacort in the management of distal ureter stones. Urology. 2000;56:579–82.
7. Tzortzis V, Mamoulakis C, Rioja J, Gravas S, Michel MC, de la Rosette JJ. Medical expulsive therapy for distal ureteral stones. Drugs. 2009;69:677–92.
8. Tatemichi S, Kobayashi K, Maezawa A, Kobayashi M, Yamazaki Y, Shibata N. α1-Adenoceptor subtype selectivity and organ specificity of silodosin (KMD-3213). Yakugaku Zasshi. 2006;126:209–16.
9. Jadad AR. Randomised controlled trials. London: BMJ Publishing Group; 1998.
10. Higgins JPT, Green S, editors: Cochrane handbook for systematic reviews of interventions, v.5.1 [updated March 2011]. Cochrane Collaboration Web site. http://handbook.cochrane.org/.
11. DerSimonian R, Laird N. Meta-analysis in clinical trials. Control Clin Trials. 1986;7:177–88.
12. Higgins JP, Thompson SG, Deeks JJ, Altman DG. Measuring inconsistency in meta-analyses. BMJ. 2003;327:557–60.
13. Itoh Y, Okada A, Yasui T, Hamamoto S, Hirose M, Kojima Y. Efficacy of selective α1A adrenoceptor antagonist silodosin in the medical expulsive therapy for ureteral stones. Int J Urol. 2011;18:672–4.
14. Tsuzaka Y, Matsushima H, Kaneko T, Yamaguchi T, Homma Y. Naftopidil vs silodosin in medical expulsive therapy for ureteral stones: a randomized controlled study in Japanese male patients. Int J Urol. 2011;18:792–5.
15. Gupta S, Lodh B, Singh AK, Somarendra K, Meitei KS, Singh SR. Comparing the efficacy of tamsulosin and silodosin in the medical expulsion therapy for ureteral calculi. J Clin Diagn Res. 2013;7:1672–4.
16. Dell'Atti L. Silodosin versus Tamsulosin as medical expulsive therapy for distal ureteral stones: a prospective randomized study. Urologia. 2014;82:54–7.
17. Sur RL, Shore N, L'Esperance J, Knudsen B, Gupta M, Olsen S, et al. Silodosin to Facilitate Passage of Ureteral Stones: A Multi-institutional, Randomized, Double-blinded, Placebo-controlled Trial. Eur Urol. 2014;67:959–64.
18. Kumar S, Jayant K, Agrawal MM, Singh SK, Agrawal S, Parmar KM. Role of tamsulosin, tadalafil, and silodosin as the medical expulsive therapy in lower ureteric stone: a randomized trial (a pilot study). Urology. 2015;85:59–63.
19. Sun X, He L, Ge W, Lv J. Efficacy of selective alpha1D-blocker naftopidil as medical expulsive therapy for distal ureteral stones. J Urol. 2009;181:1716–20.
20. Griwan MS, Singh SK, Paul H, Pawar DS, Verma M. The efficacy of tamsulosin in lower ureteral calculi. Urol Ann. 2010;2:63–6.
21. De SM, Autorino R, Di LG, Damiano R, Giordano D, Cosentino L. Medical expulsive treatment of distal-ureteral stones using tamsulosin: a single-center experience. J Endourol. 2006;20:12–6.
22. Sasaki S, Tomiyama Y, Kobayashi S, Kojima Y, Kubota Y, Kohri K. Characterization of α1-adrenoceptor subtypes mediating contraction in human isolated ureters. Urology. 2011;77:762.e13-17.
23. Kobayashi S, Tomiyama Y, Hoyano Y, Yamazaki Y, Kusama H, Itoh Y. Gene expressions and mechanical functions of α1-adrenoceptor subtypes in mouseureter. World J Urol. 2009;27:775–80.
24. Preminger GM, Tiselius HG, Assimos DG, Alken P, Buck C, Gallucci M, Knoll T, Lingeman JE, Nakada SY, Pearle MS, et al. 2007 guideline for the management of ureteral calculi. J Urol. 2007;178(6):2418-34.
25. Cui Y, Zong H, Zhang Y. The efficacy and safety of silodosin in treating BPH: a systematic review and meta-analysis. Int Urol Nephrol. 2013;44:1601–9.
26. Montorsi F. Profile of Silodosin. Eur Urol Suppl. 2010;491–495.
27. Imperatore V, Fusco F, Creta M, Di Meo S, Buonopane R, Longo N, et al. Medical expulsive therapy for distal ureteric stones: tamsulosin versus silodosin. Arch Ital Urol Androl. 2014;86:103–7.

30

Review by urological pathologists improves the accuracy of Gleason grading by general pathologists

Yasushi Nakai[1], Nobumichi Tanaka[1], Keiji Shimada[2], Noboru Konishi[2], Makito Miyake[1], Satoshi Anai[1] and Kiyohide Fujimoto[1*]

Abstract

Backgrounds: Urologists use biopsy Gleason scores for patient counseling, prognosis prediction, and decision making. The accuracy of Gleason grading is very important. However, the variability of Gleason grading between general pathologists cannot be overlooked. Here we evaluate the discrepancy in the Gleason grading between 2 urologic pathologists and general pathologists as well as improvement in the accuracy of Gleason grading by general pathologists as a result of review by urologic pathologists.

Methods: The subjects enrolled in the study were 755 patients who underwent prostate needle biopsy at affiliate hospitals of Nara Medical University over a period of 2 years. The biopsy samples were diagnosed by general pathologists. All biopsy samples were sent to Nara Medical University where they were diagnosed by 2 urologic pathologists. The results were then returned to the general pathologists. We compared the diagnostic accuracy of the general pathologists with that of the urologic pathologists for the parameters of no malignancy, atypical small acinar proliferation, high grade prostatic intraepithelial neoplasia and Gleason score (6, 3 + 4, 4 + 3 and 8–10). We then evaluated the concordance rate between the general and urologic pathologists for each of four consecutive 6-month periods.

Results: The overall concordance rate of urologic pathologists and general pathologists in the first, second, third and last 6-month periods was 71.8 % (140/198), 79.8 % (168/225), 89.7 % (166/185) and 89.9 % (133/148), respectively. The concordance rate of the Gleason score between urologic pathologists and general pathologists in the first, second, third and last 6-month periods was 47.5 %(38/80), 62.6 %(57/91),76.9 %(50/65) and 78.7 %(48/61), respectively, and the kappa value was 0.55, 0.68, 0.81 and 0.84, respectively. The concordance rate improved significantly over the course of each period ($P = 0.04$).

Conclusion: The concordance rate of the Gleason grading between the general pathologists and the urologic pathologists was 47.5 %. However, improvement of the concordance rate as a result of review by the urological pathologist could be seen.

Keywords: Gleason score, Prostate biopsy, General pathologist, Urological pathologist

* Correspondence: kiyokun@naramed-u.ac.jp
[1]Department of Urology, Nara Medical University, 840 Shijo-cho, Kashihara, Nara 634-8522, Japan
Full list of author information is available at the end of the article

Backgrounds

Gleason et al [1] introduced the Gleason grading system for prostate cancer in 1966 and it was modified in 1974 [2] and 1977 [3]. Gleason grading is now accepted as the international standard for pathological grading in prostate cancer. In Japan, Gleason grading was introduced for clinical and pathological studies of prostate cancer in 2001; since then, it has been the standard for the pathological classification of prostate cancer [4]. Previously reported studies demonstrated the ability of the Gleason grading system to serve as a predictor of the final pathological stage and prognosis [5–7]. Generally, urologists use biopsy Gleason scores (GS) for patient counseling, prognosis prediction, and decision making. It goes without saying that the accuracy of Gleason grading is very important; however, several studies have described interobserver variabilities [8, 9]. The variability of Gleason grading between general pathologists cannot be overlooked [8, 10]. To improve these variabilities, the International Society of Urological Pathology (ISUP) convened a consensus conference on the Gleason grading of Prostatic carcinoma at 2005 [11]. The 2005 ISUP modified Gleason system is considered as the currently accepted version of Gleason grading [12, 13].

In this study, we evaluated discrepancies in Gleason grading between urological pathologists and general pathologists. We also sought to evaluate the impact of Gleason grading by general pathologists.

Methods

Between April 2006 and March 2008, we enrolled 755 patients who underwent prostate needle biopsy at 2 hospitals affiliated to the Nara Medical University. Approval for the study was obtained from the Nara Medical University Hospital Institutional Review Board. We obtained written informed consent from each enrolled patient before biopsy. Prostate-specific antigen (PSA) levels were determined using the PSA age-specific reference range according to Ito et al. [14] The cutoff value was 3.1 ng/mL in patients aged <65 years, 3.6 ng/mL in those aged 65–70 years, and 4.1 ng/mL in those aged ≥70 years. Biopsy was performed under transrectal ultrasonography while adjusting the number (6–12 cores) on the basis of the prostate volume and age (Table 1) [14, 15]. All general pathologists in both affiliated hospitals evaluated the biopsy samples.

Table 1 Optimal number of biopsy cores based on patient age and total prostate volume

Prostate volume (mL)	Age (yrs)			
	<60	60-64	65-69	≥70
0-25	12	10	8	6
25-50	12	12	10	8
50<	12	12	12	10

All biopsy samples were subsequently sent to Nara Medical University, where a urological pathological diagnosis was made by 2 experts in prostate cancer diagnosis who were blinded to the general pathologists' evaluations. Each slide was diagnosed by 2 urological pathologists. When discrepancy between urological pathologists, they discussed with the case and determined the final diagnosis. The results were then returned to the general pathologists who reviewed the results given by the urological pathologist. The results were only described about GS, high grade prostatic intraepithelial neoplasia (HGPIN), atypical small acinar proliferation (ASAP), prostatitis, hypertrophy, or no malignancy (NM), and portion of cancer in each core. This procedure was followed for all samples. We compared the diagnostic accuracy between general and urological pathologists for the parameters of no malignancy, ASAP, HGPIN, and GS (6, 3 + 4, 4 + 3 and 8–10) at the worst GS for each patient. We then evaluated the concordance rate between general and urological pathologists for each 6-month period.

We used the Kruskal–Wallis test or chi-square test to estimate the distribution of each parameter in each term. The concordance was measured on the basis of the percentage of concordance and Cohen's Kappa. Kappa values of 0.00–0.20, 0.21–0.40, 0.41–0.60, 0.61–0.80, and 0.81–1.00 represented slight, fair, moderate, substantial, and almost perfect concordance, respectively. These statistical analyses were performed using SPSS®, version 19 (SPSS Inc., Chicago, IL). Improvement of concordance over the course of each period was estimated by the chi-square test for trend using Graph Pad Prism®, version 5.01 (Graph Pad Software, San Diego, CA). A p-value of <0.05 was considered to be significant.

Results

Table 2 shows patient characteristics for each 6-month period. No significant dispersion was noted for age, PSA level, the number of biopsy cores, or GS between the 4 groups using the Kruskal–Wallis test or the chi-square test.

In the first period, the overall concordance rate of urological pathologists and general pathologists was 71.8 % (140/198 samples; Table 3). The urological pathologists diagnosed NM in 103 samples, ASAP in 4 samples, HGPIN in 11 patients, and prostate cancer in 80 samples. For 99 of 103 samples (96.1 %) diagnosed with NM, 1 of 4 samples (25.0 %) diagnosed with ASAP and 9 of 11 samples (81.8 %) with HGPIN, the general and urological pathologists' diagnoses were in agreement. For 38 of these 80 samples (47.5 %), the general and urological pathologists' GS diagnoses were in agreement and the kappa value was 0.55. The general pathologists undergraded 35.1 % (27/80) samples and overgraded 18.1 %

Table 2 Characteristics of patients

	Overall (n = 755)	Apr./06-Sep./06 (n = 197)	Oct./06-Mar./07 (n = 225)	Apr./07-Sep./07 (n = 185)	Oct./07-Mar./08 (n = 148)	p Value
Age (median: yrs)	71 (41–90)	71 (46–94)	72 (41–85)	71 (46–91)	71 (44–90)	0.61[a]
PSA (median: ng/mL)	7.6 (0.3-5490)	7.6 (0.3–475)	7.6 (0.58–196)	7.2 (0.57–5490)	7.7 (1.0–864)	0.52[a]
No. of cores (median)	10 (6–12)	10 (6–12)	10 (6–12)	10 (6–12)	10 (6–12)	0.08[a]
GS 6 (%)	14.6 (n = 110)	17.2 (n = 34)	13.3 (n = 30)	11.9 (n = 22)	16.2 (n = 24)	0.51[b]
GS 3 + 4 (%)	11.1 (n = 84)	9.1 (n = 18)	12.0 (n = 27)	11.4 (n = 27)	8.1 (n = 12)	0.13[b]
GS 4 + 3 (%)	8.1 (n = 61)	5.6 (n = 11)	8.9 (n = 20)	7.0 (n = 13)	11.5 (n = 17)	0.23[b]
GS 8–10 %	6.6 (n = 50)	8.6 (n = 17)	6.2 (n = 14)	5.9 (n = 11)	5.4 (n = 8)	0.64[b]

PSA Prostate specific antigen, *GS* Gleason score
[a]Kruskal-wallis test. [b]chi-square test

(14/80) samples (Table 4). The general pathologists diagnosed 120 patients with NM and 5 patients with ASAP. Nine patients of patients diagnosed with NM and 2 of patients with ASAP by general pathologists were diagnosed with prostate cancer by urological pathologists.

In the second period, the overall concordance rate of urological and general pathologists was 79.8 % (168/225 samples; Table 5). The urological pathologists diagnosed NM in 126 samples, ASAP in 2 samples, HGPIN in 6 patients, and prostate cancer in 91 samples. For 118 of 126 samples (93.7 %) diagnosed with NM, 2 of 2 samples (100 %) diagnosed with ASAP and 1 of 6 samples (16.7 %) with HGPIN, the general and urological pathologists' diagnoses were in agreement. For 57 of these 91 samples (62.6 %), the general and urological pathologists' GS diagnoses were in agreement and the kappa value was 0.68. General pathologists undergraded 23.1 % (21/91) samples and overgraded 14.3 % (13/91) samples (Table 4). The general pathologists diagnosed 125 patients with NM and 13 patients with ASAP. Two

patients of patients diagnosed with NM and 4 of patients with ASAP were diagnosed with prostate cancer by urological pathologists.

In the third period, the overall concordance rate of urological and general pathologists was 89.7 % (166/185; Table 6). The urological pathologists diagnosed NM in 115 samples, ASAP in 1 sample, HGPIN in 2 patients, and prostate cancer in 65 samples. For 115 of 115 samples (100 %) diagnosed with NM, 1 of 1 sample (100 %) diagnosed with ASAP and 0 of 2 samples (0 %) with HGPIN, the general and urological pathologists' diagnoses were in agreement. For 50 out of these 65 samples (76.9 %), the general and urological pathologists' GS diagnoses were in agreement and the kappa value was 0.81. General pathologists undergraded 11.9 % (8/65) samples and overgraded 14.1 % (9/65) samples (Table 4). The general pathologists diagnosed 117 patients with NM and 2 patients with ASAP. No patient of patients diagnosed with NM and 1 of patients with ASAP were diagnosed with prostate cancer by urological pathologists.

Table 3 Concordance of the diagnosis of a needle biopsy between urological and general pathologists (Apr./06- Sep./06)

General pathologist diagnosis	Urological pathologist diagnosis								
	NM	ASAP	HGPIN	5	6	3 + 4	4 + 3	8–10	Overall
NM	99	3	9	0	9	0	0	0	
ASAP	2	1	0	0	2	0	0	0	
HGPIN	1	0	2	0	0	0	0	0	
5	0	0	0	0	2	0	0	0	
6	1	0	0	0	19	10	0	1	
3 + 4	0	0	0	0	1	4	1	2	
4 + 3	0	0	0	0	1	1	2	1	
8–10	0	0	0	0	0	3	8	13	
	103	4	11	0	34	18	11	17	197
% Exact Concordance	96.1	25.0	18.1	0	55.9	22.2	9.1	76.4	71.8
% Undergrading by UPD vs GPD					38.2	55.5	18.1	23.5	35.1
% Overgrading by UPD vs GPD					5.9	22.2	72.7	0	18.1

UPD urological pathologist diagnosis, *GPD* general pathologist diagnosis, *NM* No malignancy, *ASAP* atypical small acinar proliferation suspicious, *HGPIN* high grade prostatic intraepithelial hyperplasia

Table 4 Comparison of concordance of the Gleason score between urological and general pathologists in 4 periods

	% Exact Concordance of GS					% Undergrading by UPD vs GPD	% Overgrading by UPD vs GPD	Kappa score
	Overall	6	3 + 4	4 + 3	8–10			
Apr./06–Sep./06 (n = 80)	47.5 (38/80)	55.9 (19/34)	22.2 (4/18)	9.1 (2/11)	76.4 (13/17)	35.1 (28/80)	18.1 (14/80)	0.55
Oct./06–Mar./07 (n = 91)	62.6 (57/91)	86.7 (26/30)	66.7 (18/27)	25.0 (5/20)	57.1 (8/14)	23.1 (21/91)	14.3 (13/91)	0.68
Apr./07–Sep./07 (n = 65)	76.9 (50/65)	72.3 (16/22)	80.9 (17/21)	53.8 (7/13)	90.9 (10/11)	11.9 (8/65)	14.1 (9/65)	0.81
Oct./07–Mar./08 (n = 61)	78.7 (48/61)	87.5 (21/24)	75.0 (9/12)	70.6 (12/17)	75.0 (6/8)	16.4 (10/61)	4.9 (3/61)	0.84

UPD urological pathologist diagnosis, *GPD* general pathologist diagnosis, *GS* Gleason score

In the last period, the overall concordance rate of urological and general pathologists was 89.9 % (133/148; Table 7). The urological pathologists diagnosed NM in 85 samples, ASAP in 1 sample, HGPIN in 1 sample, and prostate cancer in 61 samples. For 84 of 85 samples (98.8 %) diagnosed with NM, 1 of 1 sample (100 %) diagnosed with ASAP and 0 of 1 samples (0 %) with HGPIN, the general and urological pathologists' diagnoses were in agreement. For 48 of these 61 samples (78.7 %), the general and urological pathologists' GS diagnoses were in agreement and the kappa value was 0.84. General pathologists undergraded 16.4 % (10/61) samples and overgraded 4.9 % (3/61) samples (Table 4). The general pathologists diagnosed 86 patients with NM and 3 patients with ASAP. One patient of patients diagnosed with NM and 1 of patients diagnosed with ASAP were diagnosed with prostate cancer by urological pathologists.

The kappa value increased with time. The concordance rate significantly improved over the course of the study across periods (p = 0.04).

Fifty three patients were diagnosed with prostate cancer by urological pathologists on one positive core and 243 patients diagnosed with prostate cancer on two or more positive cores. Discrepancy between general and urological pathologists was found in 30 patients (56.6 %) of 53 and 76 patients (31.3 %) of 243 (p < 0.01), respectively.

Discussion

Biopsy GS is an important predictor of the likelihood of various final pathological stages of radical retropubic prostatectomy [7], and it is also a significant predictor of biochemical recurrence in patients who undergo radical prostatectomy [16, 17]. Biopsy GS is also associated with biochemical failure in those who have undergone permanent brachytherapy [18] and external beam radiation therapy [19]. Biopsy GS, in combination with PSA level and clinical stage, is a very important factor in decision making for initial therapy. However, several studies have described interobserver variability in Gleason grading [8, 9]. In particular, the variability in Gleason grading between general pathologists should not be overlooked [8, 10]. Burchardt et al. demonstrated that 29 German pathologists who analyzed a series of tissue microarray images showed 45.7 % concordance with biopsy GS assigned by an expert. [20] Coard et al. reported 67 %

Table 5 Concordance of the diagnosis of a needle biopsy between urological and general pathologists (Oct./06–Mar./07)

General pathologist diagnosis	Urological pathologist diagnosis								
	NM	ASAP	HGPIN	5	6	3 + 4	4 + 3	8-10	Overall
NM	118	0	5	0	0	0	0	2	
ASAP	7	2	0	0	0	4	0	0	
HGPIN	0	0	1	0	0	0	0	0	
5	0	0	0	0	0	0	0	0	
6	1	0	0	0	26	3	0	0	
3 + 4	0	0	0	0	4	18	8	1	
4 + 3	0	0	0	0	0	1	5	3	
8-10	0	0	0	0	0	1	7	8	
	126	2	6	0	30	27	20	14	225
% Exact Concordance	93.6	100	16.7	0	86.7	66.7	25.0	57.1	79.1
% Undergrading by UPD vs GPD					0	25.9	40.0	42.9	23.1
% Overgrading by UPD vs GPD					13.3	7.4	35.0	0	14.3

UPD urological pathologist diagnosis, *GPD* General pathologist diagnosis, *NM* no malignancy, *ASAP* atypical small acinar proliferation suspicious, *HGPIN* high grade prostatic intraepithelial hyperplasia

Table 6 Concordance of the diagnosis of a needle biopsy between urological and general pathologists (Apr./07–Sep./07)

General pathologist diagnosis	Urological pathologist diagnosis								
	NM	ASAP	HGPIN	5	6	3 + 4	4 + 3	8–10	Overall
NM	115	0	2	0	0	0	0	0	
ASAP	0	1	0	0	1	0	0	0	
HGPIN	0	0	0	0	0	0	0	0	
5	0	0	0	0	0	0	0	0	
6	0	0	0	0	16	3	1	0	
3 + 4	0	0	0	0	5	17	2	0	
4 + 3	0	0	0	0	0	1	7	1	
8–10	0	0	0	0	0	0	3	10	
	115	1	2	0	22	21	13	11	185
% Exact Concordance	100	100	0	0	72.3	80.9	53.8	90.9	89.7
% Undergrading by UPD vs GPD					4.5	14.3	23.1	9.1	11.9
% Overgrading by UPD vs GPD					22.7	4.8	23.1	0	14.1

UPD urological pathologist diagnosis, *GPD* general pathologist diagnosis, *NM* no malignancy, *ASAP* atypical small acinar proliferation suspicious, *HGPIN* High grade prostatic intraepithelial hyperplasia

overall concordance between anatomical pathologists and an experienced pathologist for consensus on prostate cancer GS [10]. In the present study, the overall concordance between general pathologists and the urological pathologists was 47.5 % and the kappa score was 0.55 in the first 6-month period. This was not an acceptable concordance and was similar to the results of previous studies. These discrepancies may have been caused by (1) a sampling effect caused by tumor heterogeneity, (2) interpretational bias, or (3) the small volume of tissue for cancer biopsy [10, 21]. In the present study, patients who diagnosed with prostate cancer on one positive core tended to be misdiagnosed compared to those who diagnosed on two or more cores and another reason for

discordance may have been that the general pathologists did not refer to the 2005 ISUP consensus conference on the Gleason grading of Prostatic Carcinoma [11].

To improve this discrepancy, Mikami et al [22] used a 40-min educational lecture or a tutorial with an anatomical atlas. In a lecture group, the average concordance rates before and after the lecture were 55.7 % and 68.4 %, and the average kappa values were 0.43 and 0.67, respectively. In the atlas group, the average concordance rates before and after providing the atlas were 61.3 % and 74.5 %, and the average kappa values were 0.44 and 0.68, respectively. Allsbrook et al [8] reported that concordance between general pathologists and urological pathologists improved to 77.4 % (kappa value = 0.73) by

Table 7 Concordance of the diagnosis of a needle biopsy between urological and general pathologists (Oct./07–Mar./08)

General pathologist diagnosis	Urological pathologist diagnosis								
	NM	ASAP	HGPIN	5	6	3 + 4	4 + 3	8–10	Overall
NM	84	0	1	0	1	0	0	0	
ASAP	1	1	0	0	1	0	0	0	
HGPIN	0	0	0	0	0	0	0	0	
5	0	0	0	0	0	0	0	0	
6	0	0	0	0	21	3	0	0	
3 + 4	0	0	0	0	1	9	3	0	
4 + 3	0	0	0	0	0	0	12	2	
8–10	0	0	0	0	0	0	2	6	
	85	1	1	0	24	12	17	8	148
% Exact concordance	98.8	100	0	0	87.5	75.0	70.6	75.0	89.9
% Undergrading by UPD vs GPD					8.3	25.0	17.6	25.0	16.4
% Overgrading by UPD vs GPD					4.2	0	11.8	0	4.9

UPD Urological pathologist diagnosis, *GPD* General pathologist diagnosis, *NM* No malignancy, *ASAP* atypical small acinar proliferation suspicious, *HGPIN* High grade prostatic intraepithelial hyperplasia

web-based virtual microscopy. In Egevad's study, the proportion of correct GS improved from 70.5 % to 86.6 % after a teaching set of 40 images illustrating GS was distributed among 85 pathologists [23]. The present study demonstrated an improvement in the accuracy of general pathologists' GS after review by 2 urological pathologist. The rate of agreement and the kappa value increased with the period and improved from an initial 47.5 % (kappa score = 0.55) to a final 80.3 % (kappa value = 0.84). Furthermore in the third period, the rate of concordance was high and the high rate continued in the last period. So the appropriate time of this method for improving GS may need one year by our way.

It is well known that general pathologists tend to underestimate GS [8, 10, 20, 24]. Coard et al. reported that anatomical pathologists undergraded 25.6 % of all biopsy specimens and overgraded 6.7 % [10], whereas Burchardt et al. reported that the rates of undergrading and overgrading were 38.9 % and 15.4 %, respectively [20]. Similar to our reports, Barqawi et al. evaluated defference between outside pathologists and their institution pathologists and Gleason undergrading occurred in 46 % outside and 38 % their institution diagnosis with respect to radical prostatectomy specimens [24]. The corresponding values in the first period in the present study were 35.1 % and 18.1 %, respectively, showing that general pathologists tended to undergrade as in other reports. Undergrading was particularly common for tumors with a GS of 6 and 3 + 4 in our study. Allsbrook et al. found 47 % undergrading of tumors with GS 5–6, and 43 % undergrading of tumors with GS 7 [8]. In the present study, the undergrading of GS in 7 samples most probably resulted from mistaking Gleason pattern 4 for pattern 3, and the undergrading of GS in 6 tumors most probably resulted from mistaking pattern 3 for pattern 2. This is in accordance with the studies of Allsbrook et al. [8], Burchardt et al. [20], and Mikami et al. [22] Thus, there is a tendency for general pathologists to underestimate GS, especially in Gleason patterns 3 and 4.

However, the rate of undergrading decreased to 16.4 % in the last period after general pathologists had the experienced of review by the urological pathologists in the present study. Mikami et al. reported an improvement in the rate of undergrading from 36.3 % to 14.2 % after a lecture [22]. Egevad reported improvement of undergrading by the use of reference images [23]. It shows that the tendency for general pathologists to undergrade can improve when they study GS patterns using any of the common methods. Particular improvement in undergrading among general pathologists can be expected by preventing mistakes in identifying Gleason pattern 3 for pattern 2 and pattern 4 for pattern 3.

20 patients who diagnosed with NM and ASAP by general urologists were diagnosed with prostate cancer by urological patients. This discrepancy could be fatal. This discrepancy improved with time, 17/263 (6.5 %) in first and second period to 3/208 (1.4 %) in third and fourth period in the presents study ($p = 0.01$, chi-square test). Furthermore in 14 cases (70 %) the positive core was one. These result showed the discrepancy was caused by small cancer volume and interpretative error.

A limitation of this study was the inability to isolate the general pathologists from other educational sources associated with Gleason scoring over a period of 2 years. Therefore, any improvement seen may not necessarily be a direct result of the experience of the review by the urological pathologists.

Conclusion

The concordance rate of GS between the urological and general pathologists was initially low (47.5 %), but following the expert reviews there was a significantly improvement in concordance rate over time.

Abbreviations
ASAP: Atypical small acinar proliferation; GS: Gleason score, HGPIN, High grade prostatic intraepithelial neoplasia; ISUP: International Society of Urological Pathology; NM: No malignancy; PSA: Prostate-specific antigen.

Competing interests
The authors declare that they have no competing interests.

Authors' contributions
YN analysed and interpreted the data, and drafted the manuscript. NT conceived of the study and revised this manuscript. KS participated in this study as a urological pathologist and helped to carry out this study. NK participated in this study as a urological pathologist and provided valuable help on the study. MM and SA provided valuable help on the experiments. KF participated in its design and gave final approval of the version to be published. All authors read and approved the final manuscript.

Acknowledgements
We are very grateful to Shuji Watanabe (Saiseikai Chuwa Hospital), Yoshinori Nakagawa (Yamato Takada Municipal Hospital) and Shuya Hirao (Hirao Hospital) for their valuable cooperation in our study.

Author details
[1]Department of Urology, Nara Medical University, 840 Shijo-cho, Kashihara, Nara 634-8522, Japan. [2]Department of Pathology, Nara Medical University, 840 Shijo-cho, Kashihara, Nara 634-8522, Japan.

References
1. Gleason DF. Classification of prostatic carcinoma. Cancer Chemother Rep. 1966;50:125.
2. Gleason DF, Mellinger GT. Prediction of prognosis for prostatic adenocarcinoma by combined histological grading and clinical staging. J Urol. 1974;111:58.
3. Gleason DF. Histologic grading and clinical staging of prostatic carcinoma. In: Tannenbaum M, editor. Urologic Pathology: The Prostate. Philadelphia: Lea and Febiger; 1977. p. 171.
4. Japanese Urological Association and the Japanese Society of Pathology, editor. General rule for clinical and pathological studies on prostate cancer. 3rd ed. Tokyo: Kanahara-Shuppan; 2001.
5. Oesterling JE, Brendler CB, Epstein JI, Kimball AW Jr, Walsh PC. Correlation of clinical stage, serum prostatic acid phosphatase and preoperative Gleason grade with final pathological stage in 275 patients with clinically localized adenocarcinoma of the prostate. J Urol. 1987;38:92.

6. Epstein JI, Pizov G, Walsh PC. Correlation of pathologic findings with progression after radical retropubic prostatectomy. Cancer. 1993;71:3582.

7. Partin AW, Mangold LA, Lamm DM, Walsh PC, Epstein JI, Pearson JD. Contemporary update of prostate cancer staging nomograms (Partin Tables) for the new millennium. Urology. 2001;58:843.

8. Allsbrook WC Jr, Mangold KA, Johnson MH, Lane RB, Lane CG, Amin MB et al. Interobserver reproducibility of Gleason grading of prostatic carcinoma: urologic pathologists. Hum Pathol. 2001;32:74.

9. McLean M, Srigley J, Banerjee D, Warde P, Hao Y. Interobserver variation in prostate cancer Gleason scoring: are there implications for the design of clinical trials and treatment strategies? Clin Oncol (R Coll Radiol). 1997;9:222.

10. Coard KC, Freeman VL. Gleason grading of prostate cancer: level of concordance between pathologists at the University Hospital of the West Indies. Am J Clin Patol. 2004;122:373.

11. Epstein JI, Allsbrook WC Jr, Amin MB, Egevad LL.The 2005 International Society of Urological Pathology (ISUP) Consensus Conference on Gleason Grading of Prostatic Carcinoma. Am J Surg Pathol. 2005;29:1228.

12. Billis A, Quintal MM, Meirelles L, Freitas LL, Costa LB, Bonfitto JF, et al. The value of the 2005 International Society of Urological Pathology (ISUP) modified Gleason grading system as a predictor of biochemical recurrence after radical prostatectomy. Int Urol Nephrol. 2014;46:935.

13. Dong F, Wang C, Farris AB, Wu S, Lee H, Olumi AF, et al. Impact on the clinical outcome of prostate cancer by the 2005 international society of urological pathology modified Gleason grading system. Am J Surg Pathol. 2012;36:838.

14. Ito K, Ohi M, Yamamoto T, Miyamoto S, Kurokawa K, Fukabori Y, et al.The diagnostic accuracy of the age-adjusted and prostate volume-adjusted biopsy method in males with proatate specific antigen levels of 4.1-10.0 ng/mL. Cancer. 2002;95:2112.

15. Tanaka N1, Fujimoto K, Yoshikawa M, Tanaka M, Hirao Y, Kondo H, et al. Prostatic volume and volume-adjusted prostate-specific antigen as predictive parameters for T1c prostatecancer. Hinyokika kiyo. 2007;53:459.

16. Han M, Partin AW, Zahurak M, Piantadosi S, Epstein JI, Walsh PC. Biochemical (prostate specific antigen) recurrence probability following radical prostatectomy for clinically localized prostate cancer. J Urol. 2003;169:517.

17. Tanaka N, Fujimoto K, Hirayama A, Torimoto K, Okajima E, Tanaka M, et al. Risk-stratified survival rates and predictors of biochemical recurrence after radical prostatectomy in a Nara, Japan, cohort study. Int J Clin Oncol. 2011;16:553.

18. Potters L, Purrazzella R, Brustein S, Fearn P, Huang D, Leibel SA, et al. The prognostic significance of Gleason grade in patients treated with permanent prostate brachytherapy. Int J Radiat Oncol Boil Phys. 2003;56:749.

19. Sabolch A1, Feng FY, Daignault-Newton S, Halverson S, Blas K, Phelps L, et al. Gleason pattern 5 is the greatest risk factor for clinical failure and death from prostate cancer after dose-escalated radiation therapy and hormonal ablation. Int J Radiat Oncol Boil Phys. 2011;81:e351.

20. Burchardt M, Engers R, Müller M, Burchardt T, Willers R, Epstein JI, et al. Interobserver reproducibility of Gleason grading: evaluation using prostate cancer tissue microarrays. J cancer Res Clin Oncol. 2008;134:1071.

21. King CR, McNeal JE, Gill H, Presti JC Jr. Extended prostate biopsy scheme improves reliability of Gleason grading: implications for radiotherapy patients. Int J Radiat Oncol Biol Phys. 2004;59:386.

22. Mikami Y, Manabe T, Epstein JI, Shiraishi T, Furusato M, Tsuzuki T, et al. Accuracy of Gleason grading by practicing pathologists and the impact of education on improving agreement. Hum Pathol. 2003;34:658.

23. Egevad L. Reproducibility of Gleason grading of prostate cancer can be improved by the use of reference images. Urology. 2001;57:291.

24. Barqawi AB, Turcanu R, Gamito EJ, Lucia SM, O'Donnell CI, Crawford ED, et al. The value of second-opinion pathology diagnosis on prostate biopsies from patients reffered for management of prostate cancer. Int J Clin Exp Pathol. 2011;4:468–75.

31

Increased risk for urological cancer associated with anxiety disorder

Yung-Chan Chen[1], Li-Ting Kao[2], Herng-Ching Lin[3], Hsin-Chien Lee[1,3,4], Chung-Chien Huang[5†]
and Shiu-Dong Chung[3,6,7,8*†]

Abstract

Background: Anxiety disorders (ADs) are common with a high rate of medical comorbidities. Although the association between ADs and the overall cancer risk remains controversial, patients with ADs were found to be more likely to develop specific cancer types. Herein, we estimated the risk of developing urological cancers among patients with ADs in a 5-year follow-up period using a population-based database.

Methods: Two study cohorts were identified from the Taiwan Longitudinal Health Insurance Database 2005: patients with ADs, and comparison subjects selected by one-to-one matching for sex, age, and the year of recruitment. Follow-up was undertaken to determine whether sampled patients and comparison subjects had developed urological cancers in the subsequent 5 years.

Results: We found that urological cancers occurred among 0.54% of patients with ADs and 0.13% of comparison subjects. After adjusting for sociodemographic characteristics, medical comorbidities, and alcohol and tobacco use disorder, the stratified Cox proportional hazard regression suggested that patients with ADs were more likely to develop urological cancers relative to comparison subjects (adjusted hazard ratio, 3.67; 95% confidence interval, 2. 85 ~ 4.72). The adjusted HR for males with ADs was 3.82 (95% CI: 2.79 ~ 5.23) in comparison to males without ADs. In addition, the adjusted HR for females with ADs was 3.47 (95% CI: 2.26 ~ 5.31) than those females without ADs.

Conclusions: We concluded that during the 5-year follow-up period, there was a significantly increased risk of urological cancers among patients with ADs.

Keyword: Anxiety disorder, Urological cancer, Bladder cancer, Epidemiology

Background

Anxiety disorders (ADs), including panic disorder, generalized anxiety disorder, phobic disorder and so on, are common mental disorders within a disease category characterized by excessive worry which might affect 9.2% ~ 28.7% of the general population around the world [1, 2]. The prevalence of ADs is not only high but also strikingly increasing in Asian populations [3, 4].

ADs are shown to markedly compromise the quality of life and psychosocial functioning in several domains [5].

ADs are highly comorbid with numerous chronic medical illness including diabetes, coronary artery disease, congestive heart failure, asthma, chronic obstructive pulmonary disease, and arthritis [6, 7]. Thus, the research focus has gradually turned to the relationship between ADs and malignancies. Indeed, psychological distress was proven to have an adverse effect on cancer survival [8, 9].

Nevertheless, it is still controversial and unclear whether the existence of ADs is associated with the subsequent occurrence of cancer [8, 10–13]. Patients with ADs were found to be at increased risks of developing specific cancer types including lung, brain, and prostate cancers [11–13]. Although the underlying mechanism remains obscure, indirect relationships through a

* Correspondence: chungshiudong@gmail.com
†Equal contributors
[3]Sleep Research Center, Taipei Medical University, Taipei, Taiwan
[6]Division of Urology, Department of Surgery, Far Eastern Memorial Hospital, New Taipei City, Taiwan
Full list of author information is available at the end of the article

surveillance bias and unhealthy lifestyle behaviors were proposed to interpret this association [12, 13]. It is debatable whether these factors could contribute to the overall cancer risk instead of to certain cancer types such as prostate and other urological cancers found in previous studies.

It is possible that the weak, though significant, association seen in previous studies lends support to a direct relationship between ADs and urological cancers. Even so, there is evidence that dysfunction of the serotonin receptor pathway, crucial in anxiety disorders, might also be involved in the proliferation of urological cancer [14, 15]. This could pose a threat to both a patient's mental and physical health. Considering the biological plausibility, this study aimed to investigate the relationship between ADs and the subsequent occurrence of urological cancers using a longitudinal population-based database.

Methods

Database

The data for this retrospective cohort study were sourced from the Taiwan Longitudinal Health Insurance Database 2005 (LHID2005). The LHID2005, compiled by the Taiwan National Health Research Institute, consists of original medical claims data for 1,000,000 individuals randomly sampled from all enrollees ($n = 25.68$ million) in the Taiwan National Health Insurance (NHI) program in 2005. Since around 96% of the Taiwanese population enrolled in the NHI program, the LHID2005 provides an exclusive opportunity for researchers to follow-up the use of all medical services for nationwide, population-based sampled subjects. Hundreds of studies utilizing this dataset have been published in internationally peer-reviewed journals [16].

This study was exempt from full review by the Institutional Review Board of National Defense Medical Center since the LHID2005 consists of de-identified secondary data released to the public for research purposes.

Study sample

This study features a study cohort and a comparison cohort. The study cohort included all patients who had received one of the following ADs diagnoses between January 1, 2001 and December 31, 2008: panic disorder (ICD-9-CM: 300.01), generalized anxiety disorder (ICD-9-CM: 300.02), phobic disorder (ICD-9-CM: 300.2, 300.20 ~ 300.29), obsessive-compulsive disorder (ICD-9-CM: 300.3) and acute stress reaction & post-traumatic stress disorder (ICD-9-CM: 308, 309.81 ~ 309.83) ($n = 143,329$). In order to increase the diagnosis validity, this study only included patients with ADs who received at least two anxiety disorder diagnoses with at least one diagnosis having been made by a board-certified psychiatrist ($n = 71,065$). We assigned the date of the second

medical service utilization for ADs during the recruitment period as the index date. We then excluded patients aged under 18 years ($n = 1,961$) in order to limit the study to the adult population. Additionally, subjects who had a history of major psychiatric disorders or a substance-related disorder (ICD-9-CM codes 290 ~ 299 or 303 ~ 305) ($n = 3,236$) were excluded in order to exclude possible confounding effects of other mental illnesses on the association between ADs and urological cancers. We further excluded those subjects who were diagnosed with any type of cancer (ICD-9-CM codes 140 ~ 239) prior to the index date ($n = 7,265$). As a result, 58,603 subjects with ADs were included in the study cohort. The selection procedures were shown in Fig. 1.

We likewise extracted the comparison cohort from the LHID2005. We randomly selected one comparison subject for every study subject, matched by sex, age (18 ~ 30, 30 ~ 39, 40 ~ 49, 50 ~ 59, 60 ~ 69, and >69 years), and index year. While for the study cohort, the year of the index date was the year in which the study subjects received their first diagnosis of ADs, for the comparison

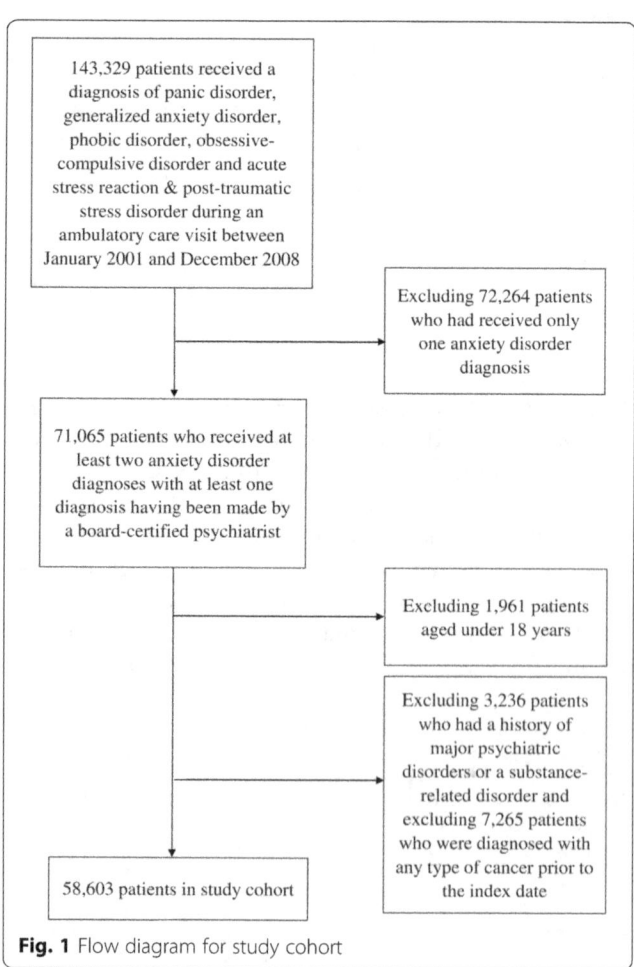

Fig. 1 Flow diagram for study cohort

cohort, the year of the index date was simply a matched year in which comparison subjects had a medical utilization. We assigned the date of their first use of medical services occurring during that matched year as the index date for the comparison cohort. We ensured that no selected comparison subjects had ever received a diagnosis of ADs since initiation of the Taiwan NHI program in 1995. We also assured that no selected comparison subjects had ever received a diagnosis of major psychiatric disorders, substance-related disorder, or any type of cancer prior to the index date.

Thereafter, each patient in the study ($n = 117,206$) was individually tracked for a 5-year period from their index date to identify whether or not they had received a diagnosis of urological cancer (ICD-9-CM code185 ~ 189). The diagnoses of urological cancers have been confirmed by the registry of catastrophic illness. For the occurrence of cancer to be reported in the registry, histological confirmation is required.

Statistical analysis

All statistical analyses were performed by the SAS statistical package (SAS System for Windows, vers. 8.2, Cary, NC, USA). We used the Kaplan-Meier method to estimate the 5-year cancer-free survival rate and the log-rank test to examine differences in the risks of urological cancer xbetween these two cohorts. We used stratified Cox proportional hazard regressions, stratified by sex, age group, and index year to calculate the cancer hazard for the study cohort relative to the comparison cohort. We adjusted for demographic and socioeconomic characteristics, medical comorbidities, and alcohol and tobacco use in the regression model. The variables of socioeconomic characteristics included monthly income (New Taiwan (NT)\$0 ~ 15,840, NT\$15,841 ~ 25,000, ≥NT\$25,001; the average exchange rate in 2011 was US\$1 ≈ NT\$29), geographical location (northern, central, eastern, and southern Taiwan), and urbanization level of each subject's residence (5 levels, with 1 indicating the most urbanized and 5 the least urbanized). NT\$15,840 was used as the first cut-off value as it is the government-stipulated minimum wage for full-time employees in Taiwan. Medical comorbidities selected in this study were hypertension, diabetes, obesity, alcohol abuse, and tobacco use disorder. All medical comorbidities were defined by using ICD-9-CM codes in LHID2005. In addition, we censored subjects who died from non-cancer causes during the 5-year follow-up period in the regression model. Of the sampled subjects, 3749 died from non-cancer causes, including 2051 from the study cohort (3.5% of study cohort) and 1698 from the comparison cohort (2.9% of the comparison cohort). The differences were considered significant with a two-sided p value of ≤0.05.

Results

Of the 117,206 study subjects, the mean age was 51.0 years (standard deviation, 16.5 years), while they were 51.1 years for the study cohort and 50.9 years for the comparison cohort ($p = 0.209$). Table 1 shows the demographic and socioeconomic characteristics of subjects with and without ADs. The overwhelming majority (61.8%) of study subjects were female, and over half were aged <50 years (about 57%). There were significant differences between the study and comparison cohorts in terms of monthly

Table 1 Subjects with anxiety disorder and a comparison group in relation to sociodemographic characteristics and medical comorbidities in Taiwan ($n = 117,206$)

Variable	Patients with anxiety disorder $n = 58,603$		Comparison cohort $n = 58,603$		p value
	No.	Percent	No.	Percent	
Sex					1.000
Male	22,394	38.2	22,394	38.2	
Female	36,209	61.8	36,209	61.8	
Age (years)					1.000
<40	19,722	33.8	19,722	33.8	
40 ~ 49	13,269	22.7	13,269	22.7	
50 ~ 59	10,654	18.2	10,654	18.2	
60 ~ 69	7,405	12.7	7,405	12.7	
>69	7,323	12.6	7,323	12.6	
Monthly income					<0.001
≤NT\$15,840	24,159	41.2	23,299	39.8	
NT\$15,841 ~ 25,000	22,503	38.4	22,108	37.7	
≥NT\$25,001	11,941	20.4	13,196	22.5	
Geographic region					<0.001
Northern	25,542	43.6	27,622	47.1	
Central	16,292	27.8	13,642	23.3	
Southern	15,574	26.6	15,797	27.0	
Eastern	1,195	2.0	1,542	2.6	
Urbanization level					<0.001
1 (most urbanized)	16,858	28.8	17,685	30.2	
2	16,235	27.7	16,224	27.7	
3	8,593	14.7	9,509	16.2	
4	9,217	15.7	8,288	14.1	
5 (least urbanized)	7,700	13.1	6,897	11.8	
Obesity	670	1.1	390	0.7	<0.001
Alcohol abuse/ alcohol dependence syndrome	790	1.4	69	0.1	<0.001
Tobacco use disorder	1,497	2.6	355	0.6	<0.001
Diabetes	6,611	11.3	5,483	9.4	<0.001
Hypertension	18,871	32.2	12,041	20.6	<0.001

Note: In 2011, the average exchange rate was US\$1 ≈ New Taiwan (NT) \$29

income, geographical location, and urbanization level of each subject's residence. In addition, subjects with ADs had a higher prevalence of medical comorbidities of hypertension, diabetes, obesity, and alcohol and tobacco use problems than subjects without ADs (all $p < 0.001$).

Table 2 presents the incidence rate for a new urological cancer diagnosis by cohort within the 5-year follow-up period. Of the 117,206 subjects, 391 (0.33%) received a diagnosis of urological cancer: 315 in the study cohort (0.54% of the subjects with anxiety disorder) and 76 in the comparison cohort (0.13% of subjects without anxiety disorder). The incidence rates of urological cancers during the 5-year follow-up period were 10.93 (9.76 ~ 12.21) per 10,000 person-years for the study cohort and 2.62 (2.07 ~ 3.28) per 10,000 person-years for the comparison cohort. The log-rank test revealed that subjects with ADs had a significantly lower 5-year urological cancer-free survival rate than comparison subjects ($p = 0.005$). Figure 2 presents results of the Kaplan-Meier survival analysis.

Results of the stratified Cox proportional regressions (stratified on sex, age group, and index year) are also presented in Table 2. The crude hazard ratio (HR) for urological cancer during the 5-year follow-up period for the study cohort was 4.16 (95% confidence interval (CI): 3.23 ~ 5.34) with respect to the comparison cohort. After adjusting for urbanization level, monthly income, geographic region, hypertension, diabetes, obesity, and alcohol and tobacco use, and censoring cases that died from non-cancer causes, the HR for urological cancer during the 5-year follow-up period for study cohort was 3.67 (95% CI: 2.85 ~ 4.72) that of comparison patients.

Table 3 presents the proportional HRs of subgroups classified by the type of urological cancers (kidney cancer, bladder cancer, prostate cancer, and others). The adjusted HRs for kidney cancer, bladder cancer, prostate cancer, and others for subjects with ADs were 2.84 (95% CI: 1.73 ~ 4.66), 2.94 (95% CI: 1.89 ~ 4.58), 4.67 (95% CI: 3.06 ~ 7.12), and 6.75 (95% CI: 2.01 ~ 22.69), respectively, relative to those without ADs.

The incidences of urological cancers within 5 years after the index date between patients with ADs and those without ADs stratified by sex are presented in Table 4. The adjusted HR for males with ADs was 3.82 (95% CI: 2.79 ~ 5.23) in comparison to males without ADs. In addition, the adjusted HR for females with ADs was 3.47 (95% CI: 2.26 ~ 5.31) than those females without ADs.

Discussion

A relationship exists between ADs and the subsequent occurrence of urological cancers, as suggested by the results herein. The findings of this study were consistent with previous reports [12, 13]. Shen and colleagues reported that male patients with generalized ADs had an increased standardized incidence ratio (SIR) for prostate cancer (2.17, 95% CI: 1.56 ~ 2.93) [13]. Since the prevalence of ADs in the general population is substantial, the observed SIR may introduce bias and cause underestimation of the true relative risk [17]. Another study by Liang and colleagues only demonstrated an increased risk of developing prostate cancer among patients with ADs older than 65 years [12]. The failure to exclude comorbid psychiatric disorders made the study group more heterogeneous which could have biased the results toward zero.

Both studies argued that the higher risk of prostate cancer could be partially explained by a surveillance bias. Patients with ADs were likely to search for medical help and thus might have received more imaging and laboratory examinations [6, 7, 18]. If true, the overall risk of cancer should also increase among patients with ADs, which was not supported by previous study results. Patients with ADs have more urological complaints [19, 20]. Liang and colleagues further validated their assumption regarding a surveillance bias by showing a higher prostate-specific antigen (PSA) screening rate among patients with ADs [12]. However, the proposed explanation is difficult to apply to the significantly increased risks of urological cancers other than prostate cancer among patients with ADs.

Another explanation stems from unhealthy lifestyles and medication use among patients with ADs. Patients with ADs tend to be overweight and physically inactive and are more likely to use alcohol and tobacco [21, 22].

Table 2 Hazard ratios (HRs) and 95% confidence intervals (CIs) of urological cancer among sampled subjects during the 5-year follow-up period from the index date

Presence of urological cancer	Total sample $n = 117,206$		Patients with anxiety disorder $n = 58,603$		Comparison cohort $n = 58,603$	
	No.	Percent	No.	Percent	No.	Percent
Yes	391 (0.33)		315 (0.54)		76 (0.13)	
Incidence rate per 10,000 person-years (95% CI)	6.76 (6.11 ~ 7.47)		10.93 (9.76 ~ 12.21)		2.62 (2.07 ~ 3.28)	
Crude HR [a](95% CI)	–		4.16*** (3.23 ~ 5.34)		1.00	
Adjusted HR[b] (95% CI)	–		3.67*** (2.85 ~ 4.72)		1.00	

Notes: [a]Stratified Cox proportional regression stratified on patients' sex, age group, and index year. [b]Adjusted for patients' monthly income, urbanization level, geographic region, hypertension, diabetes, obesity, tobacco use disorder, and alcohol abuse/alcohol dependence syndrome
***$p < 0.001$

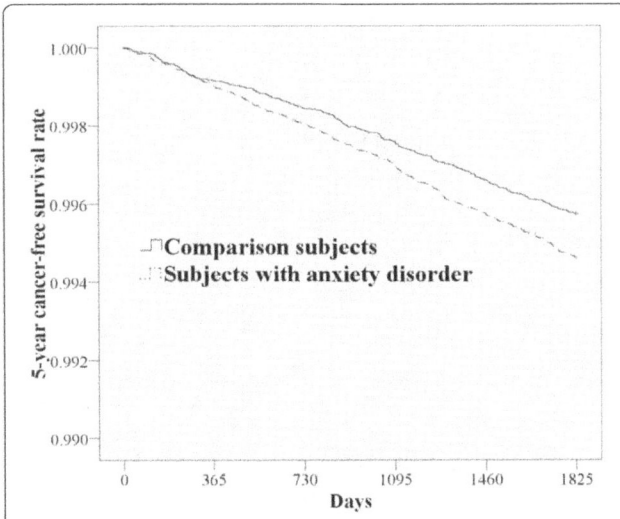

Fig. 2 Urological cancer-free survival rates for subjects with anxiety disorder and comparison subjects

In addition, a stress-prone personality and unfavorable coping styles commonly seen among patients with ADs might place them at a higher cancer risk [8]. Even so, the overall cancer risks were not consistently high in previous studies [11, 12].

In an earlier comprehensive review of the relationship between lifestyle issues and urological cancers, only strong connections of tobacco use with bladder and renal cancers were repeatedly supported by the literature [23]. Other lifestyle risk factors, if they existed, had only modest impacts on the development of urological malignancies. Furthermore, patients with ADs remained at a significantly high risk of developing all kinds of urological cancers after adjusting for tobacco use disorder in this study.

The long-term use of psychotropic medications, particularly benzodiazepine anxiolytics, is prevalent among patients with ADs. However, study results of the carcinogenic potential of benzodiazepine anxiolytics remain equivocal [24, 25]. Kao and colleagues reported that patients with a history of taking benzodiazepine were more likely to develop prostate and bladder/kidney cancers with respective HRs of 1.72 and 1.76 [24]. There is still no specific mechanisms or explanations which account for the observed increased risk, and their findings were challenged for failing to control numerous confounding factors [26].

The current study demonstrated that patients with ADs were more likely to develop prostate cancer after adjusting for available demographic, socioeconomic, and comorbid medical and substance use variables. A direct mechanism linking ADs itself to urological cancers should not be neglected.

As stated before, stress-related psychosocial factors can have adverse effects on cancer incidence and survival by disturbing functions of the immune system, thus enhancing the risk of carcinogenesis [27]. Lines of evidence

Table 3 Hazard ratios (HRs) and 95% confidence intervals (CIs) of urological cancer among sampled subjects during the 5-year follow-up period from the index date according to the type of urological cancer

Presence of urological cancer	Patients with anxiety disorder $n = 58,603$		Comparison cohort $n = 58,603$	
	No.	Percent	No.	Percent
Kidney cancer				
Yes	67 (0.11)		21 (0.04)	
Incidence rate per 100,000 person-years (95% CI)	23.20 (17.98 ~ 29.47)		7.24 (4.48 ~ 11.07)	
Adjusted HR[a,b] (95% CI)	2.84*** (1.73 ~ 4.66)		1.00	
Bladder cancer				
Yes	88 (0.15)		26 (0.04)	
Incidence rate per 100,000 person-years (95% CI)	30.48 (24.45 ~ 37.55)		8.97 (5.86 ~ 13.14)	
Adjusted HR[a,b] (95% CI)	2.94*** (1.89 ~ 4.58)		1.00	
Prostate cancer (men only)				
Yes	138 (0.62)		26 (0.12)	
Incidence rate per 10,000 person-years (95% CI)	12.53 (10.53 ~ 14.81)		2.35 (1.53 ~ 3.44)	
Adjusted HR[a,b] (95% CI)	4.67*** (3.06 ~ 7.12)		1.00	
Others				
Yes	22 (0.04)		3 (0.01)	
Incidence rate per 100,000 person-years (95% CI)	7.62 (4.77 ~ 11.53)		1.04 (0.21 ~ 3.02)	
Adjusted HR[a,b] (95% CI)	6.75** (2.01 ~ 22.69)		1.00	

Notes: [a]Stratified Cox proportional regression stratified on patients' sex, age group, and index year. [b] Adjusted for patients' monthly income, urbanization level, geographic region, hypertension, diabetes, obesity, tobacco use disorder, and alcohol abuse/alcohol dependence syndrome
**$p < 0.01$, ***$p < 0.001$

Table 4 Hazard ratios (HRs) and 95% confidence intervals (CIs) of urological cancer among sampled subjects during the 5-year follow-up period from the index date according to sex

Presence of urological cancer	Males				Females			
	Patients with anxiety disorder (n = 22,394)		Comparison cohort (n = 22,394)		Patients with anxiety disorder (n = 36,209)		Comparison cohort (n = 36,209)	
	No.	Percent	No.	Percent	No.	Percent	No.	Percent
Yes	209 (0.93)		49 (0.22)		106 (0.29)		27 (0.07)	
Incidence rate per 10,000 person-years (95% CI)	19.01 (16.52 ~ 21.77)		4.43 (3.27 ~ 5.85)		5.95 (4.87 ~ 7.19)		1.51 (0.99 ~ 2.19)	
Crude HR[a] (95% CI)	4.28*** (3.14 ~ 5.85)		1.00		3.93*** (2.58 ~ 6.00)		1.00	
Adjusted HR[b] (95% CI)	3.82*** (2.79 ~ 5.23)		1.00		3.47*** (2.26 ~ 5.31)		1.00	

Notes: [a]Stratified Cox proportional regression stratified on patients' age group and index year
[b]Adjusted for patients' monthly income, urbanization level, geographic region, hypertension, diabetes, obesity, tobacco use disorder, and alcohol abuse/alcohol dependence syndrome. ***$p < 0.001$

suggest that persistent activation of the hypothalamic-pituitary-adrenal (HPA) axis can alter the function of the neuroendocrine system, disrupt the circadian glucocorticoid rhythm, and thus promote tumor initiation and progression [28–31]. More specifically, stress-related neurotransmitters such as serotonin were proposed as being correlated with the progression of urological cancers [32, 33].

As an important monoamine neurotransmitter in the brain, serotonin plays a crucial role in the neurobiological processing of anxiety. Dysregulation of serotonin is strongly associated with the development of ADs [34]. Serotonin also serves as a messenger that controls several processes of the body including carcinogenesis. Siddiqui and colleague found that serotonin could increase the proliferation of bladder cancer cells in vitro in a dose-dependent manner and could modify the growth inhibitory effect of doxazosin on prostate and bladder cancer cells [15, 35]. Based on relevant findings, serotonin was proposed to be a prognostic marker for urological cancer [36]. Although the majority of previous studies were conducted in vitro and clinical applications remain controversial [37]. We argue that dysregulation of the serotonin receptor pathway might contribute to the relationship between ADs and urological cancers.

Lines of evidence support that traumatic experience may alter core physiological systems and even cause carcinogenesis through DNA breakage [38]. Traumatic experience, even early childhood maltreatment, may increase the risk of ADs [39]. On the other hand, effective treatment such as psychotherapy could reverse DNA damage [40]. There could be a remote and common cause for both ADs and urological cancers. The strength of this study comes from it utilizing a large, population-based sample. Still, the results should be interpreted in light of potential methodological limitations. First of all, the use of non-standardized diagnoses made by different physicians is an inherent problem with population-based studies. By restricting our analyses to two visits with a diagnosis of

ADs with at least one having been made by a board-certified psychiatrist, we enhanced the specificity of the psychiatric diagnoses. Further, we chose a broad approach to a diagnosis of ADs in order to reduce misclassification. Second, information about certain risk factors for urological cancer including environmental exposure, amount of tobacco and alcohol use, body mass index and family cancer history is not available in the database. Information on traumatic events and critical life events is also unavailable. We adjusted for the geographical location and urbanization level of each subject's residence in the study. The diagnoses of tobacco and alcohol use disorders, which represent the most severe form of tobacco and alcohol use, were also considered in our analyses. In addition, the LHID2005 provides no information about serotonin levels or the serotonin axis. Consequently, we could not demonstrate the notion whether serotonin is important in patients with ADs developing bladder cancer. Still, a potential bias could exist. And last, a 5-year follow up period was chosen to ensure an adequate time window for the development of urological cancers among subjects at risk. Some subjects might have had a more-insidious onset and could not be identified within the 5-year follow-up period.

Conclusions

Despite these limitations, we found that during the 5-year follow-up period, the risk of developing urological caner was much higher among patients with ADs, compared to their counterparts without ADs, and this association was totally independent from comorbid hypertension, diabetes, obesity, and registered alcohol and tobacco use disorders. Clinicians should be aware of the increased risk of developing urological cancer among patients with ADs and are encouraged not to neglect relevant urological complaints.

Abbreviations
ADs: Anxiety disorders; HR: hazard ratio; LHID2005: Longitudinal health insurance database 2005; NHI: National health insurance; SIR: Standardized incidence ratio.

Acknowledgements
This study is based in part on data from the *National Health Insurance Research Database* provided by the Bureau of National Health Insurance, Department of Health, Taiwan and managed by the National Health Research Institutes. The interpretations and conclusions contained herein do not represent those of the Bureau of National Health Insurance, Department of Health, or the National Health Research Institutes.

Funding
None.

Authors' contributions
YC participated in the design of the study and helped to draft the manuscript. HCLin, HCLee and LT performed the statistical analysis and helped to draft the manuscript. SD conceived of the study, participated in its design and coordination and helped to draft the manuscript. CC helped to revise the manuscript critically for important intellectual content and made substantial contributions to analysis and interpretation of data. All authors reviewed the manuscript.

Competing interests
The authors declare that they have no competing interests.

Author details
[1]Department of Psychiatry, Shuang Ho Hospital, Taipei Medical University, New Taipei City, Taiwan. [2]Graduate Institute of Life Science, National Defense Medical Center, Taipei, Taiwan. [3]Sleep Research Center, Taipei Medical University, Taipei, Taiwan. [4]Department of Psychiatry and Medical Humanities, School of Medicine, College of Medicine, Taipei Medical University, Taipei, Taiwan. [5]School of Health Care Administration, Taipei Medical University, Taipei, Taiwan. [6]Division of Urology, Department of Surgery, Far Eastern Memorial Hospital, New Taipei City, Taiwan. [7]Graduate Program in Biomedical Informatics, College of Informatics, Yuan-Ze University, Chung-Li, Taiwan. [8]Department of Surgery, Far Eastern Memorial Hospital, No.21, Sec. 2, Nanya S. Rd., Banciao Dist, New Taipei City 220, Taiwan.

References
1. Somers JM, Goldner EM, Waraich P, Hsu L. Prevalence and incidence studies of anxiety disorders: a systematic review of the literature. Can J Psychiatry. 2006;51:100–13.
2. Marques L, Robinaugh DJ, LeBlanc NJ, Hinton D. Cross-cultural variations in the prevalence and presentation of anxiety disorders. Expert Rev Neurother. 2011;11:313–22.
3. Faravelli C, Guerrini Degl'Innocenti B, Giardinelli L. Epidemiology of anxiety disorders in Florence. Acta Psychiatr Scand. 1989;79:308–12.
4. Chen CN, Wong J, Lee N, Chan-Ho MW, Lau JT, Fung M. The Shatin community mental health survey in Hong Kong. II. Major findings. Arch Gen Psychiatry. 1993;50:125–33.
5. Mendlowicz MV, Stein MB. Quality of life in individuals with anxiety disorders. Am J Psychiatry. 2000;157:669–82.
6. Marciniak MD, Lage MJ, Dunayevich E, Russell JM, Bowman L, et al. The cost of treating anxiety: the medical and demographic correlates that impact total medical costs. Depress Anxiety. 2005;21:178–84.
7. Katon W, Lin EH, Kroenke K. The association of depression and anxiety with medical symptom burden in patients with chronic medical illness. Gen Hosp Psychiatry. 2007;29:147–55.
8. Chida Y, Hamer M, Wardle J, Steptoe A. Do stress-related psychosocial factors contribute to cancer incidence and survival? Nat Clin Pract Oncol. 2008;5:466–75.
9. Hamer M, Chida Y, Molloy GJ. Psychological distress and cancer mortality. J Psychosom Res. 2009;66:255–8.
10. Aro AR, De Koning HJ, Schreck M, Henriksson M, Anttila A, et al. Psychological risk factors of incidence of breast cancer: a prospective cohort study in Finland. Psychol Med. 2005;35:1515–21.
11. Goldacre MJ, Wotton CJ, Yeates D, Seagroatt V, Flint J. Cancer in people with depression or anxiety: record-linkage study. Soc Psychiatry Psychiatr Epidemiol. 2007;42:683–9.
12. Liang JA, Sun LM, Su KP, Chang SN, Sung FC, et al. A nationwide population-based cohort study: will anxiety disorders increase subsequent cancer risk? PLoS One. 2012;7:e36370.
13. Shen CC, Hu YW, Hu LY, Hung MH, Su TP, et al. The risk of cancer in patients with generalized anxiety disorder: a nationwide population-based study. PLoS One. 2013;8:e57399.
14. Siddiqui EJ, Shabbir M, Thompson CS, Mumtaz FH, Mikhailidis DP. Growth inhibitory effect of doxazosin on prostate and bladder cancer cells. Is the serotonin receptor pathway involved? Anticancer Res. 2005;25:4281–6.
15. Siddiqui EJ, Shabbir MA, Mikhailidis DP, Mumtaz FH, Thompson CS. The effect of serotonin and serotonin antagonists on bladder cancer cell proliferation. BJU Int. 2006;97:634–9.
16. Chen YH, Yeh HY, Wu JC, Haschler I, Chen TJ, Wetter T. Taiwan's National Health Insurance Research Database: administrative health care database as study object in bibliometrics. Scientometrics. 2011;86:365–80.
17. Jones ME, Swerdlow AJ. Bias in the standardized mortality ratio when using general population rates to estimate expected number of deaths. Am J Epidemiol. 1998;148:1012–7.
18. McLaughlin TP, Khandker RK, Kruzikas DT, Tummala R. Overlap of anxiety and depression in a managed care population: Prevalence and association with resource utilization. J Clin Psychiatry. 2006;67:1187–93.
19. Chung SD, Lin HC. Association between chronic prostatitis/chronic pelvic pain syndrome and anxiety disorder: a population-based study. PLoS One. 2013;8:e64630.
20. Chung KH, Liu SP, Lin HC, Chung SD. Bladder pain syndrome/interstitial cystitis is associated with anxiety disorder. Neurourol Urodyn. 2014;33:101–5.
21. Lykouras L, Michopoulos J. Anxiety disorders and obesity. Psychiatrike. 2011;22:307–13.
22. Sabourin BC, Hilchey CA, Lefaivre MJ, Watt MC, Stewart SH. Why do they exercise less? Barriers to exercise in high-anxiety-sensitive women. Cogn Behav Ther. 2011;40:206–15.
23. Sommer F, Klotz T, Schmitz-Drager BJ. Lifestyle issues and genitourinary tumours. World J Urol. 2004;21:402–13.
24. Kao CH, Sun LM, Su KP, Chang SN, Sung FC, et al. Benzodiazepine use possibly increases cancer risk: a population-based retrospective cohort study in Taiwan. J Clin Psychiatry. 2012;73:e555–60.
25. Pottegard A, Friis S, Andersen M, Hallas J. Use of benzodiazepines or benzodiazepine related drugs and the risk of cancer: a population-based case–control study. Br J Clin Pharmacol. 2013;75:1356–64.
26. Selaman Z, Bolton JM, Oswald T, Sareen J. Association of benzodiazepine use with increased cancer risk is misleading due to lack of theoretical rationale and presence of many confounding factors. J Clin Psychiatry. 2012;73:1264.
27. Cohen S, Herbert TB. Health psychology: psychological factors and physical disease from the perspective of human psychoneuroimmunology. Annu Rev Psychol. 1996;47:113–42.
28. Sephton S, Spiegel D. Circadian disruption in cancer: a neuroendocrine-immune pathway from stress to disease? Brain Behav Immun. 2003;17:321–8.
29. Reiche EM, Nunes SO, Morimoto HK. Stress, depression, the immune system, and cancer. Lancet Oncol. 2004;5:617–25.
30. Antoni MH, Lutgendorf SK, Cole SW, Dhabhar FS, Sephton SE, et al. The influence of bio-behavioural factors on tumour biology: pathways and mechanisms. Nat Rev Cancer. 2006;6:240–8.
31. Eismann EA, Lush E, Sephton SE. Circadian effects in cancer-relevant psychoneuroendocrine and immune pathways. Psychoneuroendocrinology. 2010;35:963–76.
32. Dizeyi N, Bjartell A, Nilsson E, Hansson J, Gadaleanu V, et al. Expression of serotonin receptors and role of serotonin in human prostate cancer tissue and cell lines. Prostate. 2004;59:328–36.
33. Shinka T, Onodera D, Tanaka T, Shoji N, Miyazaki T, et al. Serotonin synthesis and metabolism-related molecules in a human prostate cancer cell line. Oncol Lett. 2011;2:211–5.

34. Akimova E, Lanzenberger R, Kasper S. The serotonin-1A receptor in anxiety disorders. Biol Psychiatry. 2009;66:627–35.
35. Siddiqui EJ, Thompson CS, Mikhailidis DP, Mumtaz FH. The role of serotonin in tumour growth (review). Oncol Rep. 2005;14:1593–7.
36. Jungwirth N, Haeberle L, Schrott KM, Wullich B, Krause FS. Serotonin used as prognostic marker of urological tumors. World J Urol. 2008;26:499–504.
37. Ronkainen H, Soini Y, Vaarala MH, Kauppila S, Hirvikoski P. Evaluation of neuroendocrine markers in renal cell carcinoma. Diagn Pathol. 2010;5:28.
38. Schury K, Kolassa IT. Biological memory of childhood maltreatment: current knowledge and recommendations for future research. Ann N Y Acad Sci. 2012;1262:93–100.
39. Green JG, McLaughlin KA, Berglund PA, Gruber MJ, Sampson NA, Zaslavsky AM, et al. Childhood adversities and adult psychiatric disorders in the national comorbidity survey replication I: associations with first onset of DSM-IV disorders. Arch Gen Psychiat. 2010;67(2):113–23.
40. Morath J, Moreno-Villanueva M, Hamuni G, Kolassa S, Ruf-Leuschner M, Schauer M, et al. Effects of psychotherapy on DNA strand break accumulation originating from traumatic stress. Psychother Psychosom. 2014;83(5):289–97.

32

Diagnostic outcome of ureteroscopy in urothelial carcinoma of the upper urinary tract: Incidence of later cancer detection and its risk factors after the first examination

Norihiro Murahashi[1], Takashige Abe[1]*, Nobuo Shinohara[1], Sachiyo Murai[1], Toru Harabayashi[2], Ataru Sazawa[3], Satoru Maruyama[1], Kunihiko Tsuchiya[1], Naoto Miyajima[1], Kanako Hatanaka[4] and Katsuya Nonomura[1]

Abstract

Background: To determine the incidence of later cancer detection and its risk factors after the first diagnostic ureteroscopy.

Methods: One hundred and sixty-six patients undergoing diagnostic ureteroscopy based on the suspicion of urothelial carcinoma of the upper urinary tract (UC of the UUT) between 1995 and 2012 were included. We examined the diagnostic outcome of the initial ureteroscopy. Thereafter, we collected follow-up data on patients who had not been diagnosed with UC of the UUT at the first examination, and evaluated the incidence of later cancer detection and its risk factors using Cox hazard models.

Results: Of the 166 patients, 76 (45.8 %) were diagnosed with UC of the UUT at the first diagnostic ureteroscopy. The remaining 90 (54.2 %) were diagnosed with other malignancies (n = 22), non-malignant disorders (n = 18), or without disorders (n = 50). Of these 90 patients, follow-up data were available in 65 patients (median: 41 months, range: 3–170). During the follow-up, carcinoma was detected in 6 patients (6/65, 9.2 %) at a median of 43.5 months (range: 10–59). Episodes of gross hematuria (p = 0.0048) and abnormal cytological findings (p = 0.0335) during the follow-up and a male sex (p = 0.0316) were adverse risk factors.

Conclusion: Later cancer detection of UC of the UUT was not uncommon after the first examination. The risk analysis revealed the aforementioned characteristics.

Background

Based on recent advances in medical equipment, ureteroscopy has become a powerful tool for the diagnosis and endoscopic treatment of patients with urothelial carcinoma (UC) of the upper urinary tract (UUT) [1–6]. The combination of direct visual examination and tumor biopsy by endoscopic cold forceps has led to marked diagnostic accuracy. However, there are potential limitations, such as the endoscopic view can be easily compromised by bleeding, and tissue samples obtained using endoscopic forceps are too small to yield a definitive diagnosis regarding the presence or absence of malignancy. In that situation, subsequent follow-up would be necessary. Data regarding these issues have not been reported. In the present study, we evaluated diagnostic outcomes of ureteroscopy and collected follow-up data on patients who were not considered to have UC of the UUT at the first examination. The aim of this study was to clarify the incidence of later cancer detection and its risk factors after the first examination.

Methods

After obtaining the approval of Institutional Review Board of Hokkaido University Hospital for Clinical Research to

* Correspondence: takataka@rf6.so-net.ne.jp
[1]Department of Urology, Hokkaido University Graduate School of Medicine, North-15, West-7, North Ward, Sapporo 060-8638, Japan
Full list of author information is available at the end of the article

access patient data, the medical records of patients undergoing ureteroscopy under general or lumbar anesthesia at Hokkaido University Hospital between 1995 and 2012 were reviewed. During this period, 208 patients underwent ureteroscopic procedures. For the present analyses, patients undergoing ureteroscopy mainly for endoscopic treatment for UC of the UUT, urolithiasis, or other diseases were excluded (n = 16). In addition, because of the special circumstances, patients undergoing ureteroscopy through an antegrade approach, an ileal conduit, or ureterocutaneostomy were excluded (n = 16). Patients under 18 years old (n = 2), those undergoing ureteroscopy for the removal of a migrated stent (n = 3), those with failure on ureteroscopy (n = 4), and a patient undergoing ureteroscopy for suspicion of recurrence after conservative treatment of UC of the UUT at the previous hospital were also excluded. Finally, 166 patients undergoing diagnostic ureteroscopy to obtain a diagnosis of UC of the UUT were included. Regarding the indication of diagnostic ureteroscopy, patients with abnormal radiological findings, such as hydronephrosis, a solid mass within the urinary tract, gross hematuria originating from the upper urinary tract, or positive urine cytology with a normal bladder mucosal appearance were considered to be candidates. In patients with apparent imaging findings and positive urinary cytology, we generally proceeded with radical surgery without diagnostic ureteroscopy.

Details of procedure

Before ureteroscopy, almost all patients underwent cystoscopy, CT, and voided urine cytology at our outpatient clinic. Under general (n = 86) or lumbar (n = 80) anesthesia, we initially performed cystoscopy and, thereafter, observed the upper urinary tract using a semi-rigid ureteroscope. Since 1998, flexible ureteroscopy has also been available in our hospital. Although, during the study period, several models of ureteroscopes were used due to the introduction of new models or simply the wear and tear of equipment, a semi-rigid ureteroscope of Richard Wolf (size: 6.0-7.5 Fr, working channel: 4 Fr) and a flexible ureteroscope of Olympus (size: 5.3-8.4, working channel: 3.6 Fr) were mostly used. With the use of 3 Fr forceps, biopsy of any suspicious region was performed, and samples were processed in formalin fixative. Washing urine samples were also collected. In patients with abnormal cytological findings without apparent abnormal radiological findings, random biopsy of the bladder mucosa was also conducted.

In the present study, we examined the diagnostic outcome at the initial ureteroscopy. Thereafter, we collected follow-up data on patients who had been diagnosed without UC of the UUT, and evaluated the incidence of later cancer detection and associated risk factors.

Statistical analysis

Cox proportional hazard model addressed the association between the clinical characteristics and later cancer detection. Survival probabilities were estimated using Kaplan-Meier methods, and survival distributions were compared with the log-rank test. All calculations were performed using JMP version 11. P-values < 0.05 were considered significant.

Results

Table 1 shows the patients' characteristics. The median age was 67.5 years (range: 22–89). Of the 166 patients, 118 (71.1 %) underwent diagnostic ureteroscopy based on abnormal radiological findings, 76 (45.8 %) based on abnormal cytology findings, and 78 (47.0 %) due to macrohematuria (there were overlaps among the groups). In the present cohort, 55 (33.1 %) patients had a concurrent or previous history of bladder cancer.

Figure 1 summarizes the diagnostic outcomes of initial examinations. Of the 166 patients, UC of the UUT was detected in 76 (45.8 %) patients. After the diagnosis, 42 patients underwent nephroureterectomy, 2 underwent nephroureterocystectomy, 2 underwent partial ureterectomy, 1 patient with bilateral UC of the UUT underwent nephroureterectomy and contralateral partial ureterectomy, and 5 underwent endoscopic conservative surgery. Pathological examination after surgery revealed that 49 patients had UC of the UUT, while 3 patients did not show evidence of carcinoma in the surgical specimens. The remaining 24 patients underwent non-surgical

Table 1 Patients' characteristics

	n = 166
Age, years	Median: 67.5 (range: 22–89)
Sex male/female	
Male	107 (64.5 %)
Female	59 (35.5 %)
Side evaluated by ureteroscopy	
Unilateral	143 (86.1 %)
Bilateral	23 (13.9 %)
Reason for undergoing ureteroscopy	
Abnormal radiological finding only	39 (23.5 %)
Abnormal cytological finding only[a]	21 (12.7 %)
Macrohematuria only	13 (7.8 %)
Multiple reasons any of the above 3 indications	83 (50 %)
Missing information	10(6 %)
Concurrent or previous history of bladder cancer	
Yes	55 (33.1 %)
No	111 (66.9 %)

[a]Abnormal cytological finding means malignant, suspicious, or atypical cells

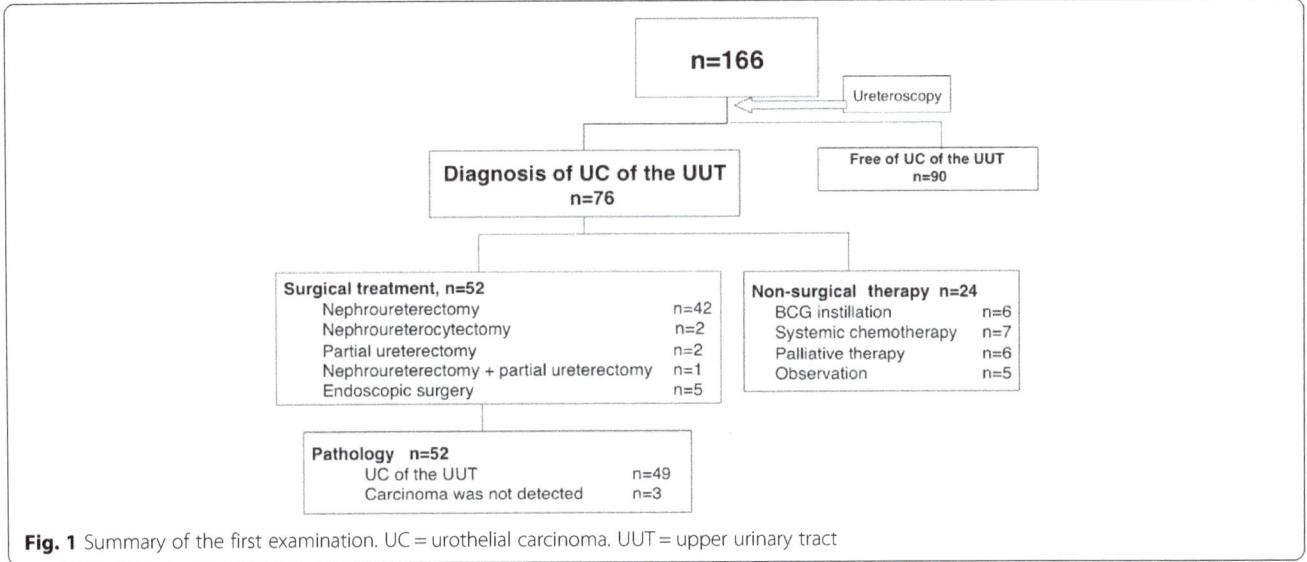

Fig. 1 Summary of the first examination. UC = urothelial carcinoma. UUT = upper urinary tract

treatment (BCG instillation into upper urinary tract: n = 6, systemic chemotherapy: n = 7, palliative therapy: n = 6, and observation: n = 5). Figure 2 summarizes the diagnostic outcomes of the remaining 90 patients without UC of the UUT at the first examination. Fifty patients, in whom no apparent tumor was observed on ureteroscopic evaluation or pathological evaluation, and washing cytology did not lead to a definitive diagnosis of UC, were considered to be without malignancy or urological disorder. In 22 patients, malignant diseases other than UC of the UUT (bladder cancer: n = 16, renal cell carcinoma: n = 2, other malignancies n = 4) were detected. In addition, non-malignant disorder was detected in 18 patients (ureteral stricture: n = 10, benign tumor: n = 4, urolithiasis: n = 2, others: n = 2). Regarding the complications among the 166 patients, major ureteral injury

occurred in one patient with a ureteral stone and severe hydronephrosis, which later resulted in nephrectomy. Minor ureteral injury occurred in 7 patients, which was resolved by ureteral stent placement. No urosepsis occurred after ureteroscopy.

After the first ureteroscopy, follow-up data were available in 65 patients with a median 41-month (range: 3–170 months) follow-up duration, while 25 patients were lost to follow-up. During the follow-up period, 11 patients underwent a second ureteroscopy, and UC of the UUT was detected in 5 patients. An additional patient developed metastatic urothelial carcinoma 33 months after the first examination (case No. 6 in Table 2). Therefore, UC of the UUT was detected in a total of 6 patients (6/65, 9.2 %) at a median of 43.5 months (range: 10–59 months) after the first ureterosopy (Fig. 2 and

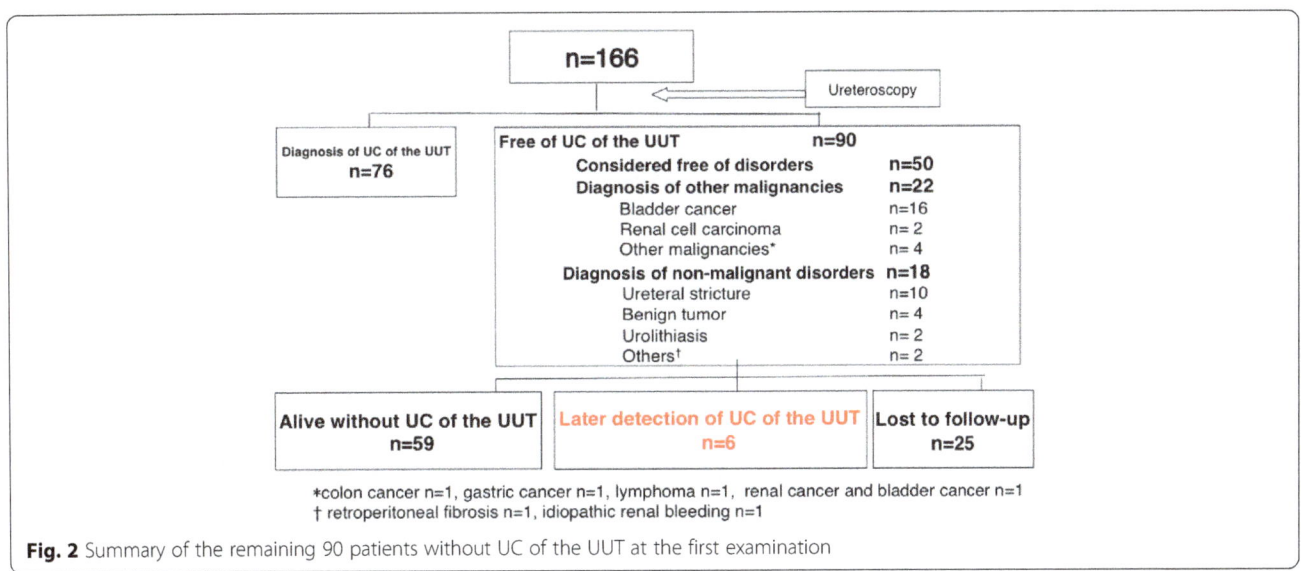

Fig. 2 Summary of the remaining 90 patients without UC of the UUT at the first examination

Table 2 Summary of the 6 patients with later detection of UC of the UUT

Case No.	Age, years	Sex	Side of first examination	Mucosa appearance of upper urinary tract at first examination	Washing cytology at first examination	Ureteral biosy at first examination	Diagnosis at first examination
1	55	Male	L	normal	not performed	not performed	bladder cancer
2	71	Male	R	normal	negative	negative	free of disorders
3	82	Male	R	normal	atypical	not performed	bladder cancer
4	68	Male	R	irregular	negative	negative	bladder cancer
5	70	Male	L	normal	negative	not performed	free of disorders
6	85	Male	L	normal	atypical	negative	free of disorders

Case No.	Side of subsequent cancer	Episode of gross hematuria after first examination	Urine cytology after first examination	Diagnostic method	Interval between first examination and cancer detetion	Treatment	Pathology
1	L	No	negative	ureteroscopy	57	nephroureterectomy	UC,G3 > 2,pT3
2	R	Yes	negative	ureteroscopy	10	nephroureterectomy	UC,G1 > 2,pT2
3	R	No	negative	ureteroscopy	60	nephroureterectomy	UC,G3,pT3
4	R	Yes	suspicious	ureteroscopy	28	BCG	UC, G2 > G3, pTa
5	B	Yes	positive	ureteroscopy	55	BCG for CIS of UUT	-
6	L	Yes	suspicious	CT	33	palliative therapy	-

Table 2). Table 3 summarizes the results of uni- and multivariate analyses of risk factors for later cancer detection. Episodes of gross hematuria (p = 0.0048) and abnormal cytological findings (p = 0.0335) during the follow-up and a male sex (p = 0.0316) were adverse risk factors of later cancer detection. When using a multivariate model adjusting for episodes of gross hematuria and abnormal cytological findings, episodes of gross hematuria remained significant (hazard ratio: 7.84, 95 % confidence interval: 1.32-61.7, p = 0.0239).

Discussion

In the present study, 76 (45.8 %) of the 166 patients were diagnosed with UC of the UUT at the first examination. Although the detection rate of UC of the UUT was lower than in previous studies [5, 6], we consider

Table 3 Univariate and multivariate analysis of risk factors for later cancer detection

Factor	No. of patients	Univariate hazard ratio (95 % confidence interval)	P-value	Multivariate hazard ratio (95 % confidence interval)	P-value
Age, year					
continuous	65	1.07 (0.99-1.18)	0.0807		
Gross hematuria after first examination					
Yes	13	11.3 (2.15-82.8)	0.0048	7.84 (1.32-61.7)	0.0239
No	50	1		1	
Cytology after first examination					
Positive/suspicious/atypical	9	6.6 (1.18-37.0)	0.0335	4.58 (0.689-31.3)	0.112
Negative	47	1		1	
Concurrent or previous history of bladder cancer					
Yes	22	3.09 (0.6-22.4)			
No	43	1	0.177		
Smoking history					
Yes	32	4.08 (0.66-78.1)			
No	26	1	0.142		
Sex		5-year cancer-free survival rate, %			
Male	40	73			
Female	25	100	0.0316		

that it is strongly influenced by the indication of diagnostic ureteroscopy at each institution. As aforementioned, we proceed directly to radical surgery without ureteroscopy in patients showing apparent imaging findings with a positive urinary cytology, and this would contribute to our lower detection rate. The incidence of urinary stones was low in our cohort, because patients requiring stone treatment were usually referred to our teaching hospitals.

At the initial diagnosis, UC of the UUT was not detected in surgical specimens in 3 patients (5.8 %, 3/52). The final pathology revealed dysplasia in one patient and the remaining two patients had neither carcinoma nor dysplasia. Of these three patients, one was diagnosed with a pelvic tumor due to positive washing cytology. This patient had concurrent bladder carcinoma, and contamination by carcinoma cells from bladder cancer would lead to a misdiagnosis. The remaining two patients were diagnosed by mucosal biopsy, which would suggest the difficulty of pathological diagnosis using small biopsy samples. Tsivian et al. reported a similar rate of misdiagnosis (not UC based on final pathologic findings), whereby it was 2.1 % (1/48) with routine ureteroscopic assessment [5]. Interestingly, they reported that the rate of misdiagnosis was 15.5 % (9/58) before routine ureteroscopic evaluation, which suggested improvement of the diagnostic accuracy due to ureteroscopy.

After the first ureteroscopy, follow-up data were available in 65 patients with a median of 41 months (range: 3–170 months), and UC of the UUT was detected on second ureteroscopy in 5 patients. Because one additional patient developed metastatic urothelial carcinoma detected by CT, UC of the UUT was detected in a total of 6 patients (6/65, 9.2 %) at a median of 43.5 months (range: 10–59 months) after the first ureteroscopy, which was an unexpectedly high detection rate. Regarding Case 2 in Table 2, because the interval between the first ureteroscopy and definitive diagnosis was relatively short (10 months), we considered that UC of the UUT carcinoma might be missed at the first examination. In the remaining 5 patients, because UC of the UUT was diagnosed after more than two years (range: 28–60 months), these carcinomas might be de novo development rather than being missed at the first examination. Cases 1, 3, and 4 had concurrent bladder cancer, and it is well-known that patients with bladder cancer are at risk of upper urinary tract recurrence. Picozzi et al. reported in their meta-analysis that the incidence of upper urinary tract recurrence after cystectomy ranged from 0.75 to 6.4 % [7]. However, interestingly, the laterality of the carcinoma was the same as that observed at the first examination in all 6 cases, although we could not clarify the

precise mechanism. At present, we consider our observations to suggest that later cancer detection of UC of the UUT was not uncommon after the first examination, but this should be verified in another cohort.

Regarding the risk factors of later cancer detection, the univariate model identified episodes of gross hematuria (p = 0.0048) and abnormal cytological findings (p = 0.0335) during the follow-up and a male sex (p = 0.0316) as adverse risk factors. Regarding the sex difference, previous epidemiologic studies revealed conflicting observations of a male [8–10] or a female [11] predominance in the incidence of UC of the UUT. Alternatively, a difference in accessibility to the upper urinary tract between males and females, due to differences in the urethral length, may influence the outcome. In the present study, the hazard ratio of males to females could not be calculated due to the absence of later cancer detection in the female cohort. When adjusting for episodes of gross hematuria and abnormal cytological findings in the multivariate model, episodes of gross hematuria remained significant (hazard ratio: 7.84, 95 % confidence interval: 1.32-61.7, p = 0.0239).

This study had several limitations, including its retrospective design, small sample size, and variations in ureteroscopies, as well as each surgeon's experience and proficiency during the study periods. In addition, we could not follow all patients after the first examination and did not have a uniform follow-up protocol, such as an indication for repeat ureteroscopy. Nevertheless, we consider that several important findings were yielded by the present study.

Conclusion

Later cancer detection of UC of the UUT was not uncommon after the first examination. Risk analysis revealed that episodes of gross hematuria (p = 0.0048) and abnormal cytological findings (p = 0.0335) during the follow-up and a male sex (p = 0.0316) were adverse risk factors.

Abbreviations
UC: Urothelial carcinoma; UUT: Upper urinary tract.

Competing interests
The authors declare that they have no competing interests.

Authors' contributions
NM and TA drafted the manuscript. SM, KT, and NM collected the follow-up data. TA and SM conducted statistical analysis. TH and AS contributed to the study design. NS and KN revised this manuscript. All authors read and approved the final manuscript.

Author details
[1]Department of Urology, Hokkaido University Graduate School of Medicine, North-15, West-7, North Ward, Sapporo 060-8638, Japan. [2]Department of Urology, Hokkaido Cancer Center, Sapporo, Japan. [3]Department of Urology, Obihiro-Kosei General Hospital, Obihiro, Japan. [4]Department of Surgical Pathology, Hokkaido University Hospital, Sapporo, Japan.

References

1. Thompson RH, Krambeck AE, Lohse CM, Elliott DS, Patterson DE, Blute ML. Elective endoscopic management of transitional cell carcinoma first diagnosed in the upper urinary tract. BJU Int. 2008;102(10):1107–110.

2. Cutress ML, Stewart GD, Wells-Cole S, Phipps S, Thomas BG, Tolley DA. Long-term endoscopic management of upper tract urothelial carcinoma: 20-year single-centre experience. BJU Int. 2012;110(11):1608–17.

3. Hara I, Hara S, Miyake H, Nomi M, Gotoh A, Kawabata G, et al. Usefulness of Ureteropyeloscopy for diagnosis of upper tract tumors. J Endourol. 2001;15(6):601–5.

4. Takao A, Saika T, Uehara S, Monden K, Abarzua F, Nasu Y, et al. Indications for ureteropyeloscopy based on radiographic findings and urine cytology in detection of upper urinary tract carcinoma. Jpn J Clin Oncol. 2010;40(11):1087–91.

5. Tsivian A, Tsivian M, Stanevsky Y, Tavdy E, Sidi AA. Routine diagnostic ureteroscopy for suspected upper tract transitional-cell carcinoma. J Endourol. 2014;28(8):922–5.

6. Vashistha V, Shabsigh A, Zynger DL. Utility and diagnostic accuracy of ureteroscopic biopsy in upper tract urothelial carcinoma. Arch Pathol Lab Med. 2013;137(3):400–7.

7. Picozzi S, Ricci C, Gaeta M, Ratti D, Macchi A, Casellato S, et al. Upper urinary tract recurrence following radical cystectomy for bladder cancer: a meta-analysis on 13,185 patients. J Urol. 2012;188(6):2046–54.

8. Shariat SF, Favaretto RL, Gupta A, Fritsche HM, Matsumoto K, Kassouf W, et al. Gender differences in radical nephroureterectomy for upper tract urothelial carcinoma. World J Urol. 2011;29(4):481–6.

9. Puente D, Malats N, Cecchini L, Tardón A, García-Closas R, Serra C, et al. Gender-related differences in clinical and pathological characteristics and therapy of bladder cancer. Eur Urol. 2003;43(1):53–62.

10. Munoz JJ, Ellison LM. Upper tract urothelial neoplasms: Incidence and survival during the last 2 decades. J Urol. 2000;164(5):1523–5.

11. Chou YH, Huang CH. Unusual clinical presentation of upper urothelial carcinoma in Taiwan. Cancer. 1999;85(6):1342–4.

33

The role of flower pollen extract in managing patients affected by chronic prostatitis/chronic pelvic pain syndrome

Tommaso Cai[1]*[iD], Paolo Verze[2], Roberto La Rocca[2], Umberto Anceschi[1], Cosimo De Nunzio[3] and Vincenzo Mirone[2]

Abstract

Background: Chronic prostatitis/chronic pelvic pain syndrome (CP/CPPS) is still a challenge to manage for all physicians. We feel that a summary of the current literature and a systematic review to evaluate the therapeutic efficacy of flower pollen extract would be helpful for physicians who are considering a phytotherapeutic approach to treating patients with CP/CPPS.

Methods: A comprehensive search of the PubMed and Embase databases up to June 2016 was performed. This comprehensive analysis included both pre-clinical and clinical trials on the role of flower pollen extract in CP/CPPS patients. Moreover, a meta-analysis of available randomized controlled trials (RCTs) was performed. The NIH Chronic Prostatitis Symptom Index (NIH-CPSI) and Quality of Life related questionnaires (QoL) were the most commonly used tools to evaluate the therapeutic efficacy of pollen extract.

Results: Pre-clinical studies demonstrated the anti-inflammatory and anti-proliferative role of pollen extract. 6 clinical, non-controlled studies including 206 patients, and 4 RCTs including 384 patients were conducted. The mean response rate in non-controlled studies was 83.6% (62.2%-96.0%). The meta-analysis revealed that flower pollen extract could significantly improve patients' quality of life [OR 0.52 (0.34-.0.81); $p = 0.02$]. No significant adverse events were reported.

Conclusion: Most of these studies presented encouraging results in terms of variations in NIH-CPSI and QoL scores. These studies suggest that the use of flower pollen extract for the management of CP/CPPS patients is beneficial. Future publications of robust evidence from additional RCTs and longer-term follow-up would provide more support encouraging the use of flower pollen extracts for CP/CPPS patients.

Keywords: Chronic pelvic pain syndrome, Inflammatory chronic pelvic pain syndrome, Prostatitis syndrome, Chronic prostatitis symptom index, Pollen extract

* Correspondence: ktommy@libero.it
[1]Department of Urology, Santa Chiara Regional Hospital, Trento, Italy
Full list of author information is available at the end of the article

Background

Chronic prostatitis has been described as one of the most common illnesses in men aged <50 year [1] with differing clinical presentations [2]. According to the classification of the National Institute of Health (NIH) [3], class III chronic prostatitis/chronic pelvic pain syndrome (CP/CPPS) is the most frequent category [4]. Symptoms such as pelvic pain, painful voiding and ejaculation and disturbed sexual functioning are common, often resulting in a significant impact on quality of life [5]. Recently, it has been established that the annual cost of a patient affected by prostatitis exceeds that of a patient with type 1 diabetes and that his quality of life is analogous to a patient with a heart attack or acute Crohn's disease [5]. Available therapies for CP/CPPS are not highly effective and require further in-depth analysis and consideration of such alternate strategies [6]. The traditional treatment of CP/CPPS is known as the "three A's": antibiotics, anti-inflammatory medications, and alpha blockers. The use of antibiotics remains controversial, especially due to the fact that bacteria cannot be isolated from the urogenital samples of CP/CPPS patients [7]. On the other hand, even if anti-inflammatory medications, aspirin or other NSAIDs such as ibuprofen can decrease pain, they can only be taken for a limited period of time due to their high prevalence of drug-related adverse effects. In other words, the standard treatment for CP/CPPS has not yet been definitively established [7]. In this scenario, even if phytotherapeutics seems to be an interesting option because of their generally low side effects, demonstrated efficacy, and high treatment compliance by patients, few compounds have been subject to scientific scrutiny and prospective controlled clinical trials [8, 9].

Over the last few years, interest in the use of flower pollen extract in the management of CP/CPPS has increased. Several clinical experiments show that flower pollen extract preparations may allow for a durable and marked symptom reduction in young men with CP/CPPS with improvement in semen quality and a significant reduction in the National Institutes of Health-Chronic Prostatitis Symptom Index (NIH-CPSI) score [10–13]. The most common pollen extracts used in clinical trials is Graminex® (Graminex® LLC, 95 Midland Road, Saginaw, MI 48638) that is a mixture of standardized extracts of rye grass pollen (Secale cereal), corn pollen (Zea mays), and timothy pollen (Phleum pretense). However, up to the present no comprehensive analysis of the current literature has been made so as to evaluate the tolerability and clinical efficacy of flower pollen extract in the management of patients affected by CP/CPPS.

Aim of the present review

Herein we aim to analyse all published data on flower pollen extract's role in the management of patients affected by CP/CPPS both in a pre-clinical and clinical setting, with particular attention given to the randomized clinical trials. Moreover, we aim to analyse all published studies in order to identify all clinical, laboratory and instrumental characteristics that are able to predict patients' clinical response to the treatment.

Research questions

We put forth two research queries:

1. Is flower pollen extract able to obtain significant pre-clinical data in order to justify its clinical use in the management of patients affected by CP/CPPS?
2. Is flower pollen extract able to improve overall and disease-specific quality of life of patients affected by CP/CPPS?

Methods

Types of studies

We have included pre-clinical studies regarding the effects of flower pollen extracts as a background and narrative review. Moreover, we have included clinical trials, randomized controlled trials, cohort, and case-control studies for our systematic review and meta-analysis. Editorials, commentaries, and review articles were used only for the background and the narrative review.

Outcome measures

The primary outcome of the study was the improvement of disease-related quality of life in terms of clinical response to the treatment as defined by the investigators. Clinical response to the treatment was generally evaluated in terms of NIH-CPSI and SF-36 questionnaires. Moreover, the improvement of symptoms [urinary and sexual symptoms, in terms of the International Prostatic Symptoms Score (IPSS)] and other questionnaires were also considered as outcome measures, if used by the investigators.

Risk of bias assessment

The risk of bias was performed by using the Newcastle-Ottawa Scale for risk of bias assessment [14].

Search strategy and research methods

We performed a search of literature up to June 2016 using the Medline computerized database of the US National Library of Medicine. The Google Scholar database was used, too. The Medline search was carried-out using Medical Subject Headings and free text terms as follows: 'pollen extract', or "flower pollen extract" and 'prostate' (exploded) were combined with the terms: 'treatment' and 'therapy'. Abstracts were not considered when full articles focusing on the same studies were available. Due to the limited number of pre-clinical studies published, we also included all non-English language papers as well. In cases of non-English language papers, the paper was included if the abstract was written in English and informative. Overlapping experiments have not been included because they were considered redundant. We considered as background information and as a comparative paper the latest review about the role of flower pollen extract in CP/CPPS patients by Wagenlehner FM published in 2011 [15]. From an initial literature search with pollen extract and prostatitis, a total of 23 extended papers were screened and 15 were selected and included in the present review. Finally, 10 clinical trials and 5 pre-clinical studies were analysed and are discussed in this review (Fig. 1). The Preferred Reporting Items for Systematic Reviews and Meta-Analyses (PRISMA) and Meta-analyses of Observational studies in Epidemiology (MOOSE) guidelines for the reporting of this present study was used in order to perform an accurate research check-list and report [16, 17]. The meta-analysis was performed using Review Manager 5.3 (Copenhagen: The Nordic Cochrane Centre, The Cochrane Collaboration, 2014) software. The inverse variance technique for the meta-analysis of the hazard ratios has been used. Due to the fact that the studies' heterogeneity cannot be explained, a random-effects model has been employed which in fact involves an assumption that the effects being estimated in the different studies are not identical.

Review methodology

Two authors performed the study selection independently (TC and PV). All disagreements were resolved by the senior author (VM). Titles and abstracts were used to screen for initial study inclusion. Full-text review was used where abstracts were insufficient to determine if the study met

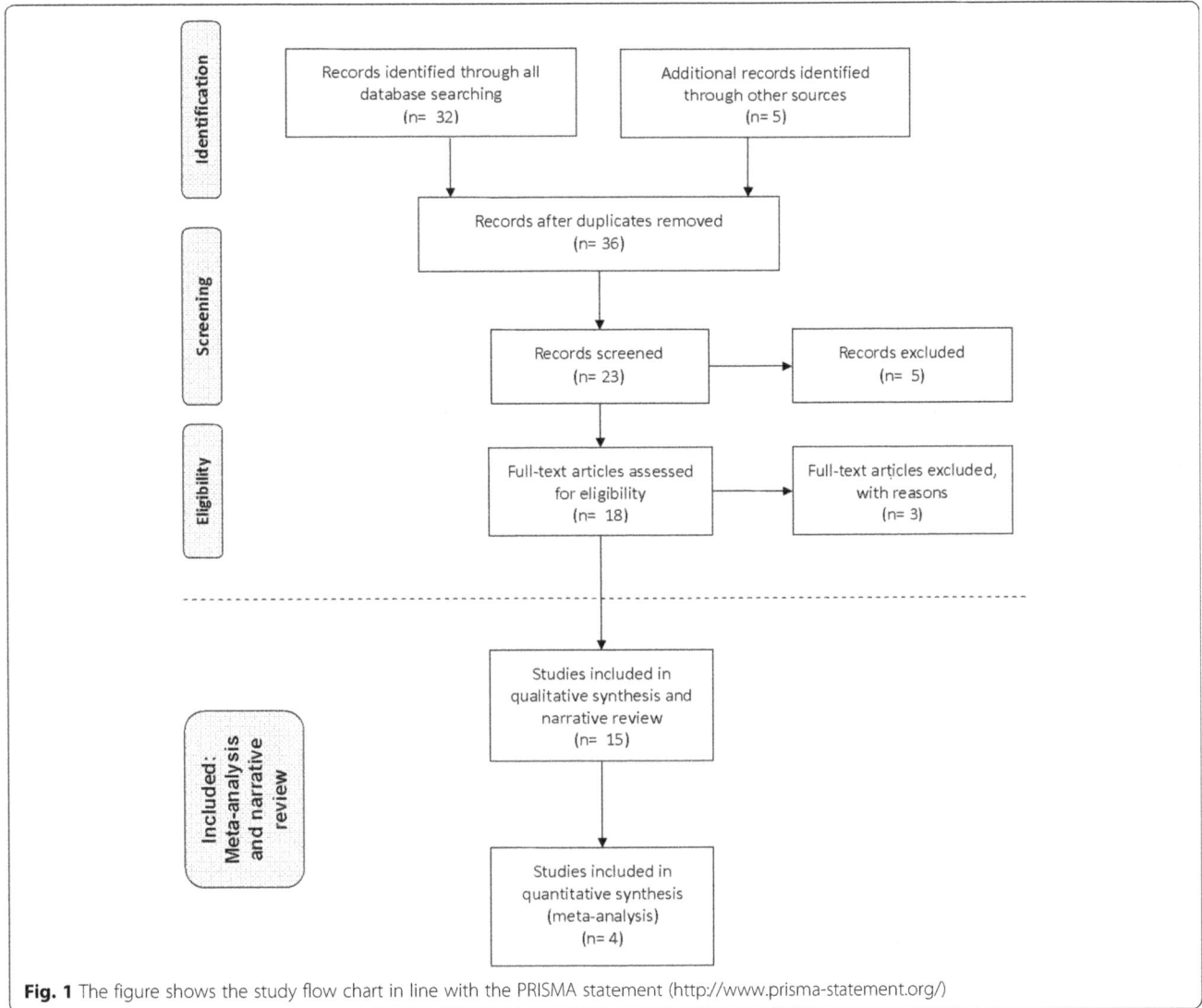

Fig. 1 The figure shows the study flow chart in line with the PRISMA statement (http://www.prisma-statement.org/)

inclusion or exclusion criteria. Two authors (TC and PV) independently performed all data abstraction including evaluation of study characteristics, risk of bias, and outcome measures with independent verification performed by the senior author (VM). The limited number of the studies collected did not require any other authors.

Results

Pre-clinical evidence

Our literature search identified 5 pre-clinical studies (Table 1). Three "in vitro models" [18–20] and three animal models [12, 21, 22] were used. All the studies demonstrated/confirmed that pollen extracts show two important pharmacological effects: anti-inflammatory and anti-proliferative. Loschen et al. demonstrated that rye pollen is able to inhibit the synthesis of prostaglandin and leukotriene performing an anticongestive and anti-inflammatory effect on the prostate tissue [20]. Another aspect to take into account is the possible effect of pollen extract on other tissues that differ from those of prostate glands. In fact, Wagenlehner highlighted another pharmacological effect of pollen extract that can be considered as a therapeutic mechanism of this compound: its effect on smooth muscles [15]. In conformity with Wagenlehner [15], Nagashima demonstrated in an animal model that consecutive administration of flower pollen extracts increased significantly maximum pressure during micturition to promote micturition reflex [22].

Anti-inflammatory effect

It was concluded that pollen extracts are able to inhibit prostaglandin and leukotriene synthesis and this effect is

comparable to that of diclofenac and indomethacin and approximately 10 times higher than that of aspirin [20].

Anti-proliferative effects

Several animal models showed that pollen extract has a possible effect on the prostate via the androgen metabolism [21]. Talpur and co-workers demonstrated that pollen extract decreased the size of the prostate in androgen-induced prostatic enlargement in rats [21]. The effect of pollen extract on prostate enlargement is due to the fact that a fraction of this compound is a powerful mitogenic inhibitor of fibroblastic and epithelial proliferation [15]. Moreover, Kamijo and co-workers found that pollen extract protects acinar epithelial cells and inhibits stromal proliferation in association with enhanced apoptosis [12]. Finally, several in vitro studies demonstrated that pollen extract is able to inhibit prostate cancer cell growth, as found by Habib [18]. This effect is even more pronounced in hormone-independent models, suggesting that there might be a place for pollen extract in the control of abnormal growth of hormone-insensitive cells [18].

Clinical evidence and meta-analysis

We identified 10 clinical studies (Table 2) and selected 6 clinical non randomized trials [10, 11, 23–26] and 4 RCTs [13, 27–29]. All trials demonstrated that pollen extracts significantly improved total symptoms, pain, and QoL in patients with inflammatory CP/CPPS without severe side-effects. Cai et al. used Graminex® (Graminex® LLC, 95 Midland Road, Saginaw, MI 48638) in association with B vitamins for the treatment of inflammatory and non-inflammatory CP/CPPS [11, 27]. Wagenlehner used Cernilton for the treatment of inflammatory CP/CPPS [13], while Elist used Prostat/Poltit that contains

Table 1 Summary of all pre-clinical studies

Author, year [reference]	Study type	Model	Compound used	Main study finding
Habib FK, 1990 [18]	In vitro study	Human prostate cancer cell line	pollen extract	- pollen extract is able to inhibit the prostate cancer cell growth (hormone-independent model)
Habib FK, 1995 [19]	In vitro study	Human prostate cancer cell line (DU145)	pollen extract	- pollen extract V-7 fraction is able to inhibit the prostate cancer cell growth
Kamijo T, 2001 [12]	Animal model	Rats	pollen extract	- pollen extract protects acinar epithelial cells and inhibits stromal proliferation in association with enhanced apoptosis
Loschen G, 1991 [20]	In vitro study	Microsomes (RBL-1 cells)	pollen extract	- pollen extract shows an anti-inflammatory and anti-proliferative therapeutic effect
Talpur N, 2003 [21]	Animal model	Rats	pollen extract vs serenoa repens	- pollen extract is able to influence prostatic hyperplasia via effects on androgen metabolism
Nagashima A, 1998 [22]	Animal model	Rats	pollen extract	- pollen extract increases the maximum pressure during urination to promote the urination reflex

Table 2 Summary of all clinical studies

Author, year [reference]	Study design	Patients number (response rate)	Controls Number (response rate)	Comparator	Outcomes measured
Buck AC. 1989 [23]	Prospective trial (phase II)	15 (86.6)	-	-	- pollen extract effective in the treatment of chronic prostatitis and prostatodynia.
Cai T. 2013 [11]	Prospective trial (phase II)	20 (90.0)	-	-	- pollen extract significantly improved total symptoms, pain, and QoL in patients with non-inflammatory CP/CPPS without severe side effects.
Cai T, 2014 [27]	Randomized controlled trial	41 (75.6)	46 (41.3)	ibuprofen	- pollen extract significantly improved quality of life of patients when compared with those treated with ibuprofen (treatment difference in the NIH-CPSI pain domain, -2.14 ± 0.51, P < 0.001; QoL scores, P = 0.002).
Elist J. 2006 [28]	Randomized controlled trial	30 (73.3)	28 (64.2)	Placebo	- pollen extract is superior to placebo in providing symptomatic relief in men with chronic nonbacterial prostatitis/chronic pelvic pain syndrome.
Iwamura H, 2015 [29]	Randomized placebo-controlled trial	50 (78.1)	50 (88.2)	Eviprostat (phytotherapeutic agent)	- pollen extract significantly reduced the symptoms of category III CP/CPPS without any adverse events, in terms of NIH-CPSI, IPSS, and QoL.
Jodai A, 1988 [24]	Prospective trial (phase II)	32 (75.0)	-	-	- pollen extract significantly reduced the symptoms in 75.0% of all treated patients.
Monden K. 2002 [25]	Prospective trial (phase II)	24 (91.6)	-	-	- pollen extract significantly reduced the symptoms of chronic prostatitis group
Rugendorff EW. 1993 [10]	Prospective trial (phase II)	90 (62.2)	-	-	- pollen extract significantly reduced the symptoms of category III CP/CPPS without any adverse events, in terms of urinary symptoms and QoL.
Suzuki T. 1992 [26]	Prospective trial (phase II)	25 (96.0)	-	-	- pollen extract significantly reduced the symptoms of prostatitis patients without any adverse events.
Wagenlehner FM. 2009 [13]	Randomized controlled trial	70 (70.6)	69 (49.3)	Placebo	- pollen extract significantly improved total symptoms, pain, and QoL in patients with inflammatory CP/CPPS without severe side-effects.

74 mg of highly defined extract of pollen from selected Graminae species [28]. Finally, Iwamura used an association of Cernitin T60 and Cernitin GBX [29].

Non-RCTs
As reported in Table 2, 6 clinical, non randomized trials including 206 patients were selected. The mean response rate in non-controlled studies was 83.6% (62.2%-96.0%). Cai and co-workers in a non-randomized clinical study reported a clinical response rate of 90%, demonstrating that

pollen extract in association with vitamins significantly improved total symptoms, pain, and QoL in patients with non-inflammatory CP/CPPS without severe side effects [11]. The same results, in terms of clinical efficacy, were reported by Rugendorff [10] and Buck [23] in two non-randomized trials which reported a clinical response rate of 62.2% and 86.6%, respectively. Moreover, three studies by Japanese researchers demonstrated a high clinical response rate to pollen extract treatment in patients with both class IIIa and class IIIb CP/CPPS [24–26].

RCTs and meta-analysis

The mean response rate in RCTs was 74.4% (70.6%-78.1%). The latest RCT carried out by Iwamura and co-workers demonstrated a response rate of 78.1% in 50 patients affected by CP/CPPS after 8 weeks of treatment [29]. The authors defined the clinical response as a decrease in the NIH-CPSI total score by at least 25% [29]. They did not observe severe adverse events in any patients in their study [29]. On the other hand, Cai and co-workers, in a cohort of patients randomized to pollen extract or ibuprofen, reported a response rate of 75.6% in the flower pollen extract group [27]. Both class IIIa and class IIIb CP/CPPS patients were enrolled and, moreover, it was reported that adverse events were less frequent in the pollen extract group than in the ibuprofen group [27]. In the largest study, Wagenlehner and co-workers demonstrated a clinical response rate of 70.6% [13] in 139 patients affected by inflammatory CP/CPPS and treated for 12 weeks with flower pollen extract. They concluded that the beneficial effect continued to improve after 12 weeks' treatment showing that pollen extract can be recommended for patients with inflammatory CP-CPPS for long-term treatment [13]. In 2006 Elist, by carrying out a double-blind study which included 60 patients with class IIIa or class IIIb CP/CPPS who were treated with flower pollen extract for 6 months, reported an overall clinical response of 73% [28]. All these 4 RCTs were used for the/included in our meta-analysis. We included 384 patients from 4 studies. The meta-analysis revealed that flower pollen extract could significantly improve patients' quality of life [OR 0.52 (0.34-.0.81); $p = 0.02$]. Figure 2 shows the forest plot of the effect of pollen extract on CP/CPPS patients in terms of clinical response rate, as defined by the investigators.

Sub-analysis on the basis of CP/CPPS type (class III a or b)

The analysis of the 4 RCT studies did not permit us to clearly identify which CP/CPPS sub-type was the best candidate to treat with the pollen extract. In this sense, the CP/CPPS class type is not able to predict patients' clinical response to the treatment. Only one out of four studies enrolled inflammatory CP/CPPS (class A) [13],

while the other three studies enrolled both class III a and b [27–29]. Cai and co-workers enrolled 25 patients with inflammatory CP/CPPS (type IIIa) and 62 type IIIb [27]. They found that in the pollen extract group patients affected by type IIIb CP/CPPS showed higher QoL results and a lower pain level following treatment in terms of the NIH-CPSI score (the NIH-CPSI score was 24.8 ± 1.8 at the enrolment versus 11.7 ± 1.7 at the follow-up visit; P < 0.001) when compared with type IIIa CP/CPPS patients [27]. Iwamura and co-workers enrolled 20 participants with class IIIa and 19 with class IIIb, without any reference to the difference between the two groups [29]. Finally, Elist did not report the results stratified by the CP/CPPS class [28]. In the two studies in which in which a data stratification according to class IIIa or b, 84 class A CP/CPPS and 30 class b had been treated with pollen extracts, while 80 class A CP/CPPS and 32 class b were considered as controls. The lack of data did not allow a significant analysis.

Risk of bias assessment

The 4 RCTs included showed few risk of bias. Three studies contained both class IIIa and IIIb CP/CPPS patients, thus introducing the risk of a selection bias. Moreover, the RCT by Elist showed an important risk of a selection bias due to the fact that in this study patients between 20 and 60 years were included.

Discussion

Main findings

Pollen extract is a mixture of natural components, such as amino acids, carbohydrates, lipids, vitamins, phytosterols and minerals that have been introduced in urological practice for the treatment of CP/CPPS patients [15]. In this review and meta-analysis of 4 RCTs with low-to-moderate risk of bias, we found that the use of flower pollen extracts in the management of CP/CPPS patients is associated with a high rate of clinical response without any significant adverse events. Moreover, we found that in both class IIIa and class IIIb the use of pollen extract is able to obtain significant improvements in a patients' QoL. These findings allow us to discuss

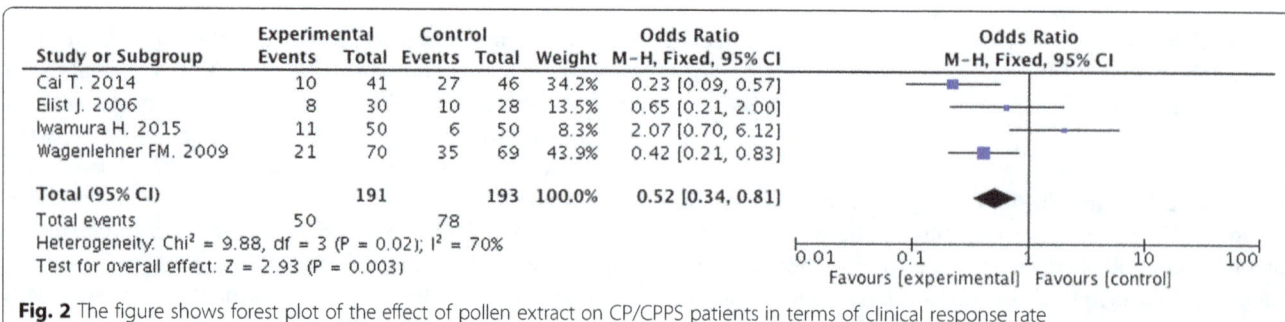

Fig. 2 The figure shows forest plot of the effect of pollen extract on CP/CPPS patients in terms of clinical response rate

several beneficial aspects of the role of pollen extract in the management of CP/CPPS patients. Firstly, upon consideration of the high clinical response rate of all included papers it was found that the mean response rate was high in both non-controlled [83.6% (62.2%-96.0%)] and in RCTs studies [74.4% (70.6%-78.1%)]. In analysing the reported encouraging results in terms of variations in NIH-CPSI and QoL scores, the following considerations should be taken into account:

- the proven anti-inflammatory, anti-proliferative effect of pollen extract
- the low rate of adverse events

All pre-clinical studies demonstrated that pollen extracts show an important anti-inflammatory effect due to the inhibition of prostaglandin and leukotriene synthesis [20]. Moreover, the dose-dependent, anti-inflammatory action of pollen extract in nonbacterial prostatitis in rats leading to decreased levels of interleukin-1b, interleukin-6 and a tumour necrosis factor, decreases glandular inflammation [15] has been demonstrated. The anti-inflammatory effect of pollen extract is approximately 10 times higher than that of aspirin [20] and did not lead to significant adverse events. This aspect is very important to highlight, due to the fact that the low prevalence of adverse effects correlates with a high patient compliance rate to the treatment. Moreover, several pre-clinical experiences demonstrated that flower pollen extract is able to inhibit 5a-reductase activity in the epithelium and stroma of the prostate in vitro, inhibiting the formation of dihydrotestosterone from testosterone [15]. This could be the reason for the improvements in urinary symptoms reported by the patients. However, the inhibition of 5a-reductase activity requires a long-term treatment as highlighted by several authors [15]. Even if a placebo effect was generally reported in patients treated with phytotherapeutic agents, in the 4 RCTs, clinically significant improvements were only observed in the pollen extract group and not in the placebo group. Finally, while Wagenlehner and co-workers found a decrease in leukocytes in post-prostate massage urine samples in both patients and controls [13], they did not find a significant difference between the two groups in terms of leukocyte number and for this reason leukocytes cannot be correlated with clinical success [13]. This aspect supports the hypothesis that the presence of inflammatory cells in the post-prostate massage urine sample is not a laboratory characteristic that is able to predict treatment response.

Strengths and limitations of the present study
In this review we excluded all studies on the effect of pollen extract on patients affected by benign prostatic hyperplasia or other urological diseases that can determine symptoms. Moreover, we excluded all studies in which the dosage of the compound was indicated in the publication. For this reason, despite the latest review by Wagenlehner we have excluded the paper by Li [30]. On the other hand, the most important limitation of this review is the lack of a pharmacokinetic evaluation of pollen extract. As highlighted by Wagenlehner, pharmacokinetic studies on the absorption, distribution, metabolism or excretion of the active components of flower pollen extracts have not been performed [15]. This is due to the fact that it is not known which compounds are primarily responsible for clinical efficacy [15].

Clinical implications
It is well known that there is no standard treatment or CP/CPPS to date. Amongst all the drugs and therapeutic approaches suggested and used, phytotherapeutic agents are those most widely prescribed in every day clinical practice with variable success. However, their use has only rarely been evaluated in suitable clinical trials. On the other hand, pollen extract has been sufficiently evaluated in preclinical and clinical studies [10, 13, 15]. Herein, we report encouraging results in terms of variations in NIH-CPSI and QoL scores in patients treated with pollen extracts indicating that the use of pollen extract appears to be safe and well tolerated by patients and, for this reason, the compliance to the treatment is high.

Conclusion
In conclusion, based upon our study analysis, pollen extracts appear to be clinically beneficial as indicated by the significant improvements in terms of the NIH-CPSI and QoL scores of patients diagnosed with CP/CPPS. Moreover, this therapeutic approach has an excellent safety profile with limited reported adverse effects. Future publications containing robust evidence from additional RCTs and longer-term follow-up would provide doctors with more confidence regarding the use of flower pollen extracts for their CP/CPPS patients.

Abbreviations
CP/CPPS: Chronic prostatitis/chronic pelvic pain syndrome; IPSS: International prostatic symptoms score; NIH: National institutes of health; NIH-CPSI: National institutes of health-chronic prostatitis symptom index; NSAIDs: Non-steroidal anti-inflammatory drugs; QoL: Quality of life; RCTs: Randomized clinical trials; SF-36: The short form (36) health survey

Acknowledgements
We are grateful to Juliet Ippolito for manuscript language revision.

Funding
None.

Authors' contributions
Study conception and design: CT, MV. Acquisition, analysis and interpretation of data: CT, AU, LRR, VP. Drafting of manuscript: Cai T. Critical revision and supervisions: DNC, MV. All authors read and approved the final manuscript.

Competing interests
Tommaso Cai, Paolo Verze and Vincenzo Mirone are consultant for and have received research support from IDIpharma.

Author details
[1]Department of Urology, Santa Chiara Regional Hospital, Trento, Italy.
[2]Department of Urology, University of Naples, Federico II, Naples, Italy.
[3]Department of Urology, Ospedale Sant'Andrea, Sapienza University of Rome, Rome, Italy.

References

1. Collins MM, Stafford RS, O'Leary MP, Barry MJ. How common is prostatitis? a national survey of physician visits. J Urol. 1998;159:1224–8.
2. Barbalias GA. Clinical and therapeutical guidelines for chronic prostatitis. From bacteriological importance to neuromuscular considerations. Eur Urol. 2000;37:116–7.
3. Workshop Committee of the National Institute of Diabetes and Digestive and Kidney Disease (NIDDK). Chronic Prostatitis Workshop, Bethesda 7–8 December, 1995.
4. Schaeffer AJ. Classification (traditional and National Institutes of Health) and demographics of prostatitis. Urology. 2002;60 Suppl 6:5–6. discussion 6–7.
5. Nickel JC. Role of alpha1-blockers in chronic prostatitis syndromes. BJU Int. 2008;101 Suppl 3:11–6.
6. Tuğcu V, Taşçi AI, Fazlioğlu A, et al. A placebo-controlled comparison of the efficiency of triple- and monotherapy in category III B chronic pelvic pain syndrome (CPPS). Eur Urol. 2007;51:1113–8.
7. Nickel JC, Downey J, Clark J, et al. Levofloxacin for chronic prostatitis/chronic pelvic pain syndrome in Men: a randomized, placebo-controlled multicenter trial. Urology. 2003;62:614–7.
8. Herati AS, Moldwin RM. Alternative therapies in the management of chronic prostatitis/chronic pelvic pain syndrome. World J Urol. 2013;31(4):761–6.
9. Shoskes DA, Zeitlin SI, Shahed A, Rajfer J. Quercetin in men with category III chronic prostatitis: a preliminary prospective, doubleblind, placebo-controlled trial. Urology. 1999;54:960–3.
10. Rugendorff EW, Weidner W, Ebeling L, et al. Results of treatment with pollen extract (Cernilton N) in chronic prostatitis and prostatodynia. Br J Urol. 1993;71:433–8.
11. Cai T, Luciani LG, Caola I, et al. Effects of pollen extract in association with vitamins (DEPROX 500®) for pain relief in patients affected by chronic prostatitis/chronic pelvic pain syndrome: results from a pilot study. Urologia. 2013;80 Suppl 22:5–10.
12. Kamijo T, Sato S, Kitamura T. Effect of cernitin pollen-extract on experimental nonbacterial prostatitis in rats. Prostate. 2001;49:122–31.
13. Wagenlehner FM, Schneider H, Ludwig M, Schnitker J, Brähler E, Weidner W. A pollen extract (Cernilton) in patients with inflammatory chronic prostatitis-chronic pelvic pain syndrome: a multicentre, randomised, prospective, doubleblind, placebo-controlled phase 3 study. Eur Urol. 2009; 56(3):544–51.
14. Wells GA, Shea B, O'Connell D, et al. The Newcastle-Ottawa Scale (NOS) for assessing the quality of nonrandomized studies in meta-analyses, 2011. http://www.ohri.ca/programs/clinical_epidemiology/oxford.asp. Accessed June 2016.
15. Wagenlehner FM, Bschleipfer T, Pilatz A, Weidner W. Pollen extract for chronic prostatitis-chronic pelvic pain syndrome. Urol Clin North Am. 2011; 38(3):285–92.
16. Moher D, Liberati A, Tetzlaff J, Altman DG, PRISMA group. Preferred reporting items for systematic reviews and meta-analyses: the PRISMA statement. Ann Intern Med. 2009;151:264–9.
17. Stroup DF, Berlin JA, Morton SC, et al. Meta-analysis of observational studies in epidemiology: a proposal for reporting, metaanalysis of observational studies in epidemiology (MOOSE) group. JAMA. 2000;283:2008–12.
18. Habib FK, Ross M, Buck AC, Ebeling L, Lewenstein A. In vitro evaluation of the pollen extract, cernitin T-60, in the regulation of prostate cell growth. Br J Urol. 1990;66(4):393–7.
19. Habib FK, Ross M, Lewenstein A, Zhang X, Jaton JC. Identification of a prostate inhibitory substance in a pollen extract. Prostate. 1995;26(3):133–9.
20. Loschen G, Ebeling L. Inhibition of arachidonic acid cascade by extract of rye pollen. Arzneimittelforschung. 1991;41(2):162–7.
21. Talpur N, Echard B, Bagchi D, Bagchi M, Preuss HG. Comparison of Saw palmetto (extract and whole berry) and cernitin on prostate growth in rats. Mol Cell Biochem. 2003;250(1-2):21–6.
22. Nagashima A, Ishii M, Yoshinaga M, et al. Effect of cernitin extract (Cernilton) on the function of urinary bladder in conscious rats. Japan Pharmacol Ther. 1998;26(11):51–6.
23. Buck AC, Rees RW, Ebeling L. Treatment of chronic prostatitis and prostatodynia with pollen extract. Br J Urol. 1989;64(5):496–9.
24. Jodai A, Maruta N, Shimomae E, Sakuragi T, Shindo K, Saito Y. A long-term therapeutic experience with cernilton in chronic prostatitis. Hinyokika Kiyo. 1988;34(3):561–8.
25. Monden K, Tsugawa M, Ninomiya Y, Ando E, Kumon H. A Japanese version of the national institutes of health chronic prostatitis symptom index (NIH-CPSI, Okayama version) and the clinical evaluation of cernitin pollen extract for chronic non-bacterial prostatitis. Nihon Hinyokika Gakkai Zasshi. 2002; 93(4):539–47.
26. Suzuki T, Kurokawa K, Mashimo T, Takezawa Y, Kobayashi D, Kawashima K, Totsuka Y, Shiono A, Imai K, Yamanaka H. Clinical effect of cernilton in chronic prostatitis. Hinyokika Kiyo. 1992;38(4):489–94.
27. Cai T, Wagenlehner FM, Luciani LG, Tiscione D, Malossini G, Verze P, Mirone V, Bartoletti R. Pollen extract in association with vitamins provides early pain relief in patients affected by chronic prostatitis/chronic pelvic pain syndrome. Exp Ther Med. 2014;8(4):1032–8.
28. Elist J. Effects of pollen extract preparation prostat/poltit on lower urinary tract symptoms in patients with chronic nonbacterial prostatitis/chronic pelvic pain syndrome: a randomized, double-blind, placebo-controlled study. Urology. 2006;67(1):60–3.
29. Iwamura H, Koie T, Soma O, Matsumoto T, Imai A, Hatakeyama S, Yoneyama T, Hashimoto Y, Ohyama C. Eviprostat has an identical effect compared to pollen extract (Cernilton) in patients with chronic prostatitis/chronic pelvic pain syndrome: a randomized, prospective study. BMC Urol. 2015;15:120.
30. Li NC, Na YQ, Guo HQ. Clinical study with prostat (Poltit) for treatment for chronic nonbacterial prostatitis. Chin J Urol. 2003;24:635–7.

34

Effect of sample time on urinary lithogenic risk indexes in healthy and stone-forming adults and children

Adrian Rodriguez[1], Concepcion Saez-Torres[1*], Concepcion Mir[1,2], Paula Casasayas[3], Nuria Rodriguez[3], Dolores Rodrigo[1,2], Guiem Frontera[4], Juan Manuel Buades[5], Cristina Gomez[6], Antonia Costa-Bauza[1] and Felix Grases[1]

Abstract

Background: The diagnosis and follow-up of stone forming patients is usually performed by analysis of 24-h urine samples. However, crystallization risk varies throughout the day, being higher at night. The main objective of this study is to evaluate the urinary crystallization risk in adults and children by calculating risk indexes based on different collection periods.

Methods: The study included 149 adults (82 healthy and 67 stone-formers) and 108 children (87 healthy and 21 stone-formers). 24-h urine was collected, divided into 12-h daytime sample (8 am to 8 pm), and 12-h overnight sample (8 pm to 8 am next morning). Solute concentrations, the calcium to citrate ratio (Ca/Cit), and the ion activity product of calcium oxalate (AP[CaOx]) and calcium phosphate (AP[CaP]) were calculated in each 12-h sample and in overall 24-h urine. Assessments were also related to stone type.

Results: Ca/Cit and AP(CaOx) were significantly higher in stone forming patients than in healthy subjects. The 12-h overnight samples had the highest values for both risk indexes, confirming a greater risk for crystallization at night. The AP(CaP) index was significantly higher in patients with pure hydroxyapatite stones than healthy controls, but was not significantly different between stone-formers overall and healthy controls.

Conclusions: The calculation of risk indexes is a simple method that clinicians can use to estimate crystallization risk. For this purpose, the use of 12-h overnight urine may be a reliable alternative to 24-h collections.

Keywords: 12-h night urine, AP(CaOx) index, AP(CaP) index, Ca/Cit ratio, Crystallization risk, Renal Lithiasis

Background

Renal lithiasis has a high prevalence in adults and is relatively rare in children, although it is increasing in all age groups [1, 2]. Up to 80% of renal stones contain different forms of calcium oxalate or calcium phosphate crystals [3, 4]. The different types of renal stones have different etiologies, which include particular features of urine composition. Thus, renal calculi consisting of calcium oxalate dihydrate (COD), pure hydroxyapatite (HAP), or admixtured COD +HAP, are more likely to form in the presence of urine with a high level of calcium and a low level of citrate [5]. On the other hand, even at relatively low levels of urinary supersaturation, injured papillary tissue can initiate the formation of papillary calcium oxalate monohydrate calculi (COMp) [6], and the presence of heterogeneous nucleating elements is related to the formation of unattached calcium oxalate monohydrate calculi (COMu) [5].

The traditional diagnosis and follow-up of stone-forming patients consists of assessment of the concentration and excretion of different solutes in 24-h urine samples (typically creatinine, calcium, magnesium, phosphate, oxalate, citrate, and uric acid), and measurements of urinary pH and volume. This approach allows diagnosis of metabolic abnormalities, such as hypercalciuria, hyperoxaluria, and hypocitraturia. However, some patients are classified as having idiopathic renal stones if there is no evidence of a metabolic abnormality. This may be because the key factor for urinary crystallization is not the absolute solute excretions but the urinary supersaturation degree, a parameter that depends on

* Correspondence: currisaez@telefonica.net
[1]Laboratory of Renal Lithiasis Research, University Institute of Health Sciences Research (IUNICS-IdISBa), University of Balearic Islands, Ctra Valldemossa, km 7.5, 07122 Palma de Mallorca, Spain
Full list of author information is available at the end of the article

urine concentration. For this reason, and due to the multifactorial characteristics of renal lithiasis, some authors have developed different risk indexes to estimate the risk of urinary crystallization [7, 8]. Several studies used these indexes, including the calcium/citrate ratio, the ion activity product of calcium oxalate (AP[CaOx]), and calcium phosphate (AP[CaP]), to compare stone-forming children and adults with healthy controls, and found significant differences [7, 9–11]. Furthermore, previous studies have shown cut off values for urinary solute concentrations that makes urine prone to crystallize in an in vitro model [12, 13].

On the other hand, when performing the metabolic evaluation of the stone forming patient, it must be considered that urinary composition varies throughout the day, leading to a higher risk of crystallization at night. More precisely, there is a 12-h high-risk period from 8 p.m. to 8 a.m. [14]. However, to our knowledge, no study has yet compared the stone risk factors in 12-h overnight samples with 12-h daytime urine samples.

Thus, the objectives of this study are to (i) evaluate the urinary crystallization risk by measuring urinary solute concentrations and calculating risk formulas in children and adults with and without a history of lithiasis, (ii) compare the results of the risk parameters in 12-h daytime, 12-h overnight, and overall 24-h urine, and (iii) examine the relationships of the different risk formulas with stone type.

Methods
Study subjects
This study examined 257 participants who were divided into four groups: 87 healthy children (4–17 years), 21 stone-forming children (4–17 years), 82 healthy adults (23–57 years), and 67 stone-forming adults (18–71 years). Healthy children were recruited from schools, both primary and secondary. Stone formers were from the pediatric nephrology unit or the urology department of our tertiary hospital. All stone-formers had a confirmed history of renal lithiasis in the previous 2 years. Subjects with a history of disorders that could affect urine chemistry (bowel disease with malabsorption, bone fracture, active urinary tract infection, chronic kidney disease, metabolic syndrome) were excluded. Medications, including diuretics and alkali citrate, were discontinued three days before urine collection. Participants were told not to change their normal diet and physical activity. We obtained approval from the local Ethics Committee (IB3152/16) and informed consent from each participant or his/her legal representative.

Renal calculi analysis
Stone analysis was performed by stereoscopic microscopy (Optomic, Madrid, Spain), scanning electron microscopy (S-530 M, Hitachi, Tokyo, Japan), X-ray microanalysis (Oxford Link Isis; Oxford, UK), and infrared spectrometry (Infrared Spectroscope Bruker IFS66; Bruker, Ettlingen, Germany).

The obtained stones were classified into 5 groups [5]: calcium oxalate monohydrate renal calculi developed on papillary tissue (COMp); unattached calcium oxalate monohydrate calculi (COMu); calcium oxalate dihydrate calculi (COD); calcium oxalate dihydrate-hydroxyapatite mixed calculi (COD+HAP); and hydroxyapatite (HAP) calculi. In recurrent stone-formers with different types of calculi, the last calculus was used for classification.

Urine collection and analysis
Twenty-four-hour urine was collected in two separate flasks with thymol. The 12-h daytime sample began at 8 a.m. (after discarding first morning urine) and ended at 8 p.m.; at this time, participants were instructed to perform a micturition in the daytime bottle. The 12-h nighttime sample began at 8 p.m. and was collected until 8 a.m. on the next day (fasting state). Sampling adequacy was determined by asking participants about the completeness of urine collection and by using the recently-reported anthropometry-based age and sex-specific reference values for 24-h urinary creatinine excretion [15, 16].

Urinary volume, pH (measured using a Crison pH-meter), and the concentrations of creatinine, calcium, phosphorus, oxalate, uric acid, citrate, and magnesium were determined. Phosphorus was measured by the ammonium molybdate reduction method, magnesium by an enzymatic assay, calcium by a colorimetric reaction with Arsenazo III calcium-sensitive dye, uric acid by the uricase method, and creatinine using the Jaffe method. These analyses were performed using an Architect C16000 Autoanalyzer (Abbott Diagnostics, Illinois, USA). Urinary citrate was measured by an enzymatic assay (Biosystems, Barcelona, Spain), and urinary oxalate was determined using the oxalate oxidase/peroxidase method (LTA, Milano, Italy). All parameters were measured separately in 12-h samples, and then calculated for the overall 24-h urine.

The crystallization risk of urine was determined by the calcium-to-citrate ratio (Ca/Cit) and two modified estimates of AP(CaOx) and the AP(CaP), as described by Tiselius [17, 18]:

$$AP(CaOx) \text{ index} = A \times Ca^{0.84} \times Ox \times Mg^{-0.12} \\ \times Cit^{-0.22} \times V^{-1.03} \tag{1}$$

in which A is 2.7 for a 12-h sample, and 1.9 for a 24-h sample.

$$AP(CaP) \text{ index} = 0.0032 \times Ca^{1.07} \times P^{0.70} \times (pH-4.5)^{6.8} \\ \times Mg^{-0.12} \times Cit^{-0.20} \times V^{-1.31} \tag{2}$$

which was only calculated for 12-h samples, because pH was not determined for 24-h samples.

Statistical analysis

Descriptive data are presented as medians and interquartile ranges. The Wilcoxon sum-rank test was used to compare groups. The Wilcoxon signed-rank test was used to compare daytime and nighttime samples. After examined the Bonferroni, Holm and Hochberg corrections, we considered a p-value of 0.001 or less as statistically significant. IBM SPSS Statistics version 22 ® for Windows was used for statistical analyses.

Results

There were 257 study participants. The healthy and stone-forming adults had similar anthropometric characteristics, as did the healthy and stone-forming children (Table 1). Among adult stone formers, 11 had COMp stones, 11 had COMu stones, 18 had COD stones, 10 had HAP + COD stones, 4 had HAP stones, and stone analysis was unavailable for 13 patients. Among stone-forming children, 9 had COD stones, 1 had HAP + COD stones, and stone analysis was unavailable for the other 11 children.

Table 2 summarizes the urinary volume and solute concentrations in 24-h urine samples. Oxalate concentration was significantly higher in stone-forming than healthy adults; calcium concentration was significantly higher in stone-forming than healthy children.

The AP(CaOx) index and Ca/Cit ratio in 24-h urine samples were significantly higher in stone-formers than in healthy subjects, among children and adults ($p < 0.001$ for both comparisons) (Fig. 1).

Measurements of risk indexes in 12-h samples are shown in Table 3 (adults) and Table 4 (children). Regarding AP(CaOx) index and Ca/Cit, significant differences between patients and healthy subjects were observed when we performed the comparisons using only the 12-h day sample or the 12-h night urine fractions ($p < 0.001$). On the contrary, for the AP(CaP) index in 12-h samples, the differences did not reach statistical significance, neither in the daytime nor in the overnight sample analysis.

Tables 3 and 4 also compare the urinary parameters of daytime and overnight samples. Healthy and stone-forming adults had significant differences in

magnesium, phosphate, urinary pH, Ca/Cit, and AP(CaP). On the contrary, healthy subjects had a lower nighttime urinary volume, and stone-formers had a greater nighttime AP(CaOx). Comparison of daytime and nighttime samples in children indicated the healthy children had significant differences in all parameters except uric acid concentration. On the contrary, in the stone forming children group, some differences did not reach significance due to the small size of the sample.

Figure 2 shows the AP(CaOx) index, AP(CaP) index, and the Ca/Cit ratio for the 12-h overnight urine samples of stone-forming adults according to calculus composition. Patients whose calculi were COD or COD + HAP had higher AP(CaOx) indexes, while patients with pure HAP calculi had higher AP(CaP) indexes. Patients with COD, HAP, and COD+HAP calculi had higher Ca/Cit ratios. The evaluation of risk indexes in relation to stone composition performed in 12-h daytime urine and in 24-h urine showed a similar pattern of differences than observed in the 12-h overnight urine, although for AP(CaP) there were more overlapping results in the daytime than in overnight samples (data not shown).

Discussion

The main findings of this study are that the AP(CaOx) and Ca/Cit values were significantly higher in the urine of stone-forming children and adults than in the corresponding healthy controls, being the results also evident by the only analysis of the 12-h overnight urine fraction. These indexes vary according to stone composition in adults. In addition, the AP(CaP) index was only elevated in adults with phosphate stones.

Previous studies have repeatedly stressed the important role of urine supersaturation in the genesis of renal calculi [8]. However, neither the European Association of Urology nor the American Urological Association includes calculation of supersaturation in their guidelines for evaluation of patient with renal lithiasis [19, 20]. In fact, some authors do not perform these measurements because they believe there is only limited evidence that monitoring of supersaturation in urine can prevent stone recurrence [21]. On the contrary, other authors have stated that assessment of urinary lithogenic risk, determined by measuring data related to the extent of supersaturation, is useful for guiding treatment and checking patient compliance [22, 23]. The use of specific easy-calculating formulas for estimation of supersaturation overcomes several methodological pitfalls of other procedures [7, 8, 10]. We found that AP(CaOx) and Ca/Cit values provided reliable estimates of the risk of renal lithiasis, in that each was significantly higher in stone-forming children and adults than the corresponding healthy controls. In the case of the AP(CaP) index, we observed differences in patients with phosphate

Table 1 Anthropometric measures of the four study groups

	Healthy adults ($N = 82$)	Stone forming adults ($N = 67$)	Healthy children ($N = 87$)	Stone forming children ($N = 21$)
% men	46	55	57	64
Age (years)	40 (10)	46 (13)	12 (3)	12 (4)
Weight (kg)	68 (13)	71 (16)	46 (14)	44 (18)
Height (cm)	170 (8)	167 (10)	151 (17)	147 (21)
BMI (kg/m²)	24 (3)	25 (4)	19 (3)	19 (9)

Results are expressed as % or mean (SD)

Table 2 Urinary volume and solute concentrations in 24-h urine samples of the four study groups

	Adults			Children		
	Healthy	Stone formers	p-value	Heatlhy	Stone formers	p-value
Volume (mL/24 h)	1573 (1189–2173)	1778 (1250–2380)	0.089	876 (672–1180)	1100 (645–1707)	0.111
Creatinine (mg/L)	919 (648–1230)	804 (571–1098)	0.106	970 (763–1294)	796 (565–1245)	0.007
Calcium (mg/L)	106 (70–179)	124 (89–174)	0.166	72 (45–120)	130 (72–231)	< 0.001
Magnesium (mg/L)	64 (44–86)	55 (43–76)	0.143	113 (77–142)	93 (52–125)	0.081
Oxalate (mg/L)	15 (12–19)	20 (14–24)	0.001	22 (17–29)	25 (22–32)	0.120
Phosphorous (mg/L)	517 (397–784)	515 (357–637)	0.207	840 (597–1063)	597 (430–768)	0.002
Uric acid (mg/L)	369 (272–513)	343 (258–481)	0.334	548 (393–691)	411 (298–606)	0.018
Citrate (mg/L)	435 (286–676)	322 (226–470)	0.003	517 (373–722)	347 (205–626)	0.005

Results are expressed as median (P_{25}-P_{75}). Statistical comparisons are between healthy and stone-forming adults, and between healthy and stone-forming children

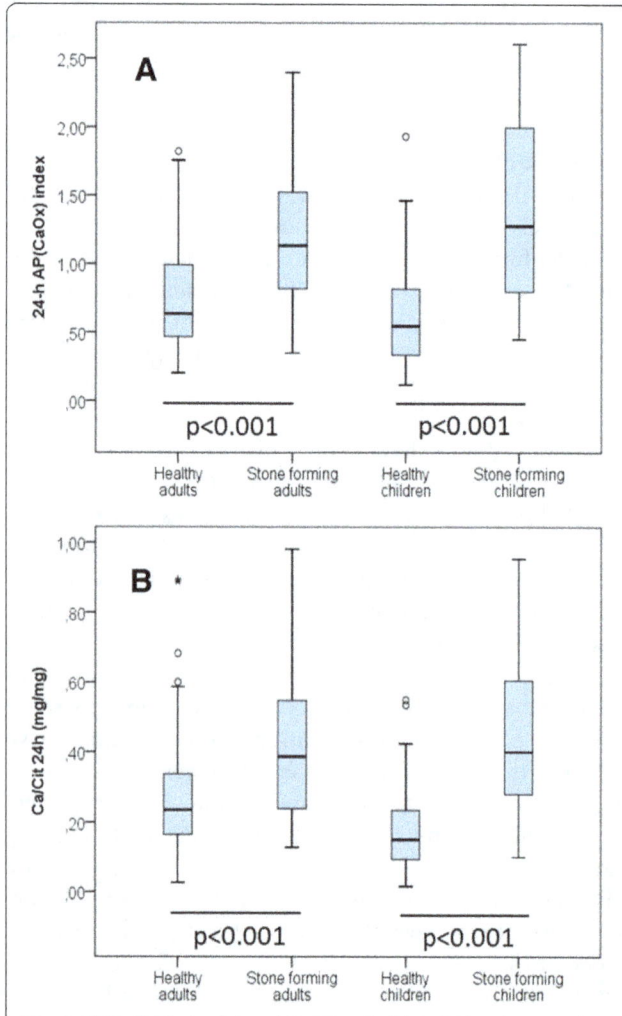

Fig. 1 AP(CaOx) index (**a**) and Ca/Cit ratio (**b**) in 24-h urine samples of the four study groups. Statistical comparisons are between healthy and stone-forming adults, and between healthy and stone-forming children

stones, but not stone-formers overall, because most subjects had calcium oxalate stones.

Use of the Ca/Cit ratio to assess the risk of renal lithiasis is widespread in the literature and in clinical practice [9]. Calculation of AP indexes allows integration of information on additional components of urine, as well as urine volume. Regarding cut-off points for the different indexes, the overlap of index values in the healthy and stone-forming groups means it is difficult to establish precise values to discriminate subjects with and without risk. Despite this, we believe these indexes provide relevant information, because higher index values indicate higher risk of crystallization in urine [24].

Some researchers have recommended that supersaturation be assessed in 24-h urine samples before treatment, 4–6 weeks afterwards, and in subsequent follow-ups [25]. However, collection of urine over 24 h can be cumbersome, so a simpler sampling method would be more convenient for patients. Our results show that the AP(CaOx) and Ca/Cit in 12-h overnight urine samples were significantly different in stone-forming and healthy individuals. Moreover, the overnight samples had higher values for both risk indexes than the 12-h daytime samples and the 24-h samples. These findings support previous evidence that averaging results from the whole day masks peaks of lithogenic risk that occur at nighttime [14, 26]. Therefore, the analysis of a 12-h overnight sample is more convenient for patients and appears to be more sensitive in detection of increased risk of crystallization of urine. Considering that the night is a period of high urinary crystallization risk, the advice of increasing fluid intake at the late evening should be strongly encouraged in order to decrease urinary supersaturation degree.

Our data on the AP(CaP) index indicated the highest values were in daytime urine. This is due to diurnal variations in pH, which strongly affects calcium phosphate solubility [27, 28]. Urinary pH increases during the day, and so does calcium phosphate supersaturation [29].

Table 3 Urinary volume, pH, solute concentrations, Ca/Cit ratio, and AP indexes in 12-h daytime and 12-h overnight urine samples of healthy and stone-forming adults

	Healthy adults (n = 82)			Stone forming adults (n = 67)		
	12-h day	12-h night	p-value	12-h day	12-h night	p-value
Volume (mL/12 h)	870 (600–1165)	650 (481–1010)	0.001	920 (700–1200)	780 (600–1135)	0.071
Creatinine (mg/dL)	940 (560–1310)	1025 (670–1563)	0.002	736 (562–1233)	946 (553–1224)	0.192
Calcium (mg/L)	90 (72–161)	133 (63–201)	0.060	123 (84–167)	142 (90–184)	0.031
Magnesium (mg/L)	52 (37–81)	79 (50–109)	< 0.001	49 (38–68)	68 (50–90)	< 0.001
Oxalate (mg/L)	15 (11–19)	16 (11–23)	0.04	18 (14–24)	21 (15–27)	0.003
Phosphorous (mg/L)	469 (353–683)	651 (442–1085)	< 0.001	473 (314–622)	581 (382–773)	< 0.001
Uric acid (mg/L)	426 (278–556)	372 (226–526)	0.259	395 (263–499)	338 (241–473)	0.031
Citrate (mg/L)	495 (315–754)	408 (232–710)	0.016	347 (223–531)	324 (205–434)	0.047
pH	6.27 (5.95–6.71)	5.64 (5.43–5.98)	< 0.001	6.12 (5.71–6.60)	5.79 (5.49–6.16)	< 0.001
Ca/Cit (mg/mg)	0.21 (0.15–0.30)	0.25 (0.18–0.42)	< 0.001	0.34 (0.21–0.44)	0.43 (0.26–0.64)	< 0.001
AP (CaOx) index	0.64 (0.49–0.90)	0.66 (0.46–1.13)	0.057	1.10 (0.66–1.54)	1.35 (0.90–1.84)	0.001
AP (CaP) index	4.85 (1.09–18.24)	0.33 (0.06–2.49)	< 0.001	3.41 (0.36–15.30)	0.93 (0.07–7.87)	0.001

Results are expressed as median (P_{25}-P_{75})

However, we think that use of overnight urine is preferable to daytime or 24-h urine for evaluation of the risk of calcium phosphate stones. Remarkably, we found that the AP(CaP) index had a much wider range in daytime than in overnight urine, and also had more overlap in relation to stone type. The influence of punctual food intake on urinary pH can explain this daytime variability. At night, fasting makes pH values decrease and stabilize [30], so the differences between patients with pure calcium phosphate stones and other types of stones were more evident.

In agreement with other studies, we observed a correlation between the indexes and renal stone type in adults. Thus, we believe that these risk indexes might be helpful in cases when analysis of calculus composition is unavailable, because the results may suggest the chemical composition of the stone.

A limitation of this study is that we only enrolled a small number of stone-forming children because renal lithiasis is very rare at this age. However, our observation of similar patterns in children and adults suggest that the findings of the larger adult group may also be applicable to children. Another limitation is that we did not have the stone composition for all patients, and that very few patients had HAP stones. However, our results provide a foundation for further studies of renal lithiasis in children and of the relationship of different indexes with stone composition. Furthermore, more data is warranted, including a higher

Table 4 Urinary volume, pH, solute concentrations, Ca/Cit ratio, and AP indexes in 12-h daytime and 12-h overnight urine samples of healthy and stone-forming children

	Healthy children (n = 87)			Stone forming children (n = 21)		
	12 h day	12 h night	p-value	12 h day	12 h night	p-value
Volume (mL/12 h)	480 (378–708)	360 (300–450)	< 0.001	650 (335–930)	530 (315–705)	0.192
Creatinine (mg/dL)	908 (686–1250)	1162 (835–1469)	< 0.001	886 (507–1393)	1000 (611–1097)	0.274
Calcium (mg/L)	57 (38–99)	86 (41–167)	< 0.001	181 (57–209)	150 (101–258)	0.082
Magnesium (mg/L)	77 (54–110)	151 (110–198)	< 0.001	79 (51–100)	128 (55–163)	0.021
Oxalate (mg/L)	20 (15–27)	26 (19–34)	< 0.001	24 (20–32)	27 (23–37)	0.244
Phosphorous (mg/L)	630 (430–872)	1060 (804–1414)	< 0.001	450 (337–664)	870 (480–1094)	0.001
Uric acid (mg/L)	597 (431–720)	529 (373–632)	0.002	454 (266–646)	396 (271–578)	0.244
Citrate (mg/L)	557 (405–737)	462 (328–668)	< 0.001	379 (250–710)	299 (208–477)	0.004
pH	6.60 (6.15–6.96)	5.79 (5.60–6.22)	< 0.001	6.36 (6.08–7.12)	5.91 (5.55–6.23)	0.001
Ca/Cit (mg/mg)	0.11 (0.07–0.17)	0.21 (0.10–0.36)	< 0.001	0.40 (0.21–0.54)	0.50 (0.33–0.94)	0.002
AP (CaOx) index	0.46 (0.29–0.65)	0.67 (0.34–1.13)	< 0.001	1.12 (0.74–1.80)	1.28 (0.87–2.55)	0.052
AP (CaP) index	8.24 (2.34–21.86)	1.09 (0.16–3.04)	< 0.001	8.85 (1.78–62.5)	3.03 (0.34–5.56)	0.014

Results are expressed as median (P_{25}-P_{75})

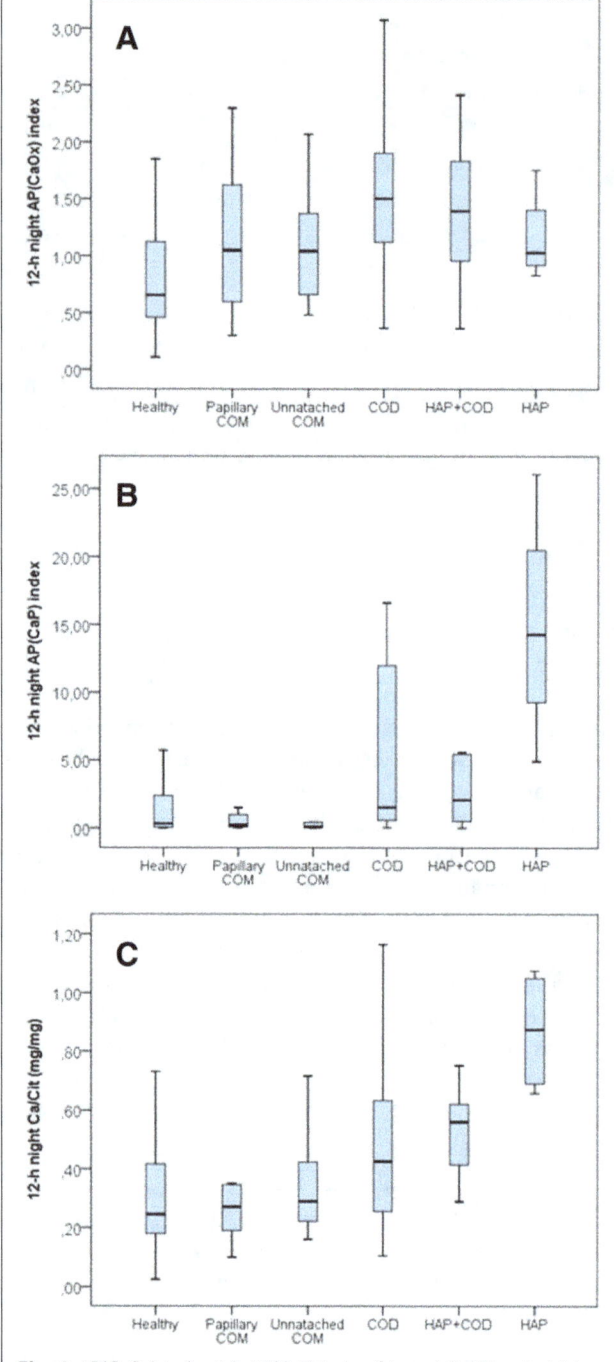

Fig. 2 AP(CaOx) index (**a**), AP(CaP) index (**b**), and Ca/Cit ratio (**c**) in 12-h overnight urine samples of adult stone-formers according to calculus composition

the results of multiple urinary parameters, have shown higher values in stone forming patients that in healthy subjects. These differences have been more evident in the 12 h overnight urine sample. Our results indicate that use of a 12-h overnight urine sample should be considered as a complementary information to that provided by the analysis of 24-h samples when evaluating lithogenic risk, because collection of the overnight sample is more convenient and has higher values in all tested indexes.

Abbreviations
AP(CaOx): ion activity product of calcium oxalate; AP(CaP): ion activity product of calcium phosphate; Ca: calcium; Cit: citrate; COD: calcium oxalate dihydrate; COMp: papillary calcium oxalate monohydrate; COMu: unattached calcium oxalate monohydrate; HAP: hydroxyapatite

Acknowledgements
A.R. is grateful to the European Social Fund and the Conselleria d'Educació, Cultura i Universitats for the fellowship FPI/1570/2013.

Funding
This work was supported by project grant AAEE42/2015 from Conselleria d'Innovació, Recerca i Turisme, Govern de les Illes Balears. The funders play no role in the design of the study and collection, analysis, and interpretation of data and in writing the manuscript.

Authors' contribution
AR: healthy subjects recruitment; data analysis; laboratory analysis and manuscript drafting. CST: healthy subjects recruitment; design protocol; manuscript drafting and revision. CM: healthy and stone-forming children recruitment and manuscript drafting. PC: Stone-forming adults recruitment and manuscript drafting. NR: Stone-forming adults recruitment and manuscript drafting. DR: healthy and stone-forming children recruitment and manuscript revision. GF: data analysis and manuscript revision. JMB: Stone-forming adults recruitment and manuscript revision. CG: Laboratory analysis and manuscript revision. ACB: conception and design and manuscript revision. FG: conception and design and manuscript revision. All authors have read and approved the final version of the manuscript.

Competing interest
The authors declare that the have no competing interests.

Author details
[1]Laboratory of Renal Lithiasis Research, University Institute of Health Sciences Research (IUNICS-IdISBa), University of Balearic Islands, Ctra Valldemossa, km 7.5, 07122 Palma de Mallorca, Spain. [2]Department of Pediatric Nephrology, Son Espases University Hospital, 07020 Palma de Mallorca, Spain. [3]Department of Urology, Son Llatzer Hospital, 07198 Palma de Mallorca, Spain. [4]Research Unit, Son Espases University Hospital, 07020 Palma de Mallorca, Spain. [5]Department of Nephrology, Son Llatzer Hospital, 07198 Palma de Mallorca, Spain. [6]Clinical Analysis Service, Son Espases University Hospital, 07020 Palma de Mallorca, Spain.

number of patients, in order to help determine a cutoff value for the studied indexes.

Conclusions
Calculation of renal lithiasis risk indexes is easy and may facilitate the decision-making process for treatment of stone-forming patients because the indexes, which integrate

References

1. Scales CD Jr, Smith AC, Hanley JM, Saigal CS. Prevalence of kidney stones in the United States. Eur Urol. 2012;62:160–5.
2. VanDervoort K, Wiesen J, Frank R, Vento S, Crosby V, Chandra M, et al. Urolithiasis in pediatric patients: a single center study of incidence, clinical presentation and outcome. J Urol. 2007;177:2300–5.
3. Cloutier J, Villa L, Traxer O, Daudon M. Kidney stone analysis: "give me your stone, I will tell you who you are!". World J Urol. 2015;33:157–69.
4. Costa-Bauza A, Ramis M, Montesinos V, Grases F, Conte A, Piza P, et al. Type of renal calculi: variation with age and sex. World J Urol. 2007;25:415–21.
5. Grases F, Costa-Bauza A, Ramis M, Montesinos V, Conte A. Simple classification of renal calculi closely related to their micromorphology and etiology. Clin Chim Acta. 2002;322:29–36.
6. Grases F, Costa-Bauza A, Bonarriba CR, Pieras EC, Fernandez RA, Rodriguez A. On the origin of calcium oxalate monohydrate papillary renal stones. Urolithiasis. 2015;43(Suppl 1):33–9.
7. Sikora P, Zajaczkowska M, Hoppe B. Assessment of crystallization risk formulas in pediatric calcium stone-formers. Pediatr Nephrol. 2009;24:1997–2003.
8. Baumann JM, Affolter B. From crystalluria to kidney stones, some physicochemical aspects of calcium nephrolithiasis. World J Nephrol. 2014;3:256–67.
9. Arrabal-Polo MA, Arrabal-Martin M, Arias-Santiago S, Garrido-Gomez J, Poyatos-Andujar A, Zuluaga-Gomez A. Importance of citrate and the calcium : citrate ratio in patients with calcium renal lithiasis and severe lithogenesis. BJU Int. 2013;111:622–7.
10. Tiselius HG. Risk formulas in calcium oxalate urolithiasis. World J Urol. 1997; 15:176–85.
11. Tiselius HG. Estimated levels of supersaturation with calcium phosphate and calcium oxalate in the distal tubule. Urol Res. 1997;25:153–9.
12. Grases F, Costa-Bauza A, Prieto RM, Arrabal M, De Haro T, Lancina JA, et al. Urinary lithogenesis risk tessts: comparison of a commercial kit and a laboratory prototype test. Scand J Urol Nephrol. 2011;45:312–8.
13. Saez-Torres C, Grases F, Rodrigo D, Garcia-Raja AM, Gomez C, Frontera G. Risk factors for urinary stones in healthy schoolchildren with and without a family hystory of nephrolithiasis. Pedriatr Nephrol. 2013;28:639–45.
14. Tiselius HG. Should we modify the principles of risk evaluation and recurrence preventive treatment of patients with calcium oxalate stone disease in view of the etiologic importance of calcium phosphate? Urolithiasis. 2015;43(Suppl 1):47–57.
15. Forni Ogna V, Ogna A, Vuistiner P, Pruijm M, Ponte B, Ackermann D, et al. New anthropometry-based age- and sex-specific reference values for urinary 24-hour creatinine excretion based on the adult Swiss population. BMC Med. 2015;13:40.
16. Remer T, Neubert A, Maser-Gluth C. Anthropometry-based reference values for 24-h urinary creatinine excretion during growth and their use in endocrine and nutritional research. Am J Clin Nutr. 2002;75:561–9.
17. Tiselius HG. Aspects on estimation of the risk of calcium oxalate crystallization in urine. Urol Int. 1991;47:255–9.
18. Bek-Jensen H, Tiselius HG. Evaluation of urine composition and calcium salt crystallization properties in standardized volume-adjusted 12-h night urine from normal subjects and calcium oxalate stone formers. Urol Res. 1997;25:365–72.
19. Skolarikos A, Straub M, Knoll T, Sarica K, Seitz C, Petrik A, et al. Metabolic evaluation and recurrence prevention for urinary stone patients: EAU guidelines. Eur Urol. 2015;67:750–63.
20. Pearle MS, Goldfarb DS, Assimos DG, Curhan G, Denu-Ciocca CJ, Matlaga BR, et al. Medical management of kidney stones: AUA guideline. J Urol. 2014; 192:316–24.
21. Hsi RS, Sanford T, Goldfarb DS, Stoller ML. The role of the 24-hour urine collection in the prevention of kidney stone recurrence. J Urol. 2017;197: 1084–9.
22. Gambaro G, Croppi E, Coe F, Lingeman J, Moe O, Worcester E, et al. Metabolic diagnosis and medical prevention of calcium nephrolithiasis and its systemic manifestations: a consensus statement. J Nephrol. 2016;29:715–34.
23. Parks JH, Coward M, Coe FL. Correspondence between stone composition and urine supersaturation in nephrolithiasis. Kidney Int. 1997;51:894–900.
24. Curhan GC, Willett WC, Speizer FE, Stampfer MJ. Twenty-four-hour urine chemistries and the risk of kidney stones among women and men. Kidney Int. 2001;59:2290–8.
25. Coe FL, Worcester EM, Evan AP. Idiopathic hypercalciuria and formation of calcium renal stones. Nat Rev Nephrol. 2016;12:519–33.
26. Porowski T, Kirejczyk JK, Zoch-Zwierz W, Konstantynowicz J, Korzeniecka-Kozerska A, Motkowski R, et al. Assessment of lithogenic risk in children based on a morning spot urine sample. J Urol. 2010;184:2103–8.
27. Wagner CA, Mohebbi N. Urinary pH and stone formation. J Nephrol. 2010; 23(Suppl 16):S165–9.
28. Grases F, Costa-Bauza A, Gomila I, Ramis M, Garcia-Raja A, Prieto RM. Urinary pH and renal lithiasis. Urol Res. 2012;40:41–6.
29. Murayama T, Sakai N, Yamada T, Takano T. Role of the diurnal variation of urinary pH and urinary calcium in urolithiasis: a study in outpatients. Int J Urol. 2001;8:525–31.
30. Firsov D, Bonny O. Circadian regulation of renal function. Kidney Int. 2010; 78:640–5.

35

Intravesical migration of female urethral dilator: a case report of a new urologic emergency in the era of e-commerce

Andrea Mogorovich*⬤, Cesare Selli, Alessio Tognarelli, Francesca Manassero and Maurizio De Maria

Abstract

Background: The introduction of foreign bodies in the female urethra for auto-erotic stimulation or in case of psychiatric disorders is not uncommon. The occurrence of intravesical migration of these objects makes it necessary to remove it shortly after insertion, since after long term permanence complications are likely to occurr.

Case presentation: A 47-year-old white female was referred at our Urology department for migration inside the bladder of a metallic urethral dilator used for sexual stimulation. An ultrasound study and an X-ray plate of the pelvis clearly visualized the presence of an object shaped like a rifle bullet located in the bladder. Twenty-four hours later, the patient reported its spontaneous emission through the urethra during micturition. This was confirmed by US and X-ray imaging.

Conclusions: The retrieval of foreign objects introduced through body orifices with purpose of sexual gratification is a known urological expertise. Curiously, in the case reported, the patient was able to manipulate the object thus facilitating its correct orientation and passage outside the bladder during micturition. To the best of our knowledge this is the first case of documented spontaneous emission through the urethra of a sizable intravesical foreign body. Sexual gratification in females though the insertion of urethral dilators is a growing practice, as demonstrated by the broad proposal of such instruments on the web. Therefore, the occurrence of accidental intravesical displacement of such kind of foreign body is increasingly likely, and the Urologists must be aware of this possibility.

Keywords: Bladder, Urethral dilator, Foreign bodies, Foreign body migration

Background

Introduction of foreign bodies in the female urethra is not uncommon, and the main reasons are auto-erotic stimulation, hygiene or psychiatric diseases. These objects may migrate inside the bladder due to the shortness of female urethra, its straight alignment and the fact that urethral meatus is usually not visible [1].

Usually, intravesical foreign bodies can be removed endoscopically shortly after their insertion, and they mostly consist in rigid objects such as pencils, ballpoint pens, pen casings, AAA batteries, paper clips with endless varieties [2].

Long term permanence leads to complications such as chronic urinary tract infection, bladder ulceration and formation of large size calculi, which can be found in patients with psychiatric disorders [3].

Emergent surgical management for injuries associated with eroticism, including the removal of foreign bodies, is increasing but still relatively uncommon, and there is a higher prevalence in men [4].

We report herein the case of a female patient who was referred at night from the Emergency Room for urologic consultation for intravesical migration of a conic-shaped urethral dilator bought on the Internet for self-gratification. The following day, before planned endoscopic extraction, she was able to self-manipulate retrogradely the dilator through the urethra outside the bladder. To our knowledge this is the first occurrence of such an event.

* Correspondence: a.mogorovich@ao-pisa.toscana.it
Urology Unit, Department of Translational Research, University of Pisa, Via Paradisa 2, 56124 Pisa, Italy

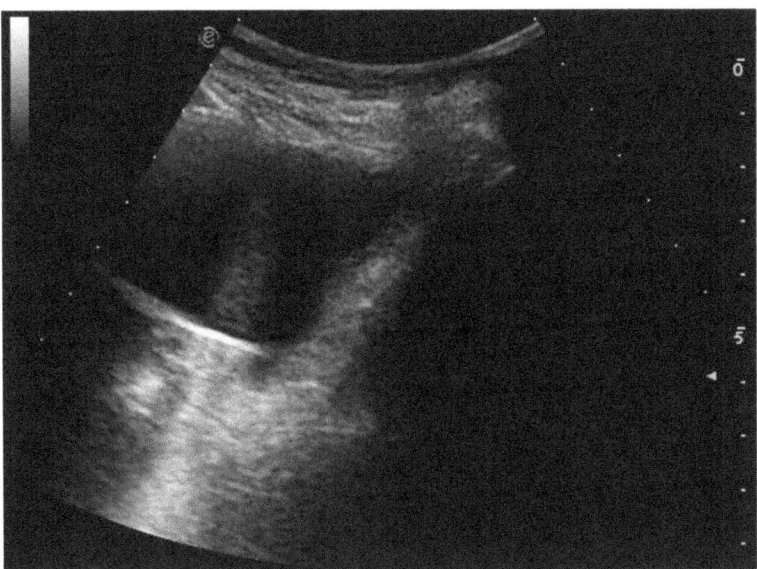

Fig. 1 US scan revealing hyperechoic linear structure within the bladder

Case presentation

A 47-year-old white female was referred at 1 AM to our Urology department from the Emergency Room for admitted migration inside the bladder of a metallic urethral dilator used for sexual stimulation. The patient stated that she had bought the object through a dedicated internet site. An ultrasound study revealed a partially full bladder with an echogenic internal structure (Fig. 1). An X-ray plate of the pelvis clearly visualized the presence of a high-density object shaped like a rifle bullet about 6 cm long, placed obliquely above the pubic symphysis.

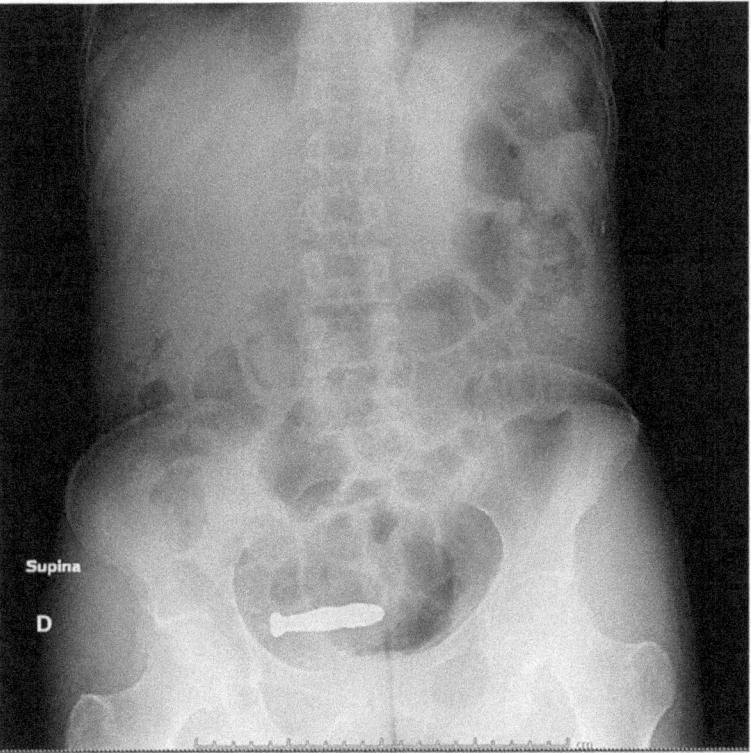

Fig. 2 X-ray plan clearly shows the presence of an intensely radiopaque bullet-shaped object above the pubic symphysis

Table 1 Summary of the clinical case

When	Patient details	Patient's concern	Management	Interventions
Initial diagnostic assessment during the night	47-yo white female reffered to our Department	Migration inside the bladder of a metallic urethral dilator during sexual stimulation	US and X-Ray	Oral antibacterial treatment, discharged...planned endoscopic removal after 2 days
After 1 day	–	The patient said was able to self-manipulate retrogradely the dilator through the urethra outside the bladder	US and X-Ray	Discharged home

It was referred by the Radiologist as "likely intrauterine device" (Fig. 2).

Since the patient had no symptoms, she opted to return home under oral antibacterial treatment with Ciprofloxacin, and endoscopic extraction was planned in 2 days time, with the program of introducing through the urethra under sedation a 24 F nephroscope and to extract the dilator placing it in line with the instrument axis and retrieving it with a 3-pronged rigid grasper.

The following day, when contacted by telephone again, the patient refused hospitalization, stating that she had be able to self-manipulate retrogradely the dilator through the urethra outside the bladder (Table 1). An US and X-ray study of the pelvis confirmed the absence of the foreign body (Fig. 3).

Discussion and conclusions

The retrieval of foreign objects introduced through body orifices with purpose of sexual gratification is a known urological expertise, and this practice is defined as polyembolokoilamania [5]. However the present case presents two points of interest.

The first one is that sexual gratification in females though the insertion inside the urethra of elongated smooth objects of tapered shape is a practice more common than previously believed, particularly in some cultures of the far East. It is not a coincidence that the largest published series comes from such a geographical area [2] and that Asian e-commerce sites under the heading "urethral dilators" offer such devices (Fig. 4). Interestingly some present at the larger end attached a

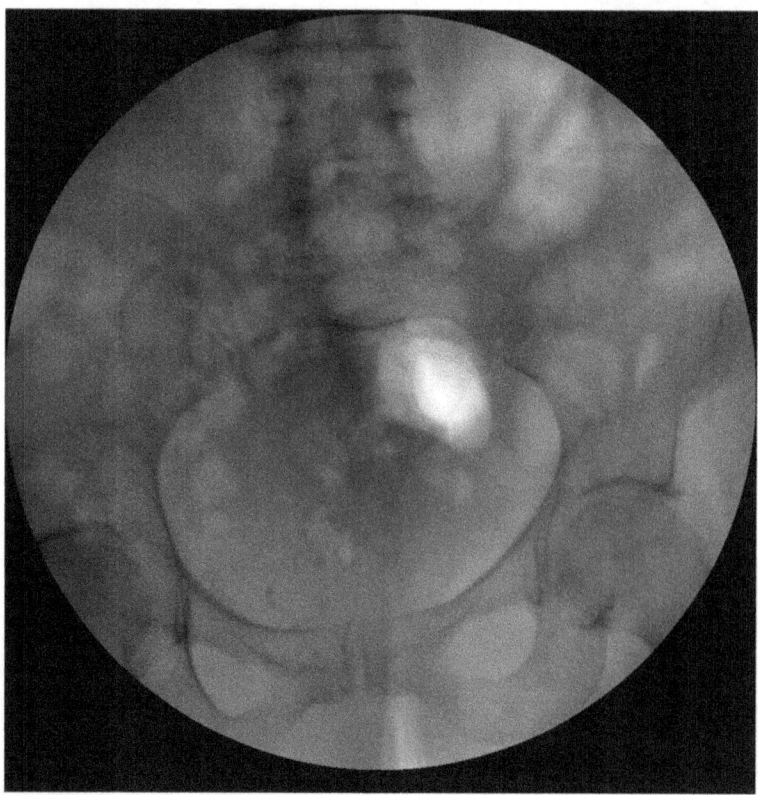

Fig. 3 X-ray of the pelvis after foreign body exit

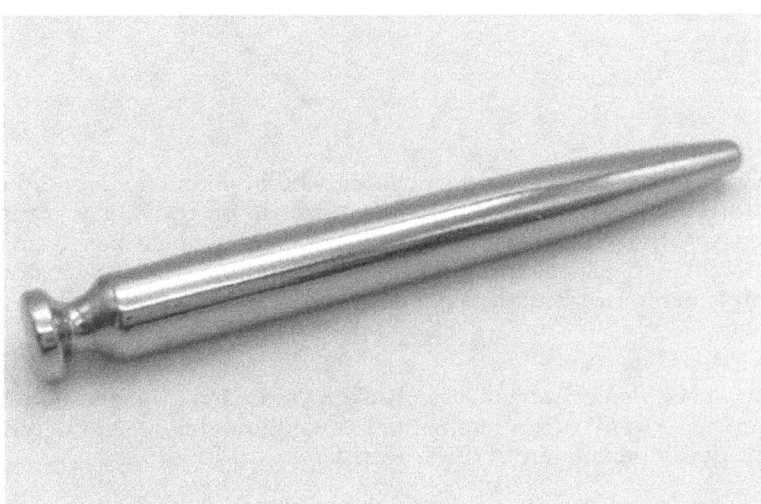

Fig. 4 Example of an urethral dilator available for purchase on e-commerce similar in shape and size to that one used in the present case report

metallic ring, evidently both for easier use and to avoid the possibility of upwards migration of the metallic object. Therefore it is likely that similar cases have occurred, but to the best of our knowledge have not been reported in the medical literature.

The second rather unique characteristic of the present case report is that the patient has been able to self-manipulate the object outside the bladder though the urethra, showing high manual dexterity. Repeated urethral dilatations evidently facilitated this uncommon maneuver, and we are unaware of such an occurrence.

Metallic bullet-shaped urethral dilators are presently available on e-commerce for sexual gratification by transurethral insertion. This increased availability makes the occurrence of accidental intravesical displacement more likely, and the Urologists must be aware of this possibility. Some of these objects have a "safety" metallic ring connected to the wider end, but should it be absent endoscopic retrieval must be performed.

Paradoxically the object weight and shape in the present case allowed its quite extraordinary extraction by the patient herself.

Authors' contributions
AM made substantial contributions to conception and design, acquisition of data; CS has been involved in drafting the manuscript and revising it critically for important intellectual content; AT made substantial contribution in drafting the manuscript and revising it; FM made contributions to conceptions and design; MDM has been involved in drafting the manuscript. All authors read and approved the final manuscript.

Competing interests
The authors declare that they have no competing interests.

References
1. Van Ophoven A, de Kernion JB. Clinical management of foreign bodies in the genitourinary tract. J Urol. 2000;164:247.
2. Kochacarn W, Pummanagura W. Foreign bodies in the female urinary bladder: 20-year experience in Ramathibodi hospital. Asian J Surg. 2008;31:130.
3. Mondaini N, Bartoletti R. Intravesical foreign body. N Engl J Med. 2007;357:588.
4. Yacobi Y, Tsivian A, Sidi AA. Emergent and surgical interventions for injuries associatedwith eroticism: a review. J Trauma. 2007;62:1522.
5. Chan G, Mamut A, Tatzel S, Welk B. An unusual case of polyembolokoilamania: urethral avulsion from foreign object use during sexual gratification. Can Urol Assoc J. 2016;10:E181.

Permissions

All chapters in this book were first published in UROLOGY, by BioMed Central; hereby published with permission under the Creative Commons Attribution License or equivalent. Every chapter published in this book has been scrutinized by our experts. Their significance has been extensively debated. The topics covered herein carry significant findings which will fuel the growth of the discipline. They may even be implemented as practical applications or may be referred to as a beginning point for another development.

The contributors of this book come from diverse backgrounds, making this book a truly international effort. This book will bring forth new frontiers with its revolutionizing research information and detailed analysis of the nascent developments around the world.

We would like to thank all the contributing authors for lending their expertise to make the book truly unique. They have played a crucial role in the development of this book. Without their invaluable contributions this book wouldn't have been possible. They have made vital efforts to compile up to date information on the varied aspects of this subject to make this book a valuable addition to the collection of many professionals and students.

This book was conceptualized with the vision of imparting up-to-date information and advanced data in this field. To ensure the same, a matchless editorial board was set up. Every individual on the board went through rigorous rounds of assessment to prove their worth. After which they invested a large part of their time researching and compiling the most relevant data for our readers.

The editorial board has been involved in producing this book since its inception. They have spent rigorous hours researching and exploring the diverse topics which have resulted in the successful publishing of this book. They have passed on their knowledge of decades through this book. To expedite this challenging task, the publisher supported the team at every step. A small team of assistant editors was also appointed to further simplify the editing procedure and attain best results for the readers.

Apart from the editorial board, the designing team has also invested a significant amount of their time in understanding the subject and creating the most relevant covers. They scrutinized every image to scout for the most suitable representation of the subject and create an appropriate cover for the book.

The publishing team has been an ardent support to the editorial, designing and production team. Their endless efforts to recruit the best for this project, has resulted in the accomplishment of this book. They are a veteran in the field of academics and their pool of knowledge is as vast as their experience in printing. Their expertise and guidance has proved useful at every step. Their uncompromising quality standards have made this book an exceptional effort. Their encouragement from time to time has been an inspiration for everyone.

The publisher and the editorial board hope that this book will prove to be a valuable piece of knowledge for researchers, students, practitioners and scholars across the globe.

List of Contributors

Jonathan Beilan, Ruth Strakosha and Diego Aguilar Palacios
University of Central Florida College of Medicine, Orlando, FL, USA

Charles J Rosser
Clinical and Translational Program, University of Hawaii Cancer Center, 701 Ilalo St, Honolulu, HI 96814, USA

Guanghua Chen, Bo Yang and Yinghao Sun
Department of Urology, Changhai Hospital, The Second Military Medical University, 168 Changhai Road, 200433 Shanghai, PR China

Tie Zhou and Huan Cao
Department of Urology, Changhai Hospital, The Second Military Medical University, 168 Changhai Road, 200433 Shanghai, PR China
Department of Urology, Haining People's Hospital, 2 QianJiang West Road, 314400 Haining City, ZheJiang Province, PR China

Emilie K Johnson, Spencer I Kozinn, Kathryn L Johnson, Sohee Kim, David A Diamond and Alan B Retik
Department of Urology, Boston Children's Hospital, 300 Longwood Ave,Boston, MA 02115, USA

Jasmir G Nayak, Darrel E Drachenberg and Elke Mau
Section of Urology, Department of Surgery, University of Manitoba, Winnipeg, Manitoba, Canada

Derek Suderman, Oliver Bucher, Pascal Lambert and Harvey Quon
CancerCare Manitoba, Winnipeg, Manitoba, Canada

Alexander Winter and Friedhelm Wawroschek
University Hospital for Urology, Klinikum Oldenburg, School of Medicine and Health Sciences, Carl von Ossietzky University Oldenburg, Rahel-Straus-Straße 10, 26133 Oldenburg, Germany

Rolf-Peter Henke
Oldenburg Institute of Pathology, Oldenburg, Germany

Adem Fazlioglu, Yilmaz Salman, Zafer Tandogdu and Fatih Osman Kurtulus
Department of Urology, Taksim Teaching Hospital, Istanbul, Turkey

Serap Bas
Department of Radiology, Gaziosmanpasa Hospital, Istanbul, Turkey

Mete Cek
Department of Urology, Trakya Medical School, Edirne, Turkey

Gong Cheng, Bianjiang Liu, Zhen Song, Aiming Xu, Ninghong Song and Zengjun Wang
State Key Laboratory of Reproductive Medicine and Department of Urology, The First Affiliated Hospital of Nanjing Medical University, Nanjing 210029, China

Babar Asma and Dodin Sylvie
Department of Obstetrics and Gynaecology, Laval University, CHU de Québec - Université Laval, 2705, boulevard Laurier, Local A1385, Québec, Québec G1V 4G2, Canada
Institute of Nutrition and Functional Foods, Laval University, 2440 Hochelaga Boulevard, Quebec City, Quebec G1V 0A6, Canada

Leblanc Vicky, Dudonne Stephanie and Desjardins Yves
Institute of Nutrition and Functional Foods, Laval University, 2440 Hochelaga Boulevard, Quebec City, Quebec G1V 0A6, Canada

Howell Amy
Rutgers University, 125A Lake Oswego Rd., Chatsworth, NJ 08019, USA

Dulcegleika VB Sartori, Hamilto A Yamamoto, Paulo R Kawano and Rodrigo Guerra
Department of Urology, Medical School of Botucatu, São Paulo State University, Botucatu, Brazil

Monica O Gameiro
Coordinator of Pelvic Floor Rehabilitation Service, Medical School of Botucat, São Paulo State University, Botucatu, Brazil

Carlos R Padovani
Department of Biostatistics, Medical School of Botucatu, São Paulo State University, Botucatu, Brazil

João L Amaro
Department of Urology, Medical School of Botucatu, São Paulo State University, Botucatu, Brazil
Department of Urology, School of Medicine, São Paulo State University (UNESP), Campus de Rubião Júnior, s/n, 18618-970 Botucatu, SP, Brazil

J Quentin Clemens
Department of Urology, University of Michigan, Ann Arbor, MI, USA

Chris Mullins, John W Kusek and Ziya Kirkali
National Institute of Diabetes and Digestive and Kidney Diseases, National Institutes of Health, Bethesda, MD, USA

Emeran A Mayer and Larissa V Rodríguez
Division of Digestive Diseases, University of California, Los Angeles, CA, USA

David J Klumpp and Anthony J Schaeffer
Department of Urology, Northwestern University, Chicago, IL, USA

Karl J Kreder
Department of Urology, University of Iowa, Iowa City, IA, USA

Dedra Buchwald
Departments of Epidemiology and Medicine, University of Washington, Seattle, WA, USA

Gerald L Andriole
Division of Urologic Surgery, Department of Surgery, Washington University School of Medicine, St Louis, MO, USA

M Scott Lucia
Department of Pathology, University of Colorado Anschutz Medical Campus, Aurora, CO, USA

J Richard Landis
Department of Biostatistics and Epidemiology, University of Pennsylvania Perelman School of Medicine, Philadelphia, PA, USA

Daniel J Clauw
Departments of Anesthesiology and Medicine, University of Michigan, Ann Arbor, MI, USA

Sigrid Carlsson
Urology Service at the Department of Surgery, Memorial Sloan-Kettering Cancer Center, 307 E. 63rd St, 2nd floor, New York, NY 10065, USA
Department of Urology, Sahlgrenska Academy at the University of Göteborg, Göteborg, Sweden

Ali Khatami, Johan Stranne, Svante Bergdahl, Pär Lodding and Jonas Hugosson
Department of Urology, Sahlgrenska Academy at the University of Göteborg, Göteborg, Sweden

Anders Berglund
Department of Surgical Sciences, Uppsala University, Uppsala University Hospital, Uppsala, Sweden

Daniel Sjoberg and Andrew Vickers
Department of Epidemiology and Biostatistics, Memorial Sloan-Kettering Cancer Center, New York, USA

Gunnar Aus
Department of Urology, Carlanderska hospital, Göteborg, Sweden

Stephan Degener, Stephan Roth and Alexander S Brandt
Department of Urology, HELIOS Medical Center Wuppertal, University of Witten/Herdecke, Heusnerstrasse 40, 42283 Wuppertal, Germany

Alexander Pohle and Jürgen Zumbé
Department of Urology, Medical Center Leverkusen, Am Gesundheitspark 11, 51375 Leverkusen, Germany

Hartmut Strelow
Institute of Hyperbaric Oxygen (HBO), University Hospital Düsseldorf, Moorenstrasse 5, 40225 Düsseldorf, Germany

Michael J Mathers
Urological Ambulatory PandaMED, Alleestrasse 105-107, 42853 Remscheid, Germany

Nancy A Robinson
Department of Biostatistics and Epidemiology, Perelman School of Medicine at the University of Pennsylvania, Philadelphia, PA, USA

David A Williams
Departments of Anesthesiology, Medicine and Psychiatry, University of Michigan, Ann Arbor, MI, USA

Adrie van Bokhoven
Department of Pathology, University of Colorado Anschutz Medical Campus, Aurora, CO, USA

Bruce D Naliboff
Departments of Medicine, Psychiatry, and Gastroenterology, University of California, Los Angeles, CA, USA

Siobhan Sutcliffe
Division of Public Health Sciences, Department of Surgery, Washington University, St Louis, MO, USA

Larissa V Rodriguez
Department of Urology, University of Southern California, Beverly Hills, CA, USA

H Henry Lai
Division of Urologic Surgery, Department of Surgery, Washington University School of Medicine, St. Louis, MO, USA

John N Krieger and Claire C Yang
Department of Urology, University of Washington, Seattle, WA, USA

Niloofar Afari
VA Center of Excellence for Stress and Mental Health, University of California San Diego, San Diego, CA, USA

Catherine S Bradley and Susan K Lutgendorf
Departments of Obstetrics and Gynecology, Urology and Epidemiology, University of Iowa, Iowa City, IA, USA

James W Griffith
Department of Medical Social Sciences, Northwestern University, Chicago, IL, USA

Barry A Hong
Departments of Psychiatry and Medicine, Washington University School of Medicine, St. Louis, MO, USA

Dedra Buchwald
Departments of Epidemiology and Medicine, University of Washington, Seattle, WA, USA

Sean Mackey
Department of Anesthesiology, Division of Pain Medicine, Stanford University School of Medicine, Palo Alto, CA, USA

Michel A Pontari
Department of Urology, Temple University School of Medicine, Philadelphia, PA, USA

Philip Hanno
Department of Urology, Perelman School of Medicine at the University of Pennsylvania, Philadelphia, PA, USA

Elisabeth M Sebesta
Columbia University College of Physicians and Surgeons, 630 W. 168th St, New York, NY 10032, USA

Hossein S Mirheydar, J Kellogg Parsons and A Karim Kader
UC San Diego Health System, 200 W. Arbor Drive #8897, San Diego, CA 92103-8897, USA
VA San Diego Healthcare System, 3350 La Jolla Village Dr. (113), San Diego, CA 92161, USA

Jessica Wang-Rodriguez
VA San Diego Healthcare System, 3350 La Jolla Village Dr. (113), San Diego, CA 92161, USA

Klaus-Peter Dieckmann, Petra Anheuser and Benjamin Soyka-Hundt
Department of Urology, Albertinen-Krankenhaus Hamburg, Hamburg, Germany

Stefan Schmidt Cord Matthies and Christian G Ruf
Department of Urology, Bundeswehrkrankenhaus Hamburg, Hamburg, Germany

Uwe Pichlmeier
Institute of Medical Biometry and Epidemiology, Universitätsklinikum Eppendorf, Hamburg, Germany

Philipp Schriefer and Michael Hartmann
Department of Urology, Universitätsklinikum Eppendorf, Hamburg, Germany

Rui-Ying Xu, Hua-Wei Liu, Ji-Ling Liu and Jun-Hua Dong
Department of Pediatrics, Qilu Hospital of Shan Dong University, Jinan 250012, China

Seung Mo Yuk
Department of Urology, Korea St. Mary's Hospital, College of Medicine, The Catholic University of Korea, Seoul, South Korea

Ju Hyun Shin, Ki Hak Song, Yong Gil Na, Jae Sung Lim and Chong Koo Sul
Department of Urology, Korea Chungnam National University Hospital, College of Medicine, Chungnam National University, Daejeon, South Korea

C. Patel, D. Loughran, R. Jones and M. Abdulmajed
Department of Urology, Wrexham Maelor Hospital, Croesnewydd Rd, Wrexham LL13 7TD, Wales

I. Shergill
Department of Urology, Wrexham Maelor Hospital, Croesnewydd Rd, Wrexham LL13 7TD, Wales
North Wales and North West Urological Research Centre, Croesnewydd Rd, Wrexham LL13 7TD, Wales

Serge P. Marinkovic, Brandi Miller, Scott Hughes, Christina Marinkovic and Lisa Gillen
Department of Urology, Detroit Medical Center, Harper Hospital, Detroit, MI 48202, USA

Larry Akoko
Muhimbili University of health and Allied Sciences, Dar es Salaam, Tanzania

Aika Shoo and Patricia Scanlan
Muhimbli National Hospital, Dar es Salaam, Tanzania

Shakilu Iumanne
Muhimbili University of health and Allied Sciences, Dar es Salaam, Tanzania College of Health Sciences, University of Dodoma, Box 339, Dodoma, Tanzania

Shenyou Sun and Dongbin Liu
Department of General surgery, Linyi People's Hospital, Shandong 276000, People's Republic of China

Ziyao Jiao
Department of Anesthesiology, Linyi People's Hospital, Shandong 276000, People's Republic of China

Hassan M. Elbiss and Nawal Osman
Department of Obstetrics and Gynaecology, College of Medicine and Health Sciences, United Arab Emirates University, Al Ain, United Arab Emirates

Fayez T. Hammad
Department of Surgery, College of Medicine and Health Sciences, United Arab Emirates University, Al Ain United Arab Emirates

Andrew Stickley
The Stockholm Center for Health and Social Change (SCOHOST), Södertörn University, Huddinge 141 89, Sweden

Ziggi Ivan Santini
The Danish National Institute of Public Health, University of Southern Denmark, Oester Farimagsgade 5A, 1353 Copenhagen, Denmark

Ai Koyanagi
Parc Sanitari Sant Joan de Déu, Universitat de Barcelona, Fundació Sant Joan de Déu/CIBERSAM, Barcelona, Spain

Tomohiro Matsuo, Yasuyoshi Miyata, Katsura Kakoki, Miki Yuzuriha, Akihiro Asai, Kojiro Ohba and Hideki Sakai
Department of Urology, Nagasaki University Graduate School of Biochemical Sciences, 1-7-1 Sakamoto, Nagasaki 852-8501, Japan

Hui Guo, Shukun Liu, Kaixuan Wang, Erpeng Liu, Faping Li and Yuchuan Hou
Department of Urology, First Hospital of Jilin University, Changchun, Jilin 130021, China

Shuaiqi Chen
Department of Urology, The First Affiliated Hospital of Xinxiang Medical University, Xinxiang, Henan 453100, China

Jiexiu Zhang, Qiang Lv, Zenjun Wang and Ming Gu
Department of Urology, The First Affiliated Hospital of Nanjing Medical University, Nanjing 210029, China

Jong Kyou Kwon and Cheol Kyu Oh
Department of Urology, Haeundae Paik Hospital, Inje University College of Medicine, Busan, South Korea

Kang Su Cho
Department of Urology, Gangnam Severance Hospital, Urological Science Institute, Yonsei University College of Medicine, Seoul, South Korea

Dong Hyuk Kang
Department of Urology, Yangpyeong Health Center, Yangpyeong, South Korea

Hyungmin Lee
Division of Epidemic Intelligence Service, Korea Centers for Disease Control and Prevention, Osong, South Korea

Won Sik Ham, Young Deuk Choi and Joo Yong Lee
Department of Urology, Severance Hospital, Urological Science Institute, Yonsei University College of Medicine, 50-1 Yonsei-roSeodaemun-gu, Seoul 120-752, South Korea

Miroslav Fajfr, Pavla Paterová, Lenka Ryšková and Helena Žemličková
Institute of Clinical Microbiology, University Hospital Hradec Kralové, Sokolska 581, Hradec Králové 50005, Czech Republic
Charles University in Prague, Faculty of Medicine in Hradec Kralové, Simkova 870, Hradec Kralove 500 38, Czech Republic

Miroslav Louda, Jaroslav Pacovský, Josef Košina and Miloš Broďák
Charles University in Prague, Faculty of Medicine in Hradec Kralové, Simkova 870, Hradec Kralove 500 38, Czech Republic
Clinic of Urology, University Hospital Hradec Kralové, Sokolska 581, Hradec Králové 50005, Czech Republic

Diandong Yang, Jitao Wu, Hejia Yuan and Yuanshan Cui
Department of Urology, Yantai Yuhuangding Hospital Affiliated to Medical College of Qingdao University, NO.20 East Yuhuangding Road, 264000 Yantai, China

Yasushi Nakai, Nobumichi Tanaka, Makito Miyake, Satoshi Anai and Kiyohide Fujimoto
Department of Urology, Nara Medical University, 840 Shijo-cho, Kashihara, Nara 634-8522, Japan

Keiji Shimada and Noboru Konishi
Department of Pathology, Nara Medical University, 840 Shijo-cho, Kashihara, Nara 634-8522, Japan

Yung-Chan Chen
Department of Psychiatry, Shuang Ho Hospital, Taipei Medical University, New Taipei City, Taiwan

Li-Ting Kao
Graduate Institute of Life Science, National Defense Medical Center, Taipei, Taiwan

Herng-Ching Lin
Sleep Research Center, Taipei Medical University, Taipei, Taiwan

Hsin-Chien Lee
Department of Psychiatry, Shuang Ho Hospital, Taipei Medical University, New Taipei City, Taiwan
Sleep Research Center, Taipei Medical University, Taipei, Taiwan
Department of Psychiatry and Medical Humanities, School of Medicine, College of Medicine, Taipei Medical University, Taipei, Taiwan

Chung-Chien Huang
School of Health Care Administration, Taipei Medical University, Taipei, Taiwan

Shiu-Dong Chung
Sleep Research Center, Taipei Medical University, Taipei, Taiwan
Division of Urology, Department of Surgery, Far Eastern Memorial Hospital, New Taipei City, Taiwan
Graduate Program in Biomedical Informatics, College of Informatics, Yuan-Ze University, Chung-Li, Taiwan
Department of Surgery, Far Eastern Memorial Hospital, No.21, Sec. 2, Nanya S. Rd., Banciao Dist, New Taipei City 220, Taiwan

Norihiro Murahashi, Takashige Abe, Nobuo Shinohara, Sachiyo Murai, Satoru Maruyama, Kunihiko Tsuchiya, Naoto Miyajima and Katsuya Nonomura
Department of Urology, Hokkaido University Graduate School of Medicine, North-15, West-7, North Ward, Sapporo 060-8638, Japan

Toru Harabayashi
Department of Urology, Hokkaido Cancer Center, Sapporo, Japan

Ataru Sazawa
Department of Urology, Obihiro-Kosei General Hospital, Obihiro, Japan

Kanako Hatanaka
Department of Surgical Pathology, Hokkaido University Hospital, Sapporo, Japan

Tommaso Cai and Umberto Anceschi
Department of Urology, Santa Chiara Regional Hospital, Trento, Italy

Paolo Verze, Roberto La Rocca and Vincenzo Mirone
Department of Urology, University of Naples, Federico II, Naples, Italy

Cosimo De Nunzio
Department of Urology, Ospedale Sant'Andrea, Sapienza University of Rome, Rome, Italy

Adrian Rodriguez, Concepcion Saez-Torres, Antonia Costa-Bauza and Felix Grases
Laboratory of Renal Lithiasis Research, University Institute of Health Sciences Research (IUNICS-IdISBa), University of Balearic Islands, Ctra Valldemossa, km 7.5, 07122 Palma de Mallorca, Spain

Concepcion Mir and Dolores Rodrigo
Laboratory of Renal Lithiasis Research, University Institute of Health Sciences Research (IUNICS-IdISBa), University of Balearic Islands, Ctra Valldemossa, km 7.5, 07122 Palma de Mallorca, Spain
Department of Pediatric Nephrology, Son Espases Universitary Hospital, 07020 Palma de Mallorca, Spain

Paula Casasayas and Nuria Rodriguez
Department of Urology, Son Llatzer Hospital, 07198 Palma de Mallorca, Spain

Guiem Frontera
Research Unit, Son Espases Universitary Hospital, 07020 Palma de Mallorca, Spain

Juan Manuel Buades
Department of Nephrology, Son Llatzer Hospital, 07198 Palma de Mallorca, Spain

Cristina Gomez
Clinical Analysis Service, Son Espases Universitary Hospital, 07020 Palma de Mallorca, Spain

Andrea Mogorovich, Cesare Selli, Alessio Tognarelli, Francesca Manassero and Maurizio De Maria
Urology Unit, Department of Translational Research, University of Pisa, Via Paradisa 2, 56124 Pisa, Italy

Index

www.ingramcontent.com/pod-product-compliance
Lightning Source LLC
Chambersburg PA
CBHW080409190526
45161CB00003B/180